MEDICAL MARIJUANA

A CLINICAL HANDBOOK

MEDICAL MARIJUANA

A CLINICAL HANDBOOK

FIRST EDITION

Samoon Ahmad, MD

Professor of Psychiatry
Department of Psychiatry
New York University Grossman School of Medicine
Attending Physician and Unit Chief Inpatient Psychiatry
Bellevue Hospital Center
New York, New York

Kevin P. Hill, MD, MHS

Director, Division of Addiction Psychiatry
Beth Israel Deaconess Medical Center
Associate Professor of Psychiatry
Harvard Medical School
Boston, Massachusetts

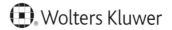. Wolters Kluwer

Philadelphia • Baltimore • New York • London
Buenos Aires • Hong Kong • Sydney • Tokyo

Acquisitions Editor: Chris Teja
Development Editor: Ariel S. Winter
Editorial Coordinator: Chester Anthony Gonzalez
Editorial Assistant: Brian Convery
Marketing Manager: Phyllis Hitner
Production Project Manager: Kim Cox
Design Coordinator: Holly McLaughlin
Manufacturing Coordinator: Beth Welsh
Prepress Vendor: SPi Global

Copyright © 2021 Wolters Kluwer

9 8 7 6 5 4 3 2 1

Printed and bound in Singapore by Markono Print Media Pte Ltd

Cataloging-in-Publication Data available on request from the Publisher

ISBN: 978-1-9751-4189-9

shop.lww.com

*Dedicated
to my wife, Kim,
and son, Daniel.*

S.A.

*Dedicated to my parents,
Anne and Larry Hill,
for making sacrifices so that I could
pursue my dreams.*

K.P.H.

Foreword

Drs. Samoon Ahmad and Kevin P. Hill—the former a Professor of Psychiatry at NYU and the latter an Associate Professor of Psychiatry at Harvard—have written a comprehensive treatise on cannabis, more commonly known as marijuana or alternatively, marihuana. It is a book that is long overdue.

The authors, an outstanding clinical psychiatrist and an addiction specialist, do much to dispel the myths and misunderstandings about cannabis, which is primarily a recreational drug but has recently been shown to have profound therapeutic effects for a great variety of medical and psychiatric disorders. Its medical use has not been available because of the many laws that prevent practitioners from prescribing it.

For example, in the United States, marijuana is an illegal drug at the federal level because of the Controlled Substance Act of 1970. Despite this, more than 33 states have created medical marijuana programs in which specially trained practitioners can recommend cannabis. Of these, 11 states also allow marijuana to be used as a recreational substance as well. Clearly, the tide is turning; however, the potential for conflict between state and federal laws is not yet resolved. One can only hope that books like this provide a path for the federal government to lift the draconian laws that prohibit its medical use.

The book opens with a chapter that introduces the reader to the history of cannabis and describes its use as a medicine throughout the ages with specific references to its use in China over 6000 years ago. There is also a chapter on the thorny issue of classification, which provides an overview of the different types of cannabis found throughout the world. The book also includes a chapter that describes more than 120 compounds that are found in the plant. The enormous number of compounds found in cannabis clearly accounts for the confusion about its effects on the mind and body.

The legal aspects surrounding cannabis mentioned above are discussed extensively in a chapter on the regulation of cannabis in this country. The rules have changed so much over the years—and continue to do so—that the authors suggest the reader stay up-to-date on a special Web site associated with the book that will chronicle not only these legal aspects but also the rapidly expanding medical knowledge about cannabis itself.

A large portion of the text deals with the pharmacology of cannabis, which the authors describe as "shrouded in mystery." They do an excellent job solving that mystery in a series of chapters that discuss principles of pharmacology in general and of cannabis in particular. The reader will gain an understanding of pharmacodynamics, pharmacokinetics, absorption, distribution, and other data, including the molecular action of the many drugs derived from the parent plant, including illustrations of chemical formulas.

At the heart of the book is a detailed exposition of each of the approved cannabis-based drugs: dronabinol, nabilone, and cannabidiol. The authors discuss these three drugs and provide extensive data, including specific dosages, preparations, routes of administration, and side effects. They are careful to differentiate approved therapeutic indications from off-label use, the latter accounting for improvement in several conditions otherwise resistant to therapy. Importantly, adverse effects and drug-drug interaction are discussed extensively throughout.

A unique aspect of the text is 12 chapters that are organized according to organ systems that provide a template for disorders for which cannabis might be of help. The chapter titles explain which drugs can be used in which disorders. They are easily understood and uniquely organized: gynecology, dermatology, rheumatology, ophthalmology, oncology, and internal medicine, among others. It is an impressive list.

The book ends on a subject of great concern—cannabis use disorder. Dependence upon and addiction to cannabis is a public health problem that effects almost 10% of Americans, especially those who are young. The authors describe the signs and symptoms of the disorder and offer helpful suggestions on treatment. This is a most important contribution to the text.

The authors are to be congratulated on producing a book that will appeal to a large audience. Physicians of all specialties will find it particularly useful. Others in the medical field such as nurse practitioners and physician assistants will also find it of value. Even the lay person can find this book informative. Drs. Ahmad and Hill have written a book that is a complete and thorough guide to cannabis that is most timely and highly informative.

Benjamin Sadock, MD

Prologue

Imagine two patients sitting in the waiting area of a clinic. The first is a man in his sunset years who has recently begun treatment for stage 2 lung cancer. His treatment involves the use of chemotherapy, which has significantly reduced his appetite and given him terrible bouts of nausea. The second is a woman in her 30s. She is a former competitive skater who continues to experience chronic joint pain because of injuries she suffered on the ice. She is also reluctant to use any pain medication that has even a moderate potential for abuse because she has a history of drug addiction.

The two begin to chat. As they tell one another the reasons why they are in the clinic, the man reveals that he has lost more than 5 pounds since beginning chemotherapy only a little more than a week before and that he has no idea how he will be able to last for the entire duration of the treatment. The woman attempts to comfort him by saying that her uncle experienced a similar problem when he underwent chemo. "You should ask the doctor about cannabis," she says.

"Cannabis?" the man says. "You mean marijuana—like what those hippies in California smoke?"

"Well, yes," she concedes. "But you don't have to smoke it. You can vape it, eat it, or even drink it. My uncle preferred to take it in chocolate form. He says it saved his life."

"No thanks," the man says. "I don't want to get addicted, I don't want to become schizophrenic, and I most certainly don't want to end up moving on to something like heroin just to get my fix. It's a gateway drug, you know."

The woman again shakes her head. "Cannabis and schizophrenia are not related at all. Also, it's not a gateway drug. It's completely nonaddictive and natural. It's from Mother Earth. I plan on asking for a prescription myself, but for CBD oil."

"What's CBD oil? Is that a more concentrated version?"

"No. It comes from a different species of the cannabis plant than the one that gets you high. It helps with all sorts of things, from depression to anxiety to insomnia to chronic pain to Crohn disease to psoriasis. It's also totally legal."

The man gives the woman a skeptical look, but can't respond because he has heard his name called. The person at the desk repeats his name when they spot one another, and then adds: "The doctor will see you now."

The two patients part ways and see their respective doctors. Each describes their symptoms to their doctor, and each is told that cannabis could be used to help with their symptoms. They also discover that a large percent of what they believe about cannabis is almost comically inaccurate.

The above scenario is meant to illustrate three things. The first is that there is no shortage of misinformation about cannabis. This is particularly true when one is researching the subject on the Internet. Some Web sites claim that it is a sacred plant that can cure virtually any ailment. Others begrudgingly acknowledge that it may be beneficial but only in limited circumstances and maintain that it is too dangerous to be made widely available.

The second is that much of this misinformation exists because cannabis has been used as a standard in a culture war that has managed to drag on for 50 years. Consequently, opinions about cannabis are often shaped by one's political leanings and rarely rely on data or scientific analysis, though medicinal cannabis seems to have won nearly universal acceptance in the past few years. A Quinnipiac poll from 2018 found that 93% of Americans support allowing patients' access to medical cannabis.[1]

The third and final point to take away is that the chemistry of cannabis is anything but straightforward and that its complexity has only served to fuel more misinformation.

This latter point deserves greater clarification.

Cannabis is a genus of flowering plant in the family Cannabaceae. Though most Web sites and recreational cannabis users will claim that there are three different species of *Cannabis* (*C sativa*, *C indica*, and *C ruderalis*), there is still a lively debate among scientists about the proper classification of cannabis, and many argue that that *C indica* and *C ruderalis* are subspecies of *C sativa*. A more precise classification of the genus is not necessary for our purposes at this time and will be explored in Chapter 3 (The Classification of Cannabis). However, this opportunity should be taken to note that unless otherwise noted, the blanket term "cannabis" will refer to any (sub) species of the *Cannabis* genus herein described.

This is not to say that all cannabis is the same. Far from it.

[1] Quinnipiac University. "Do you support or oppose allowing adults to legally use marijuana for medical purposes if their doctor prescribes it?" Quinnipiac University Poll Question 36 of 50, April 26, 2018 https://poll.qu.edu/national/release-detail?ReleaseID=2539. Accessed February 11, 2020.

The cannabis plant is known to contain an immense number of compounds that interact either directly or indirectly with the body's endocannabinoid system—a physiologic web of enzymes, receptors, and ligands that runs throughout the bodies of humans and other animals (see Chapter 6: The Endocannabinoid System). Compounds that interact with the endocannabinoid system may be synthesized within the body or they may be synthesized by plants like cannabis. Those created by the body are known as endocannabinoids. When they are found in flora, they are known as phytocannabinoids. There is evidence to suggest that phytocannabinoids are not unique to cannabis.[2]

Within cannabis, there are more than 120 phytocannabinoids. Most occur in trace amounts, and their pharmacological uses have not been sufficiently explored at this time, but others occur in large enough concentrations to have attracted considerable attention. The most well-known phytocannabinoid is Δ^9-tetrahydrocannabinol (THC). When THC is ingested in sufficient quantities, it produces the intoxicating "high" for which cannabis is famous. THC has also been shown to effectively treat a myriad of conditions that will be explored throughout this book.

Most other cannabinoids, such as cannabidiol (CBD), are nonintoxicating, and research has suggested that they have pharmaceutical profiles that are distinct from THC. CBD in particular has received a great deal of attention in the media because preliminary studies have shown it to have anti-inflammatory, antiepileptic, anxiolytic, and antipsychotic[3] properties. It appears that CBD may also counteract some of the unwanted effects of THC, though not enough studies have been conducted at this time to make a conclusive statement about the matter.[4]

For a variety of reasons that will be explored in the first few chapters of the book, there are two distinct kinds of cannabis. Historically, they have served vastly different purposes and the distinctions between the two have only grown more apparent as breeding techniques have become more sophisticated. The first, industrial hemp (or hemp), was traditionally grown primarily for its seeds or fibers, which were then used to make textiles, paper, ropes, and a wide variety of other products. By definition, within section 10113 of the 2018 Farm Bill, industrial hemp contains less than 0.3% THC.[5] While low in THC, concentrations

[2]Gertsch J, Pertwee R, Di Marzo V. Phytocannabinoids beyond the Cannabis plant—do they exist? *Br J Pharmacol*. 2010;160(3):523-529. doi: 10:1111/j.1476-5381.2010.00745.x.

[3]Bridgeman MB, Abazia D. Medical cannabis: history, pharmacology, and implications for the acute care setting. *P T*. 2017;42(3):180-188.

[4]Niesink RJ, van Laar MW. Does cannabidiol protect against adverse psychological effects of THC? *Front Psychiatry*. 2013;4:130. doi: 10.3389/fpsyt.2013.00130.

[5]Hudak J. The farm bill, hemp legalization and the status of CBD: an explainer. Brookings Institute. Published December 14, 2018. https://www.brookings.edu/blog/fixgov/2018/12/14/the-farm-bill-hemp-and-cbd-explainer/. Accessed February 11, 2020.

of CBD can be quite high. Consequently, many hemp cultivars are now grown primarily for their CBD content.

Marijuana, the other type of *C sativa* as defined by the federal government, has levels of THC that meet or exceed 0.3% THC. Due to its high THC content, it has been used primarily as an intoxicant. As cultivars with higher levels of THC have historically fetched a higher price among those who use cannabis recreationally, many cultivars now contain percentages of THC that would have been unheard of only a few decades ago. One study found that average THC potency had jumped from 4% to 12% just between 1995 and 2014.[6] Conversely, by breeding marijuana with high THC levels, this led to a major reduction in CBD concentration, and the results are staggering. The typical ratio between THC and CBD in 1995 was 14:1. By 2014, the ratio had grown to 80:1.[6]

Despite the importance of THC and CBD to the use of cannabis as a medicine, focusing solely on the concentrations of these two phytocannabinoids in an attempt to predict user experience produces an incomplete picture. They are the figurative tip of the iceberg. On top of containing more than 120 phytocannabinoids that can alter the effects of either CBD or THC felt by patients, cannabis also contains a host of additional compounds (such as terpenes, terpenoids, and flavonoids, which will be explored in Chapter 4 [The Constituents of Cannabis]) that are common to the plant world and may indirectly interact with the endocannabinoid system.[7] Consequently, many of these compounds may not only alter a patient's subjective experience following use but they may also prove to be beneficial for certain conditions whether used in isolation or in conjunction with other cannabinoids.

As there are literally thousands of cultivars of cannabis, each with their own phytocannabinoid and terpenic profiles that may produce distinct therapeutic effects, it is misguided to speak of cannabis in monolithic terms. It is like making broad claims about soup. By understanding just how complex the chemistry of cannabis is, one gains a greater appreciation for why such a great deal of attention has been paid to this plant for millennia.

As the coming chapters will show, cannabis has a long history of use throughout the world (Chapter 2: The History of Cannabis) and was a relatively common medicine even in the United States until regulatory obstacles were put in place to criminalize its usage and to frustrate

---

[6]ElSohly MA, Mehmedic Z, Foster S, Gon C, Chandra S, Church J. Changes in cannabis potency over the last two decades (1995–2014): analysis of current data in the United States. *Biol Psychiatry*. 2016;79(7):613-619. doi: 10.1016/j.biopsych.2016.01.004.
[7]Andre CM, Hausman JF, Guerriero G. *Cannabis sativa*: the plant of the thousand and one molecules. *Front Plant Sci*. 2016;7:19. doi:10.3389/fpls.2016.00019.

attempts to study its potential therapeutic properties (as explored in Chapter 5: U.S. Cannabis Regulations From Past to Present). To this day, the federal government continues to recognize any cannabis plant that produces more than 0.3% THC as marijuana—a Schedule I drug that (officially) has no medicinal purposes whatsoever. Cannabis plants that produce less than 0.3% THC have only been recognized as being potentially useful by the federal government as of December 2018, when the most recent Farm Bill was signed into law. While the legislation makes industrial hemp legal at the federal level, states retain the right to ban its production or usage.[5]

Though research into cannabis is becoming more robust, its thorny legal status has been a major impediment to its study by medical researchers for several decades. Consequently, much of the literature that celebrates it as an almost magical panacea relies on anecdotal evidence or cherry-picked data from studies that, upon more thorough examination, assert only tentative conclusions about the efficacy of cannabis as a treatment for any number of symptoms. Meanwhile, much of the literature that condemns it as a public menace either ignores research that makes provisional claims about cannabis' benefits or spends far too much time focusing on the detrimental effects of excessive recreational use.

Despite the myriad inaccuracies, half-truths have a nasty habit of lingering around like unwanted house guests and eventually they begin to spread. Like any game of telephone, the further one ventures from the source, the more corrupted the original message becomes. Eventually, this leads to sensational headlines and oversimplified claims about cannabis that consumers and even some medical professionals take to be accurate. This is true of both those who advocate for cannabis and for those who continue to believe that its potential benefits are far outweighed by its potential dangers. Both sides of the argument often fail to see through the fog of the culture war, and both sides are at times guilty of being more intent on winning a political argument than approaching the issue with a clear head and an agenda couched solely in the traditional of empiricism and science. This book hopes to change that.

Apart from being discouraged by the amount of misinformation I found on the subject of cannabis, a major impetus for this book is in part due to having more than 25 years of experience running the acute psychiatric inpatient unit at a New York City Hospital. Aside from the fact that I had an opportunity to evaluate and treat innumerable patients with severe mental illnesses, I also noticed a steady increase in the number of individuals who were struggling with addiction and opioid abuse. Many of these individuals had initially obtained a prescription to help them manage their pain but eventually became addicted to opioids. This sparked my interest in alternative treatment options, and specifically cannabis, with its application potential well beyond pain management and how cannabinoids in the plant could be used to benefit patients. This led me to begin my due diligence research into the history and science of cannabis, and I was amazed by what I discovered.

I approached Kevin to help with the creation of this book because I recognized in him a vast clinical expertise, as well as a desire to cut through the politics of cannabis and to arrive at an accurate depiction of what continues to be one of the most misunderstood plants on Earth. Like me, he recognized that there is far too much misinformation about cannabis in the world. Furthermore, he understood that clinicians and patients alike regularly operate on faulty assumptions based on bad or outdated science, oftentimes because it is difficult to tell fact from fiction. What was needed, we agreed, was a medical textbook on cannabis to educate medical professionals, as well as a regularly updated Web site that takes into account any new findings from more recent studies. Such a book would include only evidence-based studies on cannabis and be compiled in such a way that the busy clinician would be able to turn to it as a quick reference.

What you currently hold in your hands is that book. It is our hope that we can eliminate unwarranted stigmas that continue to hound this quirky plant and to dispel any notions that cannabis is either a miracle drug or the devil's weed. If nothing else, we hope to provide our peers in the medical community with some degree of clarity so that they can make decisions based on the best available evidence and pass on accurate information to patients like the ones described above.

Samoon Ahmad, MD

Prologue

I took a winding path to deciding to partner with Samoon on this important textbook. I described my decision to become an addiction psychiatrist in my book *Marijuana: The Unbiased Truth about the World's Most Popular Weed*; exposure to mental illness and addiction in my family played a major role. My interest in cannabis developed during my training in addiction psychiatry. I spent a portion of my training in an outpatient program for substance use disorders (SUDs) in the greater Boston area, and the drug of choice for the patients in the program was typical of most of the SUDs programs I have worked in: 40% alcohol, 40% opioids, and 20% everything else (benzodiazepines, stimulants, and, rarely, cannabis).

When asking these patients about their histories of drug use, I found that slightly more than half of these patients would describe a time in their lives when they were using cannabis daily for years, most commonly in their late teens or early 20s. At that point, I set about trying to find an effective treatment for cannabis addiction, or cannabis use disorder (CUD), with the belief that successful treatment of CUD in a patient's teens or 20s would decrease the likelihood that those patients would turn up later in SUDs treatment facilities seeking help for alcohol use disorder or opioid use disorder (OUD).

I began conducting small randomized clinical trials of behavioral interventions, pharmacotherapies, or a combination of the two as treatment for CUD. As I was directing these trials, the Commonwealth of Massachusetts prepared to vote on medical cannabis as a part of a ballot initiative in 2012. Groups who opposed the ballot initiative asked me to educate communities about the risks of cannabis use, particularly in young people. This experience was instructive in many ways. First, I saw the polarizing nature of the topic of cannabis. Some cannabis advocates said that cannabis was harmless. Others described it as a panacea, a natural treatment for a host of conditions that did not respond to traditional medications. Those opposed to cannabis at times relayed the message that if a young person was to use cannabis, they were doomed. The loudest voices in the debate were those with political skin in the game—they were often willing to distort the scientific evidence in an effort to steer voters one way or another. Second, it was clear that there was a significant gap between the science of cannabis and its public perception. Perhaps most importantly, and certainly most relevant for this book, I saw that medical professionals were clamoring for help in this controversial area. They knew that, like it or not, a liberal state like Massachusetts was likely to vote in favor of medical cannabis laws and, therefore, their patients would be asking about medical cannabis or informing them about their use of medical cannabis in a few months' time. They needed to get up to speed on the risks and benefits of cannabis and do it quickly.

Not surprisingly, Massachusetts residents voted overwhelmingly in favor of medical cannabis, and laws went into effect on January 1, 2013. It has been a bumpy ride. Those in favor of medical cannabis have said that there are not enough dispensaries at which medical cannabis can be purchased. They are also frustrated with a patient registration process that has been cumbersome at times. Those opposed to medical cannabis think that is far too easy to acquire a medical cannabis certification—in many states, there a physician can certify the use of medical cannabis for any medical condition that they deem it potentially helpful for—and that the standard of medical care in medical cannabis clinics is substandard. Unfortunately, Massachusetts' experience with medical cannabis has been repeated in many of the 30-plus states that currently have medical cannabis laws in place.

The value of balanced, evidence-based education was apparent to me as states such as Massachusetts began to implement medical cannabis policies. That was a major reason that I wrote *Marijuana*, although that book was aimed at general audiences with more of a focus on the risks of cannabis use along with a discussion of treatment for those with CUD. I learned quickly, though, that attempting to be balanced on such a controversial topic meant that I would be criticized by cannabis advocates and critics alike. It did not take long. Those who do not take the time to read my work or hear me speak on cannabis assume that I am opposed to cannabis in all forms based upon my training, research, and clinical work as an addiction psychiatrist. Sadly, in this era of social media, probably a third of the criticism I receive is from those who have extreme views, get upset after reading something that I have said or written, then dash off a response immediately without taking the effort to understand my stances on disparate topics like the therapeutic use of cannabis and cannabis addiction. Some from the anticannabis side felt that I was not emphasizing the adverse effects of cannabis enough and that my balanced style was giving young people who listened to me the "green light" to use cannabis while their brains were still in development. On a few occasions that I am aware of, cannabis critics spoke to groups that were advertising my speaking events to plead with them to replace me with speakers who used the familiar "scare tactics"—that have been shown not to be effective—when addressing this topic with young people.

Receiving criticism from both sides hopefully means that I am right where I intend to be on the issue—in the middle. Balance on cannabis is crucial from both clinical and policy perspectives. If I am asked to talk with a patient about the daily cannabis use and I toss a pile of research papers chronicling the harms of regular cannabis use at them, he or she will likely perceive me as being opposed to cannabis at all costs and he or she will be unlikely to return to receive the ongoing treatment that he or she need. Lacking balance from a clinical perspective can be costly because the window of opportunity for a patient to accept treatment may not be open for very long.

This is also where a clinical perspective is important, for working with patients creates an inherent need for balance. Patients frequently have different ideas than I do, but we have a common goal—to improve their health. As a result, clinicians must become skilled at listening to patients' perspectives and being willing to bend at times in the service of maintaining a long-term relationship with their patients. You can imagine, then, that lobbyists, politicians, or researchers who do not treat patients may be more likely to take extreme views on cannabis.

From a policy perspective, balance is also critical. In the United States, thus far, the cannabis advocates and critics have dug in their heels in state after state without compromise. Sometimes the advocates win and sometimes the critics win. The result, though, is policy that is not as strong as it should be. Cannabis policy in the United States has suffered as a result. While I have made an effort in many states to try to inform the voters on cannabis-related issues, in states that vote for cannabis policies, I am in favor of trying to give the people what they want while mitigating risk.

Many of the answers to the important questions on cannabis have turned out to be ones that we did not expect. For example, in 2011, I published a paper in *Drug and Alcohol Dependence* on the impact of cannabis use on treatment outcome in patients with OUD receiving buprenorphine. Contrary to my hypothesis formed from my clinical experience, we found that cannabis use did not adversely affect treatment outcome in these patients. Rather than attempt to perform analyses in the hopes that additional results would fit our narrative, we double-checked our analyses and published our findings.

This willingness to be open-minded has led to my current clinical practice in which I treat patients with widely varying experiences with cannabis. On one end of the spectrum are patients who meet criteria for CUD—their cannabis use has negatively affected key aspects of their lives, typically work, school, or relationships. I routinely treat patients, often young people, whose daily cannabis use has jeopardized their future. I also work with a few different special populations, including professional athletes, and I have seen some of these athletes lose multi-million dollar careers because they were unable to stop using a drug that many people feel if not addictive.

On the contrary, I also treat patients who are utilizing medical cannabis to treat debilitating medical conditions like chronic pain or muscle spasticity from multiple sclerosis. A recent patient was sent to me by her primary care doctor in order to determine her appropriateness for a medical cannabis certification for chronic pain. She had a list of 14 medications and procedures that she had tried in collaboration with her doctor; they provided limited relief. Most doctors practice only on one of these extreme ends of the spectrum on cannabis, and these doctors often do not believe that patients at the other end exist. "Cannabis physicians" are reticent to acknowledge that CUD exists and addiction psychiatrists frequently do not believe that cannabis can be a useful pharmacotherapy.

Varied clinical and research experience with cannabis has afforded me a unique perspective. This perspective is especially important for a complex topic like cannabis with so many attempting to distort the evidence. I have written papers on the therapeutic use of cannabis in an effort to describe where strong evidence exists and where there are research gaps. I have interpreted the impact of changing cannabis policy on medical cannabis and offered suggestions on how to improve current policies. In 2018, I was awarded a grant by the World Health Organization (WHO) to summarize the current state of the evidence for the therapeutic use of cannabis for the WHO Expert Committee on Drug Dependence's 40th meeting in Geneva, Switzerland.

Health care professionals are looking for evidence-based guidance on how to approach medical cannabis in their practices. Some have extreme views as advocates or critics, but many health care professionals who see patients are open to evaluating the evidence, and they are the intended audience for this book. Much of what health care professionals have heard or read about medical cannabis is either incomplete or simply untrue. The advocates and critics alike have been guilty of this at times, either cherry-picking portions of evidence to fit their narrative or ignoring major papers that offer evidence that runs counter to their beliefs. Many health care professionals have realized this and have asked for a resource like this to cut through the political chaff in order to focus on the science.

I have known for a while that a book like this was needed because I have talked to doctors and patients all over the country and beyond.

Meeting Samoon, though, provided the impetus to push forward with this book on top of my other clinical and research obligations. I had previously been approached by other publishers to write a book like this and the timing did not seem right, especially in the early stages of development of the Division of Addiction Psychiatry that I started in September 2017. Samoon contacted me with the idea to write a textbook and to create an enduring online resource that clinicians could return to as they faced new clinical challenges in the area of medical cannabis. I was struck by his energy and passion for the project, which was born out of his busy clinical practice and recognition, like mine, that we could help large numbers of clinicians and patients alike through the creation of a definitive resource on medical cannabis.

So that is what we have done. We have written a comprehensive, evidence-based textbook on medical cannabis that is aimed at the busy clinician. A textbook and accompanying Web site that will be updated over time as new research is published and accessed quickly during a harried workday seeing patients. We cover the history of medical cannabis, the basics of the endocannabinoid system and cannabis pharmacology, the risks and benefits of medical cannabis, and, most importantly, the latest evidence for the therapeutic use of cannabis for all major medical conditions for which patients are considering it for. Patients will continue to turn to medical cannabis; we want to educate health care professionals so that they are in a better position to help patients when this happens.

Kevin P. Hill, MD, MHS

Preface

Research into cannabis has exploded in recent years as states have created medical marijuana programs, and interest has surged in nonintoxicating cannabinoids like cannabidiol (CBD). In addition, research into the body's endocannabinoid system, which represents the means through which cannabis exerts its effects, has made tremendous strides. Unfortunately, many clinicians have been unaware of these advances and, consequently, are often unfamiliar with the science of cannabis, as well as its potential benefits and risks for patients.

This book, which is the first of its kind, is meant to provide an unbiased and easy to navigate guide for clinicians on cannabis. It includes background information on the biology and chemistry of cannabis, the history of its use, the evolution of cannabis regulations, the pharmacological profile of its major constituents, its effects on various bodily systems, and much more. Though it was written by clinicians for clinicians, it can also be read by individuals who simply want to learn more about cannabis and to better understand its potential use as a medicine.

We also feel that it is important to note that, though some feel as though the word "marijuana" does have a negative connotation and racist history, we decided to include it in the title for two reasons. The first is because "marijuana" is more familiar than the word "cannabis." Secondly, and perhaps more importantly, most of the states that have legalized the use of medicinal cannabis continue to issue "medical marijuana" cards and to operate "Medical Marijuana Programs."

We also recognize the ongoing debate on the correct usage of the spellings of "marijuana" vs "marihuana" since many state licensures still use "marihuana" while scientific literature has gravitated more toward "marijuana." For the purpose of this book and in line with scientific community, we have chosen to use the variant "marijuana."

Acknowledgments

We wish to thank several individuals for their tremendous support. My deepest thanks go to Benjamin J. Sadock, MD, Menas S. Gregory Professor of Psychiatry. His encouragement fueled my participation in and contributions to several books in the Kaplan & Sadock series and, ultimately, to this book. I am immensely thankful to Ben for being a mentor, a teacher, and a lifelong friend.

Immeasurable thanks go to Jay Fox, my research and editorial assistant. His due diligence, dedication, and critical eye for detail are second to none.

Maryanne Badaracco, MD, Director and Chief of Psychiatry, Bellevue Hospital, has been a constant source of support and reinforced my pursuit of academic excellence. Finally, I extend my thanks to Charles Marmar, MD, Lucius R. Littauer Professor and Chair of the Department of Psychiatry at New York University Grossman School of Medicine, whose support and encouragement of all my academic accomplishments are highly appreciated.

Last but not the least, I would like to thank my coauthor Kevin P. Hill, MD. It has been a pleasure to collaborate with him on this important work.

Samoon Ahmad, MD
New York University Grossman School of Medicine
New York, New York

I would like to thank William Greenberg, MD, Chief of the Department of Psychiatry at Beth Israel Deaconess Medical Center for supporting my efforts on projects like this. My wife, Debbie, and my daughters, Hannah and Sophie, continue to motivate me to become a better clinician, investigator, and educator. I often joke that my mother, Anne Hill, writes my biographical paragraphs, but she has had unwavering faith in me since the beginning, and for that I am eternally grateful. Finally, it has been fun to team up with Samoon Ahmad, MD, on this book. His passion for the topic is inspiring.

Kevin P. Hill, MD, MHS
Harvard Medical School
Boston, Massachusetts

Table of Contents

1

Cannabis: An Introduction

1.1 Introduction

Cannabis sativa has been cultivated for millennia. *Cannabis* can be broken down into two broad categories: fiber-type plants and drug-type plants. Fiber-type plants, known as hemp, have historically been selected for their fibers and not their drug content. These fibers can be used for textiles, cordage, and other industrial purposes. Fiber-type plants also produce some nonintoxicating cannabinoids, most notably cannabidiol (CBD), that may be used for medicinal purposes. The second broad group, drug-type plants, is not used for their fibers, but instead for recreational or religious purposes, as they cause intoxication when consumed. The primary intoxicant in drug-type plants is Δ-9-tetrahydrocannabinol (typically referred to as THC), which is found in extremely low concentrations in fiber-type plants (<0.3%). Concentrations vary among drug-type plants.

The story of cannabis is a complicated matter. Misrepresentations and outright contradictions are pervasive in literature and on Web sites that document the constituents and effects of cannabis. Even the correct nomenclature for individual parts of the plant runs rife. As noted in the prologue, such misinformation is problematic, especially when one is using or considering using cannabis for medicinal purposes. Providing inaccurate information, like neglecting to specify that certain effects of CBD are discernible only when individual terpenes or terpenoids, or combinations of the two, are present in large enough concentrations, is misleading and potentially harmful. Terpenes and terpenoids are organic hydrocarbons found in plants, including cannabis, that give them their unique smell and taste. More will be said on terpenes and terpenoids in Chapter 4 (Constituents of Cannabis).

In this day and age, false information can be disseminated easily, and such misinformation has caused tremendous misunderstandings and misperceptions about cannabis. We hope to untangle this confusion before examining the benefits and risks of cannabis use.

One story is particularly illustrative.

In the late 1990s, a cosmetics company introduced a line of products that included hemp oil, which is derived from the seeds of industrial hemp plants, as an ingredient. While this has become commonplace in recent years, it was somewhat novel at the time, even though these plants had been a staple throughout Europe until the early 20th century. Such plants were traditionally used for their fiber to make cordage and cloth and produce only trace amounts of THC.

However, the French police in Aix-en-Provence evidently did not know this. On August 28, 1998, they raided the shop in town and confiscated all the products containing hemp oil, as well as any in-store advertising materials for the products.[1] The police believed that these products were illegal and that the shop was promoting and even encouraging the illicit use of cannabis.

The irony, of course, was that the hemp seed oil found in the products had been produced in France—the largest producer of hemp in Europe.[2] Furthermore, weedy varieties of cannabis are frequently found in drainage channels throughout the agricultural heartlands of Russia, Canada, the United States, and France.

This kind of confusion has played out in countless scenarios and stems from the fact that the

nomenclature surrounding cannabis comes from
a hodgepodge of sources that have been jumbled
together to create a single cannabis lexicon. This
lexicon emerged from the morass organically and
unscientifically, and the degree of nuance one must
employ to accurately speak about cannabis can be
taxing. Oftentimes, a single word will take on significantly different meanings depending on context.
Indica, for example, can refer to cultivars (often
referred to as strains) of cannabis that produce specific types of intoxication characterized by relaxation
and appetite stimulation. Depending on which taxonomic schema one subscribes to, *indica* can also
refer to either a species within the genus *Cannabis*
(*C. indica*) or a subspecies or variant of the species *C.
sativa* (*C. sativa* subsp. *indica* or *C. sativa* var. *indica*).

Conversely, the law often sees cannabis in
monochrome. For the police in the above scenario,
for example, the operating logic was as follows: The
plant must be illegal because it produces the street
drug marijuana. However, in France, *Cannabis
sativa* is not necessarily illegal. Some cultivars of
cannabis will produce significant concentrations
of THC, thereby giving those who consume it the
"high" for which cannabis is so notorious. These
drug-type plants are illegal. THC does not occur in
high enough concentrations in all cannabis cultivars

to effect humans in any meaningful way, and, since the dawn of agriculture, fiber-type plants have been grown in France and have been cultivated from Japan to the British Isles for myriad purposes.

The word "ganja" presents another example of the semantic difficulties one encounters with cannabis. Within Western cannabis culture, *ganja* is a generic term for cannabis that is high in THC and that is often associated with the unique cannabis culture of Jamaica.

In the Indian subcontinent, this would not be the case. THC-rich cannabis is consumed in this region for ceremonial, recreational, and spiritual purposes in three distinct forms. The first, *bhang*, is the least potent. It consists of dried cannabis leaves and can be smoked, eaten, or mixed with spices, milk, sugar, and tea to create an intoxicating beverage (Fig. 1.1). The second, *ganga*, is stronger, it is typically smoked, and it is made from the dried flowers and leaves of female cannabis plants, which are left unpollinated by male plants, thereby increasing their potency for reasons that will be discussed below (Fig. 1.2). Finally, there is *charas*, which is extremely potent and consists of resin collected from cannabis plants that has been purified and molded into discs, blocks, or sticks (Fig. 1.3). Charas can be smoked in a water pipe, crumbled up and mixed with tobacco, or consumed in beverage form.

In the mid-19th century, indentured laborers were brought from India to Jamaica by the British to cut sugar cane and they brought cannabis with them.[3] Some of that cannabis culture was eventually adopted by the black working class already living on the island. This is how "ganga" became "ganja."

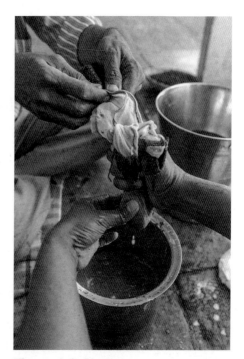

Figure 1.1 Bhang.

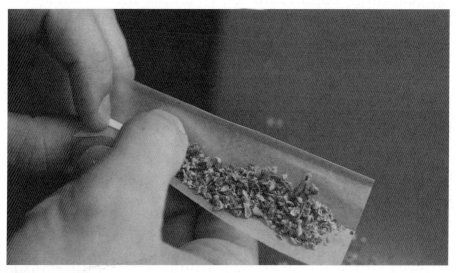

Figure 1.2 Ganga.

The takeaway is that numerous words within the parlance of drug culture are often appropriated from other cultures or scientific research and are then used in nonliteral meanings until the literal meanings become forgotten. To untangle this mess, we must first examine some of the words and

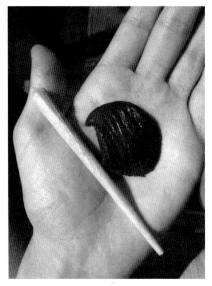

Figure 1.3 Charas.

how they have been used. This will lead us into a discussion of cannabis' classification, its morphology, and, finally, its constituents.

1.2 Folk Terminology

For our purposes in this book, "cannabis" will be used as a generic term to refer to plants found within the genus *Cannabis*. Within this genus, there exists distinct types, though it is debatable whether they constitute separate species, subspecies, or variants. Within folk terminology, cannabis is typically separated into two broad categories: hemp and marijuana.

Hemp is a type of cannabis that is primarily grown for its fibers, which have been used to make cordage, textiles, and other items for millennia. As we will see in Chapter 2 (The History of Cannabis), it has been in use since before the dawn of civilization (Fig. 1.4). Hemp is also the name of the fibers that are extracted from the plant—similar to cotton and contrary to flax (the fibers of which are known as linen). Guttenberg's first Bible was written on paper made of hemp, and paper made from hemp or flax with a mixture of recycled cloth was common well into the 19th century.[4,5]

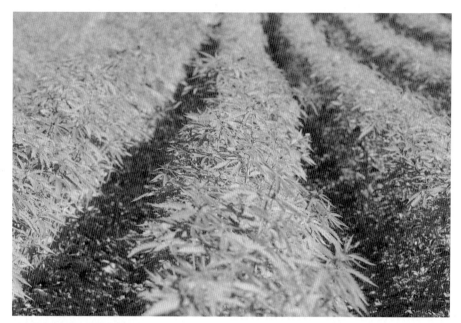

Figure 1.4 Industrial Hemp Field.

Hemp has also been used as a folk remedy for a laundry list of ailments, even though it does not produce an intoxicating effect because of its extremely low levels of THC. It does contain CBD and other compounds that have potential medicinal uses.[6] The medicinal properties of the plant extend from its roots to its seeds. The latter have also been consumed for their dense nutrient content or be pressed for oil that can be used to make things like cosmetics.

In this book, we will refer to plants that are grown for their fibers, seeds, or oil as *fiber-type plants*.

The other folk name for cannabis, *marijuana*, refers to both cannabis plants that generate enough THC to produce an intoxicating effect and is also the name of the dried *flower* and leaves of such cultivars. Though its etymology is murky, it was clearly popularized in Mexico during the second half of the 19th century. During the first half of the 20th century, it (or the variant "marihuana") became popular in the United States because demagogues linked its proliferation to Mexican immigrants and claimed that even moderate usage could lead one into a murderous rampage. Both were meant to foment xenophobic sentiments, which is why some currently consider the term to be objectionable.[7]

Within this text, plants that are rich in THC will be referred to as *drug-type plants*.

Drug-type cultivars of cannabis have been used for religious, ceremonial, and recreational purposes for millennia in certain cultures—particularly those in more equatorial climates. While not scientific by any means, the north/south, hemp/marijuana divide is a relatively accurate depiction of how cannabis has been used historically.

The hemp/marijuana distinction has even been adopted by the federal government to assert that, legally speaking, hemp and marijuana are not the same. According to H.R. 2 (also known as the Agriculture Improvement Act, or the "Farm Bill" of 2018), "hemp" is defined as: "...The plant *Cannabis sativa* L. and any part of that plant, including the seeds thereof and all derivatives, extracts, cannabinoids, isomers, acids, salts, and salts of isomers, whether growing or not, with delta-9 tetrahydrocannabinol concentration of not more than 0.3% on a dry weight basis."[8] Any cannabis plant that produces a greater concentration of THC is considered to be marijuana (or "marihuana") and, therefore, is considered a Schedule I drug. According to the United States Drug Enforcement Administration, "Schedule I drugs, substances, or chemicals are defined as drugs with no currently accepted medical use and a high potential for abuse."[9]

A history of the prohibition of cannabis in the United States, as well as a detailed examination of its current legal status will follow at length in Chapter 5 (U.S. Cannabis Regulations from Past to Present). As legalization efforts for both the recreational and medicinal use of cannabis are ongoing, it is recommended that readers consult our Web site for periodic updates.

1.3 A Note on Slang

An entire volume could be dedicated to documenting all the slang terms that have arisen in cannabis culture. For our purpose, we will highlight the most common terms as we tread through the history of cannabis and include them in a glossary found in Appendix A. The definitions of most slang terms can be deduced without deviations from the core narrative of the following chapters.

1.4 Classification

Cannabis has been classified in numerous ways throughout history. By exploring the numerous schemas developed over the centuries, it becomes evident that the plant can and has served a wide variety of purposes across different cultures.

that have adapted to colder environments enter into their flowering stage independently of photoperiod—a phenomenon that has come to be known as *autoflowering*.[14]

Following germination, the initial sprout will contain a root that will give it access to water and nutrients from the soil, as well as a single cotyledon (seed leaf) that will give the plant access to light. It will convert the light into energy via photosynthesis. It will then enter the seedling stage, a transitionary period between germination and the vegetative stage that lasts just a few weeks. Upon entering the vegetative stage, the cannabis plant will produce a green and hollow stalk that is cylindrical and longitudinally ridged with secondary branches that produce palmate leaves (often called fan leaves). These leaves typically contain between 5 and 11 lobes.

During the vegetative stage, the plant will grow at an extremely brisk pace (hence the reason it is commonly referred to as *weed*). Some varieties are capable of increasing in height at a rate of 10 cm per day.[12]

The root system is relatively small when compared to other annuals. On average, the roots make up only between 8% and 9% of the plant's total biomass, though the main root can grow to a depth of over 2 m. Secondary roots tend to grow between 10 and 60 cm deep.[2]

Until the vegetative stage begins to conclude, it is virtually impossible to distinguish between male and female plants without examining each plant's DNA.[15] This changes as the vegetative stage comes to an end and the plant begins to put less energy into producing fan leaves and more energy into reproduction. At this point, nascent flowers will begin to appear at nodes along the main stalk of the plant.

Differences in sex become apparent at this time. At the very onset of the flowering stage, male plants will produce small papillae at the base of the stem. These will become sepals out of which will arise the primordial stamens. The fully matured male flower will contain loose clusters of five segmented perianth and five stamens that open to reveal anthers, the part of the flower that contains pollen (Fig. 1.7).[16] Following anthesis and the release of its pollen, the male plant dies. This may often be between 1 and 3 weeks prior to full maturation of the female plant.[11]

The female inflorescence of the cannabis plant is more tightly clustered (Fig. 1.8). Within the nomenclature of cannabis culture, they are known as *buds* or *nugs*. An examination of the inflorescence will reveal a plethora of small, single-leaflet leaves

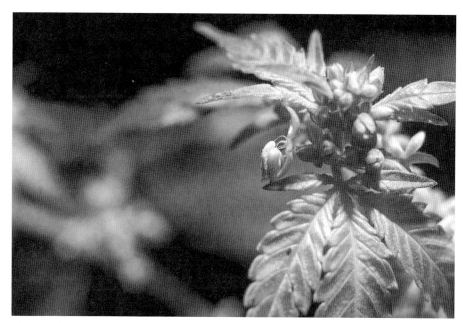

Figure 1.7 Male cannabis flower.

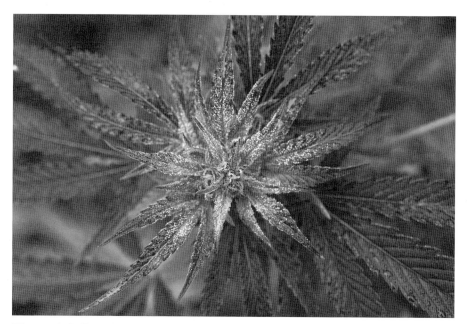

Figure 1.8 Female cannabis flower.

that are perigonal bracts (an enclosure of specialized leaves). The ovule is found within the bract. From the ovule extend two stigmas that protrude from the bract. These stigmas (often called *hairs*) capture the pollen released by male plant. In wild varieties, they tend to be about 3 mm in length, but some illicitly grown cultivars can produce stigmas that are up to 8 mm in length.[17] Initially white in color, stigmas can darken to taken on vivid yellow, orange, or red hues. As the flowering stage progresses, small, unifoliolate leaves will be produced. They tend to become larger as one travels down the flowering axis proximally toward the stalk.[11]

If the female flower is pollinated by the male, the ovule will produce a single seed (technically an achene) that will expand within the bract. Pollinated plants will dedicate considerable amounts of energy to the development of these seeds. After ~3-6 weeks, the seed (achene) will mature, at which point it can be harvested or will fall to the ground. It may measure anywhere from 2 to 6 mm in length and 1 to 4 mm in diameter.[12]

If left unpollinated, the plant will continue to expend energy producing a larger and more robust inflorescence, as well as more cannabinoid-rich trichomes (see below). Consequently, cultivators of drug-type plants go to great lengths to keep their females unpollinated. Unpollinated, seedless female inflorescences are known as *sinsemilla* (or *sin semillas* [Spanish for "without seeds"]). Sinsemilla fetches a far higher price than pollinated flowers, which are often derided by cannabis users as being *"seeds and stems."*

Bracts contain the highest concentration of trichomes. When viewed through a microscope, trichomes have an appearance similar to enoki mushrooms (the mushrooms that are typically found in miso soup [Fig. 1.9]). With the naked eye, they may give cannabis something of frosted look, which is why the unifoliolate leaves that grow among the bracts are referred to as *sugar leaves* (Fig. 1.10).

Trichomes are the resin glands of the cannabis plant. They produce and contain the highest concentration of terpenes and the ~140 cannabinoids that have been discovered as of this time (of which THC and CBD are the most well known). The importance of these cannabinoids and terpenes cannot be stressed highly enough. They are the active ingredients in both recreational and medicinal cannabis. Consequently, *trichomes are the single most important part of the cannabis plant* when viewed through either a recreational or medicinal lens.

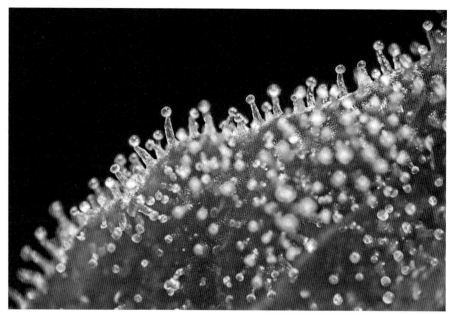

Figure 1.9 Trichomes.

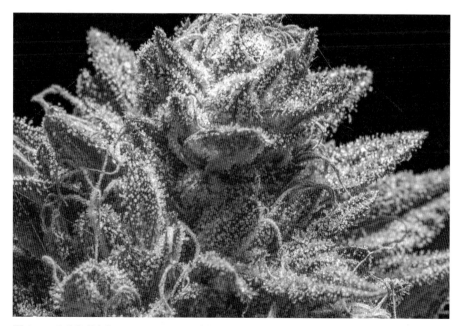

Figure 1.10 Trichomes on cannabis.

Because male plants produce far fewer trichomes (and therefore far fewer cannabinoids and terpenes) than female plants, they are not as highly regarded for their cannabinoid content. Furthermore, the pollination of a female plant by a male plant will lead it to produce seed instead of putting greater energy into producing more trichomes. Consequently, they are often treated as something almost akin to a pest by cultivators.

Trichome content varies from cultivar to cultivar, with significant differences between fiber-type plants and drug-type plants—the former containing higher concentrations of CBDA (cannabidiolic acid), the latter containing higher concentrations of THCA-A (Δ-9-tetrahydrocannabinol acid A).[6] Through decarboxylation, CBDA and THCA-A become the more familiar CBD and THC. Both CBDA and THCA-A are carboxylic acids that have a single precursor—cannabigerolic acid (CBGA).[6] One of the fundamental differences between fiber-type cultivars and drug-type cultivars is an allelic variation where one favors the biosynthesis of CBGA into CBDA (fiber type), while the other favors the biosynthesis of CBGA into THCA-A (drug type).[11] Because CBDA synthase has a higher affinity for CBGA than THCA-A synthase, more CBGA is converted into CBDA when the CBDA synthase allele and THCA-A synthase allele are both active. Drug cultivars have an active THCA-A synthase allele and a nonfunctional CBDA synthase allele, thereby meaning almost all the CBGA becomes THCA-A through biosynthesis.[13] NLD biotypes produce significantly higher concentrations of THCA-A, while BLD biotypes produce high concentrations of both THCA-A and CBDA.[13]

1.5.1 Morphology of Fiber-Type Plants

Depending on conditions, mature plants can reach a height of anywhere from 2 to 4 m in height.[18] Fiber-type plants prefer temperate climates with moist conditions, though some cultivars have been bred to survive colder conditions and even light frosts. While optimal seed germination is in temperatures of 24°C [75°F],[11] and germination tends to occur within 3-7 days,[12] mature Siberian cultivars have been known to survive in extremely frigid temperatures (−10°C [14°F]).

The stalks of fiber-type plants have a diameter averaging between 1 and 3 cm. Within the stalks are found two classes of fibers: The phloem (also known as the "bast" or "bark") that occurs in the outer stem and the xylem, which is often called the "woody core," hurd, or shiv of the stalk.[11] The phloem has historically been considered more valuable as a form of cordage and as the base for textiles. The xylem was often used as animal bedding,[6] though it can also be mixed with a lime-based binder to create a building material known as "hempcrete."[19] Both the phloem and xylem have been shown to have antibacterial properties, as they contain both free and esterified sterols and triterpenes that include β-sitosterol and β-amyrin.[6] There are numerous additional applications for hemp products that are not discussed at this time (Fig. 1.11).[6]

Fiber-type plants have historically been bred to increase the ratio of phloem to xylem. In cultivars of cannabis that are grown specifically for fiber, less than half of the stalk will be made up of xylem, whereas the stalk of drug-type and wild plants may be up to 75% woody core.[11] Furthermore, some fiber-type plants have been bred to increase the space between nodes to maximize the length of primary fibers and to limit seed productivity, as this draws energy away from the production of fiber.

Male fiber plants tend to be taller and thinner than their female counterparts. The quality of their fiber is also thought to be

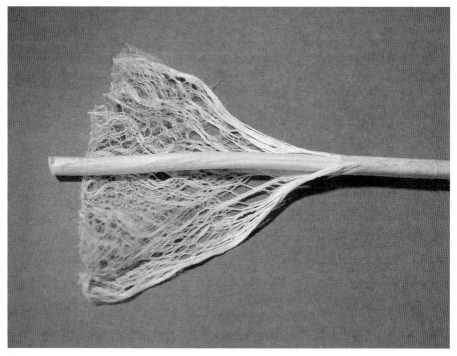

Figure 1.11 Separation of phloem and xylem.

superior to female plants. However, as noted before, female plants do produce more trichomes than males, meaning they are of far greater importance to cultivators interested in extracting non-THC cannabinoids.

The cannabinoid content of fiber-type plants varies. European cultivars usually have much <1% THC. As noted above, U.S. law requires fiber-type plants to contain <0.3% THC. Some Asiatic, broad-leaflet cultivars grown in subtropical climates, however, have THC contents approaching 3%.[11] Similarly, CBD content varies from cultivar to cultivar.

REFERENCES

[1]Cooper G. Police raid a drag for Roddick. The Independent website. https://www.independent.co.uk/news/police-raid-a-drag-for-roddick-1174448.html. Published August 28, 1998. Accessed June 4, 2019.

[2]Bouloc P. Hemp: a plant with a worldwide distribution. In: Bouloc P, ed. *Hemp: Industrial Production and Uses*. Boston, MA: CAB International; 2013:1-3.

[3]Rubin V. The "Ganga Vision" in Jamaica. In: Rubin V, ed. *Cannabis and Culture*. Chicago, IL: Aldine Publishing Company; 1975:257-268.

[4]Sen T, Reddy HNJ. Various industrial applications of hemp, kinaf, flax and ramie natural fibers. *Int J Innov Manag Technol*. 2011;2(3):192-198. doi: 10.7763/IJIMT.2011.V2.130.

[5]Valente AJ. Changes in print paper during the 19th century. Proceedings of the Charleston Library Conference. 2010. https://docs.lib.purdue.edu/cgi/viewcontent.cgi?article=1124&context=charleston. Accessed October 10, 2019.

[6]Andre CM, Hausman JF, Guerriero G. *Cannabis sativa*: the plant of the thousand and one molecules. *Front Plant Sci*. 2016;7:19. doi: 10.3389/fpls.2016.00019.

[7]Halperin A. Marijuana: is it time to stop using a word with racist roots? The Guardian website. https://www.theguardian.com/society/2018/jan/29/marijuana-name-cannabis-racism. Published January 29, 2018. Accessed June 4, 2019.

[8]H.R.2—Agriculture Improvement Act of 2018. Congress.gov. https://www.congress.gov/bill/115th-congress/house-bill/2/text. Updated December 20, 2018. Accessed June 4, 2019.

[9]Drug Scheduling. United States Drug Enforcement Administration website. https://www.dea.gov/drug-scheduling. Accessed June 4, 2019.

[10]Booth M. *Cannabis: A History*. New York, NY: Picador; 2003:3.

[11]Small E. Classification of *Cannabis sativa* L. in relation to agricultural, biotechnological, medical and recreational utilization. In: Chandra S, et al., eds. *Cannabis sativa L.—Botany and Biotechnology*. Cham, Switzerland: Springer International Publishing; 2017:1-62.

[12]Clark RC, Merlin MD. Natural origins and early evolution of *Cannabis*. In: *Cannabis: Evolution and Ethnobotany*. Berkeley, CA: University of California Press; 2013:35-71.

[13]Clarke RC, Merlin MD. Cannabis domestication, breeding history, present-day genetic diversity, and future prospects. *Crit Rev Plant Sci*. 2016;35(5-6):293-327. doi:10.1080/07352689.2016.1267498.

[14]Potter DJ. Cannabis horticulture. In Pertwee RG, ed. *Handbook on Cannabis*. New York, NY: Oxford University Press; 2013:65-88.

[15]Mandolino G, Carboni A, Forapani S, Faeti V, Ranalli P. Identification of DNA markers linked to the male sex in dioecious hemp (*Cannabis sativa* L.). *Theor Appl Genet*. 1999;98(1):86-92. doi: 10.1007/s001220051043.

[16]Reed J. Morphology of *Cannabis sativa* L. Master's thesis. Iowa City, IA: The University of Iowa; 1916. https://ir.uiowa.edu/cgi/viewcontent.cgi?article=3898&context=etd. Accessed June 4, 2019.

[17]Raman V, Lata H, Chandra S, Khan IA, ElSohly MA. Morpho-anatomy of marijuana (*Cannabis sativa* L.). In: Chandra S, et al., eds. *Cannabis sativa L.—Botany and Biotechnology*. Cham, Switzerland: Springer International Publishing; 2017:123-136.

[18]Chabbert B, Kurek B, Beherec O. Physiology and botany of industrial hemp. In: Bouloc P, ed. *Hemp: Industrial Production and Uses*. Boston, MA: CAB International; 2013:27-47.

[19]Elfordy S, Lucas F, Tancret F, Scudeller Y, Goudet L. Mechanical and thermal properties of lime and hemp concrete ("hempcrete") manufactured by a projection process. *Constr Build Mater*. 2008;22(10):2116-2123. doi: 10.1016/j.conbuildmat.2007.07.016.

2

The History of Cannabis

2.1 The History of Cannabis: An Overview

Cannabis has been used and cultivated by myriad cultures since before recorded history. Not only is it difficult to track down a precise location where humans first discovered cannabis and began to explore means of utilizing this multipurpose plant, it is also unlikely that such a singular event ever occurred. In fact, it is more plausible that numerous cultures spread throughout the Eurasian landmass began using cannabis independently of one another and that its proliferation, consequently, cannot be traced to a single source.

Perhaps more importantly, it seems likely that the distinction between varieties of cannabis existed long before humanity's first contact with the plant, and that, consequently, different cultures have found different uses for cannabis depending on what variety they first encountered. Fiber-type plants were utilized for their fibers; cultivars with larger seeds were utilized as a food source; and drug-type plants were utilized for their drug content. All three possessed potential medicinal purposes that were likely explored, as well.

As cultivation techniques became more sophisticated during the Neolithic Revolution, these disparities became more pronounced, albeit inadvertently. Fiber cultivars were selectively bred to produce better fiber; seed cultivars were bred to produce larger seeds; and drug cultivars were bred to produce more potent plants. Furthermore, wild cultivars were eschewed in favor of their domesticated counterparts, as the former possessed characteristics that were deemed more desirable. This selective process accelerated the disparities not only among the three aforementioned types but also their ruderal counterparts.

Eventually, cannabis fell out of favor as a food source and was replaced by more familiar cereals (barley, rice, wheat, etc.), and cannabis seeds became what was known as a "famine food." Fiber cultivars, however, continued to be cultivated from Japan to Europe to make ropes, fabric, and even paper. From ancient times until the advent of modern shipping, hemp was used to make the sails and cordage that allowed for maritime trade and exploration. As cotton became king following the invention of the cotton gin, hempen fabric became less common. Additional technological advancements caused industrial hemp production to wane during the 19th and 20th centuries, though it still enjoys widespread cultivation, particularly in China and, to a lesser extent, France.

The history of industrial hemp parallels the medicinal use of cannabis in many ways. Once a common folk remedy for a variety of ailments, cannabis' role as a medicinal drug was eventually eclipsed by synthetic pharmaceuticals in the late 19th and early 20th centuries. Interest in the medicinal value of cannabis resurged by the end of the 20th century, though, by this time, the United States government had created a regulatory labyrinth due to the passage of the Marihuana Tax Act of 1937 and the Controlled Substances Act of 1970, as well as the subsequent War on Drugs, that made medical research on cannabis exceptionally difficult. Because of these pieces of legislation and until 2018, the federal government conflated fiber-type and drug-type cultivars. Consequently, access to even fiber-type plants was difficult to obtain.

While cannabis declined as a crop for seed or fiber during the 20th century, its use as a recreational drug in the West has become increasingly widespread over the past century. Currently, cannabis is the most popular illicit drug in the world; however, recreational usage is nothing new.* It first became common among the inhabitants of Central Asia and the Indian subcontinent before the dawn of recorded history. Usage then spread through the Middle East, into Africa, and from there into the New World via the slave trade. While it was used by slaves in South America, Central America, and North America, as well as some indigenous peoples, those of European ancestry remained largely unaware of or opposed to its use. This was in keeping with the European idiosyncrasy of abstaining from recreational cannabis from Antiquity and into the Modern Era, despite evidence that scholars were aware of drug-type plants that possessed psychotropic qualities. The general population of Europe seems to have only had contact with fiber-type plants until the 19th century.

With the rise of imperialism and colonization in Asia and Africa, many soldiers, administrators,

---

*Though the use of cannabis, whether for recreational, religious, or medicinal purposes, has become legal or at least more accepted in many jurisdictions, far more states and countries continue to prohibit its use to some degree. As the effort to legalize cannabis progresses, it is likely that far more states and nations will sanction its use under the aegis of either a medicinal or a recreational program. At this time, however, it remains an illicit substance.

and scientists were introduced to drug-type cultivars of cannabis. While stationed in North Africa,
the Middle East, or the Indian subcontinent, they
typically consumed it in the form of hashish, which
is produced by harvesting the tetrahydrocannabinol (THC)-rich resin that collects on the surface
of drug-type cultivars. Pharmacists in Europe and
North America eventually began to carry products
made from hashish, but it does not appear that it
enjoyed widespread use. Conversely, in Mexico and
other parts of the New World, marijuana (a drug
consisting of the dried flowers and leaves of female
drug-type cultivars that is far less potent than hashish) grew in popularity during the late 19th century
as both a recreational intoxicant and a medicine.

Due to the turmoil of the Mexican Revolution,
which began in 1910 and lasted for approximately a decade, many Mexicans moved north
into the United States, where they continued to
use marijuana. Eventually, it was introduced to
other denizens within working class communities
throughout the southern region of the country. Its
use then spread to jazz musicians and was adopted
as a symbol of defiance by members of the white
countercultural movements of the 1950s and the
1960s. A reaction to all three, be it due to xeno-
phobia, racism, or the desire to restore a sense of

order among rebellious young people, resulted in increasingly strict laws against its use for any purpose, even medical research in the United States, which will be described at length in Chapter 5 (U.S. Cannabis Regulations From Past to Present).

2.2 Origins of Cannabis and First Contact

Evidence suggests that *Cannabis* diverged from its two closest taxonomic relatives, *Celtis* (the hackberry) and *Humulus* (the hop), and began evolving into a separate genera ~20 million years ago.[1] Where and how cannabis evolved following that divergence has been the subject of intense debate.

When searching for the geographical origin of a plant that has been cultivated by humans for so long, it would seem sensible to begin by looking to where feral plants thrive in the wild. This, unfortunately, is extremely difficult with cannabis for three codependent reasons.

The first is that cannabis can thrive in a wide variety of environments—from the foothills of the Himalayas to the vast steppe of Central Asia and Eurasia to any temperate or subtropical riparian zone. It prefers a warm, continental climate with significant rainfall in the spring and early summer followed by a dry and cool autumn and rarely can survive in colder regions or areas with excessive humidity. Its growth cycle corresponds with the increasing and diminishing day length that progresses from spring to fall in nontropical latitudes.[2] It is also particularly fond of the nutrient-rich dump heaps in areas cleared for temporary settlement by iterant peoples and would have followed these nomads, thereby making it what is known as a "camp follower." Nikolai Vavilov, the esteemed Soviet botanist who traveled throughout Central Asia to conduct research, noted that cannabis—both the weedy variety and the "wild" variety—seemed to trail nomads wherever they went.[3] He also noted that thick stands of weedy cannabis grew in the waste areas in and around Yarkand, a city in Xinjiang province of China, as well as in ravines, marshes, and the edges of forests.

The second is that cannabis was quite popular with prehistoric humans because it was a multipurpose plant—it has industrial, religious, recreational, and dietary uses. The archeological record suggests that humans from Japan to Europe were already using

No matter the purpose cannabis served, it would have been readily available because it grows prolifically in so many climates and it also would have been found nearby the basecamps of early humans. As mentioned before, this "camp follower" thrives in newly cleared habitats and in soils rich in nitrogen compounds like those within proximity to dump heaps. Had just a few seeds been dropped inadvertently near a settlement, cannabis would have been able to quickly colonize the open area.[†]

Regardless of which type was first discovered and exploited, the archeological record tells us that the roots of the relationship between humans and cannabis run extremely deep. In some cultures, its use predates the Neolithic Revolution and the transition from a foraging economy to a farming economy, which is thought to have begun in several independent sites more than 10 000 years ago.[4] As these cultures developed independently of one another, many developed their own uses for and beliefs about cannabis.

2.3 Cannabis in China

As humans settled into permanent camps and began to establish agrarian communities, cannabis continued to be exploited as a vital resource. One of the first locations where such communities formed was China, along the Yangtze River and the Yellow River, as well as one of its tributaries, the Wei. Evidence suggests that cannabis was enjoying widespread usage as an economic crop by 4500 BCE.[9]

When the cultivation of cannabis began in China is far less clear. The oldest hemp rope to be discovered in the area dates to between 6000 and 7000 years ago. Pottery that may be even more ancient depicts clothing made of hemp cloth.[10] Hemp ropes were also embedded into pottery as a form of decoration. Evidently, this practice was widespread, as shards of such pottery have been discovered near Taipei on the island of Taiwan at the Yangmingshan archeological site that date back to between 12 000 and 5000 years ago.[11] Traditional lacquerware items were also frequently made with hemp.[12]

Artisans were not the only ones to make use of hemp in ancient Chinese culture. The *Xia Xiao Zheng*, an agricultural treatise

---

[†] This would seem to give credence to Edgar Anderson's "dump-heap" theory, which is both a fascinating notion and too far beyond the scope of our purposes here to be fully investigated.[8]

assumed to have been written in the 16th century BCE, describes cannabis as a major crop.[13] It was regarded as one of the five primary grains along with rice, barley, millet, and soy beans but eventually fell out of favor and was replaced by other staple crops sometime after the 6th century CE.[13] Despite being relegated to an inferior position, thousands of years of selective breeding produced a large-seeded variety of fiber-type cannabis that continues to grow in northern China.[14] Furthermore, hemp seeds are still enjoyed as a snack food throughout China, they are considered a "longevity" food in parts of the Guangxi province in the country's southeastern corner, and beverages made from hemp seeds are extremely popular in Hong Kong. Even major corporations produce such beverages.[15]

Cannabis was also being used as a medicine in China. Shennong (also known as Shen-Nung), the father of traditional Chinese medicine and one of the primordial rulers of China, is said to have studied the medicinal properties of the flora throughout his kingdom during a reign that is said to have predated the Xia dynasty (c. 2070-c. 1600 BCE) by several hundred years. The *Pen Ts'ao Ching*, the first Chinese pharmacopeia, is attributed to Shennong, though the earliest known version only dates to the first century CE.[12] According to the text, cannabis had multiple medicinal applications. It was used to treat absentmindedness, rheumatic pains, constipation, and disorders afflicting the female reproductive system.[7] A type of "hemp elixir" also was used to treat other conditions, including gout and malaria.[12]

Later physicians also made use of cannabis cocktails. The founder of Chinese surgery, Hua Tuo (c. 140-208 CE), created an anesthetic known as *Ma-fei-san* ("bubbling-drug medicine"), which was a decoction of wine and herbs that is said to have included cannabis.[7] It was potent enough that it allowed him to conduct major invasive surgeries. Unfortunately, because Hua Tuo's recipes and writings have been lost, it is unclear if THC was an active ingredient, if he made use of inflorescence or seeds, or if it even contained cannabis at all. The use of the word *ma*,[13] which is Chinese for hemp, seems to be a strong indicator that *ma-fei-san* did contain cannabis, but there is no firm evidence to support the claim.

Other sources are clearer about the usage of cannabis inflorescence (translated as *mahua*, *mafen*, or *mabo*) as a means of treating pain. A formula for *shui sheng san* ("sagacious sleep powder") dating to either the 12th or 13th century is comprised of datura flower and the flower of cannabis (*mahua*), while a text from the 17th century claims that it can be used as an aesthetic.[15] As recently as 1935, the *Yao Wu Tu Kao* ("*Illustrated Analysis of Medical Substances*") recommended *mafen* for headache, itching, convulsions, anemia, dry coughing, and was also prescribed to treat menstrual irregularities.[15]

Practitioners of traditional Chinese medicine also made and continue to make use of cannabis' seeds. They have been prescribed as both a laxative and to combat diarrhea, as an antidiabetic, an emmenagogue, and to treat obstinate vomiting. The *Tu Jing Ben Cao* ("*Illustrated Classic of Materia Medica*"), which dates to 1070 CE, cites an earlier formula made from the powder of roasted seeds in wine to relieve severe pain.[15] Seeds have also been used topically as a thick porridge that can be applied to the skin to treat ulcers, wounds, and fungal diseases. This porridge was also used to prevent hair loss.[7]

Chinese physicians also made use of roots, leaves, and stalk. The latter was described as a diuretic and was evidently mixed with other drugs to aid in the excretion of kidney stones.[7]

Significantly less was written about the psychoactive or intoxicating effects of cannabis, though several sources do make mention of them. The *Pen Ts'ao Ching* notes that cannabis had the power to cause hallucinations (literally "seeing devils") and, when taken over a long period of time, would allow one to communicate with spirits. It also said that cannabis caused a lightness of the body.[7] The *Kai Bao Ben Cao* ("The *Materia Medica of the Kaibao Era*"), which dates from the late 10th century CE, states that "cannabis causes happiness in the heart." Other sources seem to indicate that cannabis was used to treat some mental illnesses, though it is unclear if the historical texts were referring to types of behavior that could be described as erratic or if they were referring to physical convulsions.[15]

Some saw cannabis in a less felicitous light. Writing in the 5th century CE, a Taoist priest noted that cannabis was used by "necromancers, in combination with ginseng, to set forward time in order to reveal future events."[7] Li Shizhen, author of the 16th century *Ben Cao Gang Mu* ("*Compendium of Materia Medica*"), said that this was an exaggeration, though he did write that it induces a form of drunkenness.[15] He also believed it could be used to treat malaria.

Suffice to say, it is evident that at least some Chinese physicians were familiar with the psychotropic qualities of cannabis, though there is no evidence to suggest that cannabis was used as an intoxicant by the people who lived under the various empires of ancient China, particularly those of the Han Chinese ethnic group, despite its widespread use as an industrial crop, which continues to this day. It became especially important for industry after Cai Lun, the director of the Imperial Workshops of Luoyang, created a form of paper made from hemp fibers in 105 CE (though a growing body of research indicates that a less durable form of hempen paper was already in existence in China by that time).[16]

Though members of the Han ethnic group did not use cannabis for its drug content, shamanistic and nomadic cultures within modern-day China did. These cultures would have existed in the northernmost and westernmost regions of modern China and would have extended into the Eurasian Steppe. Physical evidence of the use of cannabis among these cultures was found in a tomb excavated in Xinxiang, an autonomous territory in northwest China. The findings suggest that members of this culture were using cannabis ~2500 years ago for ritualistic or medicinal purposes.[17]

2.4 The Eurasian Steppe

Shamanism may have declined in China during the Han Dynasty, but it continued to be popular in the vast expanse of the Eurasian Steppe and many of those who practiced it used cannabis for religious purposes.[7] Though today it would seem strange to conflate cultures across a landmass that stretches from Mongolia to Ukraine, it does appear that cannabis use was spread by nomadic tribes throughout this transcontinental region several thousand years ago. Evidence suggests that the Sredni Stog, who flourished in Ukraine between 4500 and 3500 BCE, as well as the Yamnaya, a very early Indo-European culture that spread from what is today western Kazakhstan to northeastern Romania ~5000 year ago, were using cannabis as an intoxicant. Due to their use of horses for land transportation, they would have accelerated its proliferation.[18] Recent research has shown that there was a broad network of exchange or migration that predated the Silk Road by several thousand years and the myriad cultures from Mongolia all the way to southern Ukraine were using cannabis during the Bronze Age, if not earlier.

One of the most frequently cited pieces of historical evidence concerning cannabis use in the ancient world comes from the

Greek writer Herodotus' discussion of Scythian culture in the 5th century BCE. Herodotus notes that the Scythians, a nomadic people whose territory encompassed much of the Eurasian Steppe and stretched from Ukraine to Kyrgyzstan, had an intimate relationship with cannabis. Herodotus describes how the Massagetae—a nomadic people described as potentially being of Scythian nationality who were based in what is today eastern Turkmenistan, Uzbekistan, and southern Kazakhstan—enjoyed the fruit of a tree that he does not name specifically, though he is almost certainly describing cannabis. "When they have parties and sit around a fire, they throw some of it into the flames, and as it burns it smokes like incense, and the smell of it makes them drunk just as wine does the Greeks; and they get more and more intoxicated as more fruit is thrown on until they jump up and start dancing and singing."[19]

The Scythians of Central Asia were not the only peoples using cannabis. The excavation of ancient Bactrian sites dating back to the second millennium BCE in Margiana, which was just to the southeast of the Massagetae's territory, has shown that cannabis played an important role in their religious rites. This region would later become a satrapy of the Achaemenid (First Persian) Empire and would become known as the "Zoroastrian capital."[18] Cannabis would come to play a significant role in Zoroastrianism, the religion of Ancient Persia.[20]

Scythians living to the west enjoyed a ritual like the one described above. Herodotus claims that they enjoyed taking saunas with hemp seeds: "They take some hemp seed, creep into the tent, and throw the seed on to the hot stones. At once it begins to smoke, giving off a vapour unsurpassed by any vapour-bath one could find in Greece." He concluded: "The Scythians enjoy it so much that they howl with laughter."[21] It seems at the very least likely that these saunas also included the "fruit" of cannabis, though it cannot be known for certain.

Another ancient European writing in the first century of the common era, Pliny the Elder, described the use of gelotophyllis ("leaves of laughter") among Scythian tribes along what he called the Borysthenes River (almost certainly the Dnieper) in Ukraine. "If this be taken in myrrh and wine all kinds of phantoms beset the mind, causing laughter which persist until the kernels of pine-nuts are taken with pepper and honey in palm wine." Gelotophyllis is almost certainly cannabis. What is curious to note is that pine-nuts are said to reduce the giddiness brought on by the concoction, that pine nuts contain the terpene α-pinene, and that α-pinene has been shown to reduce the effects of cannabis intoxication in recent studies.[22] This terpene is also commonly found in many chemotypes of cannabis.

Unfortunately, the historical record does not distinguish between ceremonial, recreational, and medicinal uses for cannabis, and no archeological evidence has been uncovered to elucidate how advanced this culture's knowledge of cannabis was, but the archeological record does indicate that the above depictions of cannabis use among Scythians are accurate. The excavation of Scythian tombs in the Altai Mountains, the Caucasus Mountains, Germany, and Romania have all uncovered artifacts that corroborate the claims made by Herodotus regarding the culture's use of cannabis.[3,18,23,24]

2.5 The Indian Subcontinent

Cannabis use in Ancient India was extremely widespread, and it has been used for religious, social, ceremonial, recreational, and medicinal purposes since at least the first historical records in the region were drafted. It is likely that nomads and traders traveling south over the Himalayas introduced the use of cannabis to the region.[9]

Cannabis has a central place in the four *Vedas*, which are integral to the Hindu faith—akin to the Torah for Judaism, the four Gospels for Christianity, or the Quran for Islam. Written prior to 1000 BCE, the *Vedas* describe cannabis as one of the five sacred plants meant to "release us from anxiety."[3] Most scholars agree that cannabis was not *soma*, a ritual beverage consumed by priests and offered to the gods, though some contend that it is possible that *soma* was not one plant but a concoction made from several plants of which cannabis may have been but one ingredient.[25] According to the *Vedas*, a drop of the nectar of immortality, *amrita*, fell from heaven. From that place grew cannabis. A beverage made from cannabis became the favorite drink of Indra, the lord of the gods. When demons tried to steal it, they were driven away and, as a result, many of the names for cannabis within Hindi and Sanskrit refer to this victory or to Indra (see Table 2.1). Cannabis is also said to be the favorite food of Shiva.[26] Similarly, the Tibetan Buddhist tradition states that the Gautama Buddha, the founder of Buddhism, subsisted on one hemp seed each day in the 6 years of asceticism prior to attaining enlightenment.[7]

Table 2.1 Terms for Cannabis in India

Sanskrit or Hindi term	Meaning[a]
Ajaya	The unconquered, invincible
Ananda	The joyful, joyous, laughter moving, bliss
Bahuvadini	Causing excessive garrulousness
Bhang, bhanga	Mature cannabis leaves
Bhangini	Breaks three kinds of misery
Bharita	The green one
Capala	Agile, capricious, mischievous, scatterbrained
Capa	Lighthearted
Chapala	The lighthearted, causer of reeling gait
Charas	Cannabis resin
Cidalhada	Gives happiness to mind
Divyaka	Gives pleasure, luster, intoxication, beauty
Dnayana, vardhani	Knowledge promoter
Ganga	Seedless female cannabis flower
Ganjakini	The noisy, vibrator
Gatra-bhanga	Body disintegrator
Harshani	Joy-giver
Harshini	The exciter of sexual desire
Hursini	The exciter of sexual desire
Indrasana	Indra's food
Jaya	Victorious, the conquering
Kalaghni	Helps to overcome death
Madhudrava	Helps to excrete nectar
Madini	The intoxicator

Table 2.1 Continued

Sanskrit or Hindi term	Meaning[a]
Manonmana	Accomplishes the objects of the mind
Matulani	Wife of the datura
Matkunari	An enemy of bugs
Mohini	Fascinating
Pasupasavinaini	Liberates creatures from earthly bonds
Ranjika	Causer of excitement
Sakrasana	Food worthy of Indra
Sanvida manjari	Flower of garrulousness
Sana	Cannabis
Sarvarogaghni	That which cures all diseases
Sawi	Green-leaved
Shivbooty	Shiva's plant
Siddha	Which has attained spiritual perfection
Sidhamuli	On whose root is *siddha*
Siddhapatri	Vessel of highest attainment
Siddhi	Success giver
Siddhidi	Which endows *siddhi* on others
Sidhdi	Emancipation, fruit of worship
Suknidhan	Fountain of pleasures
Tandrakrit	Causer of drowsiness
Trailokya Vijaya	Victorious in the three worlds
Trilok kamaya	Desired in the three worlds
Ununda	The laughter mover
Urjaya	Promoter of success

(*Continued*)

Table 2.1 Continued

Sanskrit or Hindi term	Meaning[a]
Vijaya	Victorious, promoter of success
Vijpatta	The strong leaved
Virapattra	Leaf of heroes
Vrijapata	Strong-nerved

[a]Russo E. Cannabis in India: ancient lore and modern medicine. In: Mechoulam R, ed. *Cannabinoids as Therapeutics*. Boston, MA: Birkhäuser Verlag; 2005:1-22.

Cannabis is also central to the traditional medicine of the Indian subcontinent. The practice of Ayurveda medicine, which began more than 3000 years ago and continues to this day, makes use of more than 2000 drugs that are primarily found in the region's plants and herbs. Within the Ayurveda pharmacopeia, cannabis is held in an extremely high regard, and it is said to treat scores of ailments. The term *sarvarogaghni*, one of more than several dozen synonyms for cannabis in either Hindi or Sanskrit that translates into "that which cures all diseases," seems to have been taken almost literally.[20] Zoroastrian physicians in nearby Persia considered cannabis to be the most important medicinal plant.[26]

Sushruta, one of the most celebrated doctors of Ancient India who likely lived in the 6th century BCE, described cannabis as an antiphlegmatic (a substance capable of drying mucous membranes, ameliorating congestion, and, as Touw suggests, a diuretic) that would have been used to treat catarrh, diarrhea, and perhaps even mood disorders (a phlegmatic person is one who is sluggish and dull).[7] Cannabis was used as an analgesic and an aphrodisiac, suggesting that there was a greater interest in the initial phase of the drug's effects, rather than its later effects even though it was acknowledged that heavy long-term use can negate these benefits and lead one to become more phlegmatic. Conversely, Persian doctors focused on the later phase of the drug's effects and recommended it as a means of reducing one's libido.[7]

Later physicians of the Unani-Tibb (traditional Islamic) and Ayurveda systems would prescribe cannabis to improve digestion, appetite, sleep, and breathing. It was also used as an antispasmodic, antibacterial, anticonvulsive, anti-inflammatory, antirheumatic, antimalarial, antihistamine, vermifuge, and antivenin. In fact, it was used to treat everything from neuralgia and sciatica to gonorrhea and leprosy. Cannabis was also believed to have obstetric applications as a means of reducing labor pains and strengthening uterine contractions. Cannabis was typically applied topically or taken orally either as bhang or charas, though one of the more interesting means of delivery among Ayurveda physicians treating diarrhea and strangulated hernias was to blow cannabis smoke directly into the rectum.[7]

Cannabis was not merely used as a means of spiritual fulfillment or to treat disease but was also used as a recreational drug, particularly among India's working class. The Spaniard Garcia da Orta, who traveled to India in the service of Portugal in 1563, noted the casual use of bhang, a spiced beverage that contains cannabis. "Those of my servants who took it, unknown to me, said that it made them so as to not feel work, to be very happy, and to have a craving for food."[20] Bhang remains a popular means of consuming cannabis. Smoking cannabis (known as ganga) would not become popularized until after the Amerindian practice of smoking tobacco had spread to the region during the 16th century.

The use of cannabis continued unabated among India's laboring class as the British Empire expanded deeper into the Indian subcontinent, culminating in the direct rule by the British Crown in 1858. As Britain increased its presence in the area and began its administration of the British Raj, researchers from Europe came to study the flora and fauna of the region. One of these researchers, William O'Shaughnessy, became extremely interested in cannabis and conducted experiments on the plant while in the service of the East India Company during the 1830s.[27] He eventually presented his findings to the Medical and Physical Society of Bengal in 1843, which led to increased interest in the potential medicinal qualities of cannabis in Britain, continental Europe, and North America. Eventually, cannabis tinctures and even pills of hashish became rather common items found in British and American pharmacies in the second half of the 19th century. "Indian cigarettes," a combination of cannabis and tobacco, were even sold as a treatment for asthma.[28] Despite its availability, there is no evidence that it became popular as a recreational drug among more than a very small group.

This was not the case among the people of the Indian subcontinent, and attention was eventually drawn to the use of cannabis among sepoys (Indian troops employed by the British).

Some within the British press made the baseless claim that it was leading them on a path of criminality and insanity, which eventually led to a commission to study the effects of cannabis in 1871. The commission determined that it did not lead to madness or crime, and that prohibition would lead to smuggling and tax evasion. An 1877 commission reached a similar conclusion.[29]

Despite these two commissions, the matter remained unresolved, and in 1893, Lord Kimberley, the Secretary of State for India, established the Indian Hemp Drugs Commission. In 1894, the commission published its final report, which, at seven volumes and 3500 pages, continues to be one of the most thorough official studies ever done on the subject.[30] Central to the report was the testimony from doctors of the Unani-Tibb, Ayurveda, and Western traditions, who described its therapeutic uses for "cramps, spasms, convulsions, headache, hysteria, neuralgia, sciatica, tetanus, hydrophobia, ague, cholera, dysentery, leprosy, brain fever, gonorrhea, hay fever, asthma, bronchitis, catarrh, tuberculosis, piles, flatulence, dyspepsia, diabetes, delirium tremens, and impotence; as a sedative and febrifuge (substance that reduces fever); as an analgesic for toothache, tooth extraction, and many other acute or chronic pains; as an anesthetic for minor surgery including circumcision; as a diuretic, tonic, digestive, disinfectant, aphrodisiac, anaphrodisiac (substance used to decrease sexual desire), food supplement, appetite stimulant, energy-creator, cool refreshing drink to prevent malaria, cure insomnia, alleviate hunger, and ... for freedom from distress."[31]

Ultimately, the Commission concluded that no good would come from prohibition and that moderate usage of cannabis did not pose a significant danger to body, mind, or the moral glue holding society together. Excessive usage, meanwhile, was condemned as harmful to all three. It was also noted that cannabis use could pose a danger to individuals predisposed to serious mental illnesses like schizophrenia and what we today call bipolar disorder.[20]

Cannabis use would remain common throughout India into the 20th century and remains quite common to this day. Cannabis use was also common among Indian indentured laborers, and they brought their ganja with them as they were taken to places like Jamaica and South Africa to satisfy British labor demands following the end of slavery.[32] In the case of the latter, recreational cannabis was already being used by Africans for generations. There is no evidence to suggest that its use was widespread in Jamaica prior to the arrival of the Indian laborers.

2.6 The Middle East

As mentioned above, traditional physicians of the Hindu and Muslim faiths were prescribing cannabis on the Indian subcontinent. It was no different elsewhere in the Islamic world. From Persia to Morocco, doctors regularly treated a wide variety of conditions similar to those described above with cannabis. Though the Quran does forbid intoxicants, it never mentions cannabis by name and, consequently, it was widely considered permissible if used solely for medicinal purposes.

Some of these medicinal purposes were less dire than others. For example, Az-Zarkashi, a 14th century scholar based in Cairo, noted that cannabis dissolved flatulence and eliminated dandruff.[31] Conversely, Ibn al-Baytar al-Dimashqi, who practiced during the 12th century, employed cannabis to treat neuropathic pain and as a vermicide.[3] There is also the anecdotal story, purportedly from the 15th century, about a poet who provided the epileptic son of a caliph's chamberlain with cannabis. Though it cured the boy, it evidently turned him into the kind of addict depicted in the infamous propaganda film from the 1930s, *Reefer Madness* (see Chapter 5 [U.S. Cannabis Regulations From Past to Present]).

What is so interesting about this story is not only that it reveals the benefits of cannabis for treating epilepsy but it also elucidates the stigma within Islam at the time concerning cannabis use that, in many ways, echoes the way in which it was perceived by mainstream American culture during the Jazz Age and the Beat Era of the 20th century. Like their American counterparts in the 20th century, many Muslim artists during the Islamic Golden Age used cannabis recreationally. So, too, did many mystics— particularly those who practiced Sufism.[33] For them, cannabis, eaten as hashish,[‡] offered a means through which they could convene with Allah (God).

In time, ingesting hashish also became a common occurrence among the poor and destitute, thereby galvanizing the stigma against its use among the ruling classes. Though moderate rulers often turned a blind eye to the practice, more draconian leaders favored prohibition, and the punishment for using cannabis as an intoxicant was harsh.[34] In some cases, it could mean up to

---

[‡]Hashish, like charas, is prepared by collecting the resin from the cannabis plant, which contains the phytocannabinoid-producing trichomes, and compressing it into blocks, bars, or discs.

80 lashes,[31] while others were punished by having their teeth removed.[35]

As severe as these punishments were, there is no evidence that they reduced the popularity of hashish, and its use continued following the fall of the Abbasid Caliphate and other empires, while the Ottoman and Safavid took control of the region. Both disapproved of recreational hashish, but its use was widespread enough at that point that eradication was out of the question.[36]

Though it may seem reasonable to assume that much of the knowledge concerning the medicinal use and psychoactive properties of cannabis was learned from Persian and Indian physicians, at least some of this knowledge about cannabis may have come from Greek and Roman physicians such as Galen and Dioscorides, whose works Muslim scholars translated. Both Galen and Dioscorides describe some of the medicinal properties of cannabis, though it seems as though they did not know of its psychoactive effects.

There is also the possibility that a great deal about cannabis was already known, and that this knowledge did not have to be imported. In the Assyrian city of Nineveh, which sits across the Tigris River from modern-day Mosul, more than 19 000 Akkadian and Sumerian tablets were found in the Royal Library of Ashurbanipal. Some of these tablets date back to more than 4000 years ago and represent the collected wisdom of multiple cultures. Of the 19 000 tablets, ~660 were medical in nature. More to the point, many of these cuneiform tablets make mention of an herb called *azallû* in Assyrian or *A.ZAL.LA* in Sumerian that was used to create fabric; that could be psychoactive; and that was used to treat impotence, neuralgia, pulmonary congestion, depression, anxiety, and nocturnal epilepsy. After studying the potential uses of the plant, as well as the philological constructs from related languages, Reginald Campbell Thompson, who published the first comprehensive English edition of *The Epic of Gilgamesh* in 1930, determined that *azallû* and *A.ZAL.LA* were older forms of the word for cannabis, which, by the 7th century BCE, had become known as *qunnabu* in Assyrian.[3]

While not every scholar agrees with Thompson's analysis, one would be hard-pressed to find another herb with a similar pharmacological profile that can also be used to make textiles. Furthermore, it would seem at the very least plausible that an herb that, on the one hand, served as one of the most integral parts of the religious life of an adjacent civilization and, on the other, possesses so many therapeutic uses, would be of interest to the ancient Assyrians. The contrary, in fact, would seem quite bizarre.

It seems extremely likely that the knowledge of cannabis' medicinal properties was not imported into the Middle East from India or Persia subsequent to the rise of Islam, and that cannabis had been in use in the region prior to the birth of the Islamic prophet Muhammad in 570 CE, though it is difficult to establish when, how widespread usage was, and to what extent those in Western Asia knew of its psychoactive properties following the decline of Assyria in the late 7th century BCE. The philological and archaeological evidence, excluding Mesopotamian, Greek, and Roman sources, provides only scant clues.

Linguistic evidence from the Bible, for example, is less than concrete. Though the phrase "fragrant cane," transliterated as *kaneh bosm*, sounds a lot like the Greek κάνναβις (transliterated as *cannabis*), and though the root word *kan* can mean both "hemp" and "reed," the context in which "fragrant cane" is used in the Old Testament does not preclude other possibilities beyond cannabis. One such example is calamus (*Acorus calamus*), an herbaceous perennial that was frequently imported from India and used for ceremonial and medicinal purposes. It was also highly regarded for its sweet scent and continues to be used in perfumes to this day. Consequently, when God commands Moses anoint himself in a holy oil composed of myrrh, cinnamon, cassia, olive oil, and fragrant cane in Exodus 30:22-25, it is difficult to say for certain whether the "fragrant cane" is cannabis or if it is calamus. The same can be said of passages from Isiah 43:24, Jeremiah 6:20, Ezekiel 27:19, and Song of Songs 4:14. Given the context in each instance, both interpretations make sense.

The archeological evidence that cannabis enjoyed wide usage for medicinal, religious, or recreational purposes is also tenuous, though it seems clear that cultures in the region knew that cannabis could be used to create cloth. For example, hempen cloths were found in Phrygian grave mounds in Turkey dating back to the 7th century BCE.[3] Also, Herodotus mentions that the Thracians, who would have occupied parts of modern-day Romania, Bulgaria, and European Turkey, made textiles from hemp that were of very high quality.[37]

Later archeological evidence reveals that cannabis was being used for either ceremonial or medicinal purposes in the region during the late Roman Empire. In a Roman tomb ~30 km west of Jerusalem, a team of archeologists found coins from the 4th century CE and the carbonized remains of Δ-8-tetrahydrocannabinol (Δ-9-tetrahydrocannabinol's more stable relative) in a young woman's abdominal region. The skeleton of a term fetus was found in her pelvic area, as well, which suggests that she died during childbirth.[38] Unfortunately, it is unclear if the cannabis was burned for ceremonial reasons following the young woman's death or if cannabis was being used in an obstetric capacity by the individual or individuals attending to her—a common use among physicians of the Unani-Tibb and Ayurveda traditions, as noted above. The former seems unlikely. As this woman was likely Roman of some means (as we learned from electronic correspondence with Dr. Joe Zias), it stands to reason that the funerary rites observed at the time of her death would have been typical for other members of the aristocracy, meaning that carbonized Δ-8-tetrahydrocannabinol should be commonly found on or near the skeletal remains of others who possessed a similar social standing but this is not the case. In fact, this is the only instance where Δ-8-tetrahydrocannabinol has been found in the vicinity of a Roman tomb. Therefore, it seems far more likely that cannabis was used to facilitate childbirth, though, again, it is impossible to say how widespread the usage was at the time or from where the practice was learned.

2.7 Africa

Cannabis is not native to Africa, which means it had to be brought to the continent. While it is certain that it was brought into Northern Africa alongside Islam, there is the possibility that it had been brought earlier and that the medicinal properties of cannabis were known to Ancient Egyptians.

Such a premise seems entirely reliant on the belief that the Egyptian word *shemshemet* means cannabis, since archeological evidence is severely lacking. While it is true that cannabinoids were detected in the body tissues of several Egyptian mummies dating back some 3000 years ago, these same studies also found trace amounts of cocaine and nicotine.[9] As the distribution of plants containing cocaine and nicotine did not extend beyond the Americas until European contact in the 15th century, either the results of these studies were somehow contaminated or transatlantic trade networks predated Columbus by 2500 years. The former is far more likely.

From the historical record, Egyptologists have determined that *shemshemet* was used for making ropes and for medicinal purposes.

The first mention of the former dates back to the Old Kingdom, ~2350 BCE. The latter is found in numerous medical papyri during the second millennia, where it was described as a treatment for inflammation of the eyes, as well as an obstetric aid, antiparasitic, and antibacterial. The *Chester Beatty VI Papyrus*, dated to 1300 BCE, recommends using a concoction containing *shemshemet* be administered directly into the rectum to reduce diarrhea.[3] These uses match the pharmacological profile of cannabis as understood by Ayurvedic physicians. Furthermore, there were trade networks between Indian and Mesopotamia, and Mesopotamia and Egypt at this time. It stands to reason that they may have traded medical knowledge as well, though the argument that the cultures within Mesopotamia used cannabis medicinally remains controversial. More evidence is needed to support this claim.

Evidence does become significantly stronger following the rise of Islam, and cannabis use in Northern Africa has been well documented since the Islamic Golden Age. Like all practitioners of the Unani-Tibb tradition, North African doctors regularly prescribed cannabis to treat a host of conditions, as the medicinal use of cannabis was considered acceptable even under Sharia law. Recreational hashish use, meanwhile, was prohibited, though it eventually became something of an open secret during the 13th and 14th centuries and its use spread into Morocco and to Spain via the Straits of Gibraltar. As was the case throughout other parts of the Islamic world, it was begrudgingly tolerated during the reigns of less strict rulers. More conservative leaders, conversely, imposed severe penalties for its recreational use and launched campaigns to find and eradicate cannabis that was either planted in private gardens or grown on a more large-scale basis outside of urban centers.[35] This pendulous swing back and forth between tacit acceptance and overzealous prohibition continued until North Africa was conquered by the Ottomans during the first half of the 16th century.

In the 16th century, smoking cannabis became far more common, particularly in Morocco, where it was loosely chopped and mixed with dried tobacco leaves into what is known as *kaif* or *kif*.[35] It was then smoked from a long pipe known as a *sebsi*. Morocco continues to be one of the world's largest producers of cannabis to this day.[39] Though smoking quickly gained in popularity, it seems unlikely that the practice predated European interaction with Amerindians, as tobacco came from the Western Hemisphere and it is likely that the practice of pipe smoking was not known to the peoples of North Africa until they learned of it from Amerindians via European traders, though archeological evidence suggests that pipe smoking began independently of the Amerindians in sub-Saharan Africa.

While physical evidence for ancient cannabis use in sub-Saharan Africa is not strong, archeologists have uncovered smoking pipes in two sites hundreds of miles away from each other. The first, in Zambia, dates to between 1100 and 1300 CE.[18] The second set of pipes was found at a site near Lake Tana in northern Ethiopia, and they have been dated to the 14th century. It is unclear if the first were used for smoking cannabis or some other herb. The pipes found in Ethiopia did contain residual cannabis.[18]

Exactly when cannabis was introduced to Ethiopia is unclear, as trade networks between the cultures of the Mediterranean, the Arabian Peninsula, India, Northern Africa, and the areas around the Horn of Africa have existed for thousands of years. Linguistic evidence suggests that cannabis was introduced to various Bantu peoples along much of the eastern coast of Africa by either Indian or Arab merchants within the past six to eight hundred years, and that its use gradually spread inland.[31] Use of the word *"dagga,"* which is common throughout Africa, is thought to have its origins in modern-day South Africa and is of either Dutch or Khoisan origin.

Accounts by European explorers and colonists in the 19th century described both its medicinal and recreational uses among Africans. It was used to treat asthma, snakebites, malaria, and dysentery. The Sotho of southern Africa used cannabis to facilitate childbirth,[31] while Xhosa of South Africa used it as an analgesic for foot pain.[40] Cannabis became extremely popular as a recreational drug throughout Africa, whether among hunter-gatherers, shepherds, or farmers; in fishing communities; or in cosmopolitan centers like Cairo.

By the time of the French invasion of Egypt during the Napoleonic era, hashish use in cafes was a common occurrence. As alcohol was prohibited in the country, many of the French soldiers stationed in the region experimented with hashish and, upon their return to Europe, brought it back with them.[41]

2.8 Europe

Fiber-type plants have been grown throughout Europe since prehistoric times. Palynological evidence reveals that they spread from the Mediterranean during the Greek and Roman empires and into Western, Central, and Northern Europe and continued to be cultivated until industrial hemp became largely obsolete due to technological advances in the 19th and 20th centuries. There is also evidence that, prior to cultivation by the Romans and the Greeks, cannabis was brought into the Balkans by the Scythians, and it seems to have been prevalent among cultures in the area, as well as Eastern European cultures to the north. It is unclear if these eastern cultivars contained high quantities of THC or if they were used solely for industrial purposes.[18] By the Middle Ages, only fiber-type plants were being grown in Europe. No evidence has ever surfaced to support the claim that cannabis was used for recreational purposes in Europe on a large scale prior to the modern period.

As noted above, several Greek and Roman writers were aware of some of the medicinal properties of cannabis, though their knowledge seems to have been limited. Writing in the first century of the common era, Dioscorides noted that cannabis juice could treat earaches and that its seeds could "quench conception." He also believed that the roots could be used to reduce inflammation, relieve edema, and "disperse hardened matter around the joints."[42] Galen, the 2nd century physician, seems to have been more aware of its psychoactive properties, as he says that cannabis seeds, when consumed in excess, send "a warm and toxic vapor to the head."[31] He also noted that it "eliminates intestinal gas and dehydrates [the user] to such a degree that if eaten in excess it quenches sexual potency. Some squeeze juice from the green seeds and use it as an analgesic for pains caused by ear-obstruction." Both the works of Dioscorides and Galen would be translated by Muslim scholars during the European Dark Ages and rediscovered by Europeans in the Middle Ages, as was the case with many of the most brilliant minds of Antiquity. It is also noteworthy that the practice of making hemp paper was introduced to Europe by Muslims, and that the first European paper mill was established in Spain in 1150 CE.[31]

Following the decline of the Roman Empire, cannabis was still grown throughout Europe and used as a folk medicine. The juice of macerated leaves and buds was used as a vermifuge for horses, and fishermen were known to soak the ground with it to draw up worms, which were then used as bait. In the Late Middle Ages and early modern period, cannabis was used as an ointment for burns, to treat wounds, and to treat cystitis and urethritis.[40]

reports would ensue in the American media, which we will explore in greater detail in Chapter 5 (U.S. Cannabis Regulations From Past to Present).

2.10 The United States

Cannabis has been grown in the United States since Europeans began colonizing the landmass that would become the continental United States, and its cultivation mirrored that of Europe well into the 19th century. The cannabis grown in the United States was used almost solely for industrial purposes, though some evidence suggests that slaves of African descent did grow *dagga* in parts of the American south prior to the Civil War. How widespread this practice was is debatable.

Through the 19th century, only a relatively small number of Americans of European lineage experimented with products created from drug-type plants. Though easily accessible in pharmacies, as was the case in Europe, it never rose to a level of cultural significance.

American physicians, meanwhile, were intrigued by the potential benefits of cannabis and they quickly made numerous advancements that allowed them to create varieties with higher drug content and granted them the ability to standardize dosages. By the end of the century, American pharmaceutical companies were learning the methods of sinsemilla cultivation (removing male plants to encourage the growth of trichomes in unfertilized female plants) and producing plants with enough drug content to rival any cannabis in the world. By the 1930s, some leading drug manufacturers were manufacturing products that were effective at dose levels of 10 mg.[31]

Throughout the 19th and early 20th centuries, the American medical community discovered more and more potential therapeutic applications for cannabis. A clinical conference by the Ohio State Medical Society in 1860 reported that it could be used to treat stomach pain, neuralgic pain, "childbirth psychosis," chronic cough, gonorrhea, and inflammation.[31] *Sajous's Analytic Cyclopedia of Practical Medicine* of 1924, meanwhile, provided a vast list of its therapeutic uses, including as a sedative, antidepressant, analgesic, obstetric aid, and aphrodisiac. It is also said to be a treatment for delirium tremens, chorea, tetanus, rabies, hay fever, bronchitis, pulmonary tuberculosis, paralysis agitans, exophthalmic goiter, spasm of the bladder, gonorrhea, headaches, migraines, neuralgias, gastric ulcers, dyspepsia, gastralgia, wasting diseases, malaria, nervous and spasmodic dysmenorrhea, chronic inflammatory states, rheumatism, eczema, senile pruritus, dental pain, nephritis, diabetes, vertigo, and cardiac palpitation.[45]

There is no doubt that physicians at the time were aware of the potential benefits of cannabis, but interest began to wane in the late 1920s and 1930s as synthetic drugs became far more popular. Furthermore, demand for hemp was in a rapid decline and had been since the late 19th century as sailing ships were being replaced by steamships and hemp rigging was being replaced by tensile steel cable.[46] Cannabis was also becoming a dirty word politically for two distinct reasons. The first is due to the temperance movement and what could be described as the United States' first opioid crisis. The second was due to the growth of anti-immigrant sentiment, particularly against migrants from Mexico. As we will discuss in Chapter 5 (U.S. Cannabis Regulations From Past to Present), this would effectively end research into cannabis as a medicinal drug for decades to come.

REFERENCES

[1]Clark RC, Merlin MD. Cannabis and *Homo sapiens*. In: *Cannabis: Evolution and Ethnobotany*. Berkeley, CA: University of California Press; 2013:365-382.

[2]Clark RC, Merlin MD. Natural origins and early evolution of *Cannabis*. In: *Cannabis: Evolution and Ethnobotany*. Berkeley, CA: University of California Press; 2013:13-28.

[3]Russo EB. History of cannabis and its preparation in saga, science, and sobriquet. *Chem Biodivers*. 2007;4(8):1614-1648. doi: 10.1002/cbdv.200790144.

[4]Small E. Classification of *Cannabis sativa* L. in relation to agricultural, biotechnological, medical and recreational utilization. In: Chandra S, et al., eds. *Cannabis Sativa L.—Botany and Biotechnology*. Cham, Switzerland: Springer International Publishing; 2017:1-62.

[5]Pringle H. Ice age communities may be earliest known net hunters. *Science*. 1997;277(5330):1203-1204. doi: 10.1126/science.277.5330.1203.

[6]Clark RC, Merlin MD. Ethnobotanical origins, early cultivation, and evolution through human selection. In: *Cannabis: Evolution and Ethnobotany*. Berkeley, CA: University of California Press; 2013:29-58.

[7]Touw M. The religious and medicinal uses of *Cannabis* in China, India and Tibet. *J Psychoactive Drugs*. 1981;13(1):23-34. doi: 10.1080/02791072.1981.10471447.

[8]Anderson E. Dump heaps and the origin of agriculture. In: *Plants, Man and Life*. 2nd ed. Berkeley, CA: University of California Press; 1967:136-151.

[9]Fleming MP, Clarke RC. Physical evidence for the antiquity of *Cannabis sativa* L. *J Int Hemp Assoc*. 1998;5(2):80-92. https://www.druglibrary.net/olsen/HEMP/IHA/jiha5208.html. Accessed June 4, 2019.

[10]Allegret S. The history of Hemp. In: Bouloc P, ed. *Hemp: Industrial Production and Uses*. Boston, MA: CAB International; 2013:4-26.

[11]Booth M. *Cannabis: A History*. New York, NY: Picador; 2003:20.

[12]Booth M. *Cannabis: A History*. New York, NY: Picador; 2003:22.

[13]Booth M. *Cannabis: A History*. New York, NY: Picador; 2003:21.

[14]Li HL. An archaeological and historical account of *Cannabis* in China. *Econ Bot*. 1974;28(4):437-448. doi: 10.1007/BF02862859.

[15]Brand EJ, Zhao Z. Cannabis in Chinese medicine: are some traditional indications referenced in ancient literature related to cannabinoids? *Front Pharmacol*. 2017;8:108. doi: 10.3389/fphar.2017.00108. eCollection 2017.

[16]Cartwright M. Paper in ancient China. Ancient History Encyclopedia. https://www.ancient. eu/article/1120/paper-in-ancient-china/. Published September 15, 2017. Accessed June 4, 2019.

[17]Jiang HE, Li X, Zhao YX, et al. A new insight into *Cannabis sativa* (*Cannabaceae*) utilization from 2500-year-old Yanghai Tombs, Xinjiang, China. *J Ethnopharmacol*. 2006;108(3):414-422. doi: 10.1016/j.jep.2006.05.034.

[18]Merlin MD. Archaeological evidence for the tradition of psychoactive plant use in the old world. *Econ Bot*. 2003;57(3):295-323. doi: 10.1663/0013-0001(2003)057[0295:AEFTTO]2.0 .CO;2.

[19]Herodotus. *The Histories*. de Sélincourt A, trans. New York, NY: Penguin Books; 1996:80.

[20]Russo E. Cannabis in India: ancient lore and modern medicine. In: Mechoulam R, ed. *Cannabinoids as Therapeutics*. Boston, MA: Birkhäuser Verlag; 2005:1-22.

[21]Herodotus. *The Histories*. de Sélincourt A, trans. New York, NY: Penguin Books; 1996:239.

[22]Russo EB. Taming THC: potential cannabis synergy and phytocannabinoid-terpenoid entourage effects. *Br J Pharmacol*. 2011;163(7):1344-1364. doi: 10.1111/j.1476-5381.2011.01238.x.

[23]Curry A. Rites of the Scythians: spectacular new discovery from the Caucasus set the stage for a dramatic hilltop ritual. *Archaeology*. https://www.archaeology.org/ issues/220-1607/features/4560-rites-of-the-scythians. Published July/August 2016. Accessed May 9, 2019.

[24]Bennett C. The magic and ceremonial use of cannabis in the ancient world. In: Ellens JH, ed. *Seeking the Sacred With Psychoactive Substances*. Santa Barbara, CA: Praeger; 2014: 23-56.

[25]Doniger W. Humans, animals, and gods in the *Rig Veda* 1500-1000 B.C.E. In: Miles J, ed. *The Norton Anthology of World Religions*. New York, NY: W.W. Norton & Company; 2015: 83-102.

[26]Booth M. *Cannabis: A History*. New York, NY: Picador; 2003:24.

[27]Booth M. *Cannabis: A History*. New York, NY: Picador; 2003:109-113.

[28]Booth M. *Cannabis: A History*. New York, NY: Picador; 2003:116.

[29]Booth M. *Cannabis: A History*. New York, NY: Picador; 2003:138.

[30]Booth M. *Cannabis: A History*. New York, NY: Picador; 2003:139.

[31]Aldrich M. The history of therapeutic cannabis. In: Mathre ML, ed. *Cannabis in Medical Practice: A Legal, Historical and Pharmacological Overview of the Therapeutic Use of Marijuana*. Jefferson, NC: McFarland & Company, Inc., Publishers; 1997:35-55.

[32]Booth M. *Cannabis: A History*. New York, NY: Picador; 2003:141, 311.

[33]Booth M. *Cannabis: A History*. New York, NY: Picador; 2003:49-51.

[34]Booth M. *Cannabis: A History*. New York, NY: Picador; 2003:51.

[35]Nahas GG. Hashish in Islam 9th to 18th century. *Bull N Y Acad Med*. 1982;58(9):814-831. http://europepmc.org/backend/ptpmcrender.fcgi?accid=PMC1805385&blobtype=pdf. Accessed June 4, 2019.

[36]Matthee R. *The Pursuit of Pleasure: Drugs and Stimulates in Iranian History, 1500-1900*. Princeton, NJ: Princeton University Press; 2009.

[37]Herodotus. *The Histories*. de Sélincourt A, trans. New York, NY: Penguin Books; 1996: 238-239.

[38]Zias J, Stark H, Sellgman J, et al. Early medical use of cannabis. *Nature*. 1993;363:215.

[39]Blickman T. Morocco and cannabis: reduction, containment or acceptance. *Transnational Institute*. March 2017;49. https://www.tni.org/files/publication-downloads/dpb_49_eng_web. pdf. Accessed May 13, 2019.

[40]Kabelik J, Krejci Z, Santavy F. Cannabis as a medicant. *Bull Narcotics*. 1960;5-23. https:// www.unodc.org/unodc/en/data-and-analysis/bulletin/bulletin_1960-01-01_3_page003.html. Accessed June 4, 2019.

[41]Booth M. *Cannabis: A History*. New York, NY: Picador; 2003:77.

[42]Dioscorides. *De Materia Medica*. The World Digital Library. https://www.wdl.org/en/ item/10632/. Accessed June 4, 2019.

[43]Booth M. *Cannabis: A History*. New York, NY: Picador; 2003: 154-158.

[44]Campos I. 'Reefer Madness' in Mexico preceded U.S. prohibition. *O'Shaughnessy's*. Winter/Spring 2013. https://www.beyondthc.com/wp-content/uploads/2013/11/CamposPaternoism.pdf. Accessed May 13, 2019.

[45]Sajous C, Sajous M. *Cannabis indica* (Indian hemp: hashish). *Sajous's Analytic Cyclopedia of Practical Medicine*. Vol. 3, 9th ed. Philadelphia, PA; 1924:1-9. https://books.google.com/ books?id=wlQ3AQAAMAAJ&pg=PA1&source=gbs_toc_r&cad=4#v=onepage&q&f=false. Accessed May 13, 2019.

[46]Booth M. *Cannabis: A History*. New York, NY: Picador; 2003:45.

3

The Classification of Cannabis

3.1 Classification: An Overview

Cannabis has been classified in numerous ways throughout history. By exploring the numerous schemas developed over the centuries, it buttresses the larger point that the plant can and has served a wide variety of purposes across different cultures.

These purposes largely depended upon the variety available to the culture in question. Cultures based in the Eurasian Steppe and the Indian subcontinent tended to use the plant for its drug content, as the variety that was most readily accessible had high concentrations of tetrahydrocannabinol (THC) and produced fibers of relatively low quality. Cultures in East Asia and Europe, meanwhile, tended to use the plant as a source of sustenance or for industrial purposes, as the variety that was most readily accessible had low concentrations of THC and produced fibers of significantly higher quality. Regardless of THC content, all cultures seem to have used cannabis for medicinal purposes.

3.2 Ancient Classifications

Cannabis has been described by botanists, doctors, and other scientists dating back to ancient times. Most scholars from these cultures recognized only one variety of cannabis, largely because they were unable to travel widely enough to collect additional specimens, but they did notice some important distinctions even within the samples to which they had access based on the gender of the plant regardless of whether the culture under consideration used the plant for its fiber or THC content.

In China, where fiber-type plants have been grown for at least 6000 years and continue to be cultivated to this day, written evidence shows that scientists understood that cannabis was dioicous, with distinct female and male plants. Some of the earliest Chinese writings on the subject modify the character for cannabis, *ma*, to distinguish between male (*i* or *si*) and female plants (*chu* or *tsu*). The male plant was noted for its fibers, the female plant was prized for its seeds, and both appear to have been used for various medicinal purposes.[1]

Ancient Europeans distinguished between male and female plants, as well. Writing in the first century, the Greek physician and botanist Dioscorides made a distinction between *Kannabis emeros* (the female plant) and *Kannabis agria* (the male). He claimed the former was good for earaches and that its seeds could "quench conception," while the latter's roots could be used to reduce inflammation, relieve edema, and "disperse hardened matter around the joints."[2] He also said that cannabis seed, when mixed with honey, oil, and a healthy dose of dove droppings, could be used to treat carbuncles and burns.

Cultivators from the Indian subcontinent also distinguished between male and female plants, though for different reasons. As the type of cannabis that grew in the region was prized for its high

understood that the variety of cannabis found in India produced a resinous secretion and concluded that this resin, which he said was absent from European varieties, produced the various effects he observed. Despite these findings and the paper's title, he also argued that cannabis should be considered a monotype species. It has been assumed that he made the distinction in his title to emphasize the way cannabis was used among Indian physicians.[3]

Unfortunately, this was not clear to the vast majority of readers. Consequently, the name *"Cannabis indica"* remained in regular use to refer to cannabis with a high concentration of THC from the second half of the 19th century until the early 20th century.[3] This was true of European and American peddlers of tonics and other items of dubious repute, as well as manufacturers of more legitimate medicinal extracts that were also being prescribed by doctors. It is rumored that Sir John Russell Reynolds, the physician-in-ordinary for Queen Victoria, gave one such formula to the queen to relieve her menstrual cramps.[7]

The debate over whether *Cannabis* was monotypic or bitypic continued until 1924, when the Russian botanist Dmitry Janischewski made the claim that there were actually three distinct species of cannabis: *C. sativa*, *C. indica*, and *Cannabis ruderalis*, which he found growing in the wilds of Siberia and Central Asia. Janischewski argued that *ruderalis* is a unique species and described it as a moderately tall plant (typically around 1 m in height, but reaching 2 m on occasion) with small seeds. The seeds were coated by a persistent perianth (seed covering) characterized by irregular dark spots not seen on the seeds of either *indica* or *sativa*.[5] Unlike other types of cannabis, Janischewski also noted that these plants matured quicker than other cultivars.[5] Nikolai Vavilov, another Russian botanist researching in Central Asia contemporaneously, coined the taxon *C. sativa* var. *spontanea* when describing similar plants. He also advocated for additional taxonomic distinctions for varieties and forms he discovered while traveling in Afghanistan and the surrounding environs, which he labeled *afghanica* and *kafiristanica*.*

Until the 1970s, there remained a distinct cultural divide regarding the classification of *Cannabis*. In the Soviet Union, there was a clear preference for the polytypic schema of Janischewski, which included *C. sativa*, *C. indica*, and *C. ruderalis*. The Anglophone world, however, favored the monotypic *C. sativa* with

---

*These additional classifications include the variety (or form) *afghanica* and the variety *kafiristanica*, which Vavilov initially assigned to *C. sativa*, but later assigned to *C. indica*. For a more information on *Cannabis'* taxonomic history, see McPartland J, Guy GW. Models of cannabis taxonomy, cultural bias, and conflicts between scientific and vernacular names. *Bot Rev.* 2017;83:327-381.

the following variants: *C. sativa* var. *sativa*, *C. sativa* var. *indica*, and *C. sativa* var. *ruderalis*. Other parts of the world did not ascribe to the same level of cultural bias.

3.4 The Case of John Anthony van Alstyne

During the 1970s, the debate became more complex. The United States government had formally adopted the monotypic view of *Cannabis*. This meant that that only *C. sativa* was an illegal substance, as the law made no mention of *C. indica*. Some legal minds reasoned that if *C. indica* and *C. sativa* could be proven to be a unique species before a court of law, this would mean that prohibition did not apply to *C. indica* and that a person found to be in possession of *C. indica* would not be guilty of any crime. This legal theory was put to the test when John Anthony van Alstyne was arrested in California in 1973 for being in possession of cannabis he claimed was *C. indica*.

In the corner of van Alstyne was the father of ethnobotany, Richard Evans Schultes. His adversary was the Canadian botanist Ernest Small.

Small argued that cannabis, although monotypic, could be broken up into four distinct varieties based on a two-step hierarchic classification system. The first step recognized two subspecies based on the THC content of female flowers. One subspecies contained <0.3% THC. The other contained a concentration of THC that was >0.3%. The second step recognized two varieties between the two subspecies based on domestication phase. He named them:

- *C. sativa* subsp. *sativa* var. *sativa*: Low THC and cultivated;
- *C. sativa* subsp. *sativa* var. *spontanea*: Low THC and noncultivated;
- *C. sativa* subsp. *indica* var. *indica*: High THC and cultivated;
- *C. sativa* subsp. *indica* var. *kafiristanica*: High THC and noncultivated.

Small also found that there were three chemovars when analyzing THC to cannabidiol (CBD) ratios. Type I had a THC content >0.3% and a CBD content <0.5%; type II had a THC content >0.3% and a CBD content >0.5%; and type III had a THC content <0.3% and a CBD content >0.5%. Type I plants were regarded as drug-type plants with provenance in areas below the 30th parallel. Type III plants were fiber-type plants with provenance in areas above the 30th parallel. Type II was a hybrid of type I and type III.[5]

Schultes, conversely, argued that there were three species of Cannabis: *C. sativa*, *C. indica*, and *C. ruderalis*. Another witness for van

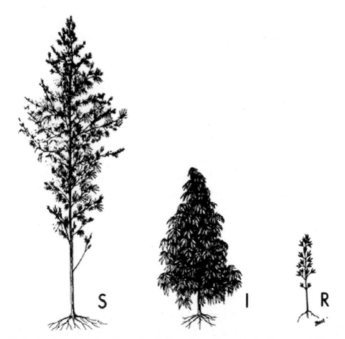

Figure 3.1 Anderson drawing depicting *C. sativa*, *C. indica*, and *C. ruderalis*.

Alstyne, Loran Anderson, supported the polytypic schema of Schultes and created a line drawing that has become a common feature on many Web sites. It shows *C. sativa* to be almost tree-like and *C. indica* to be extremely bushy. *C. ruderalis* is depicted as a runty weed (see Fig. 3.1).[5]

Ultimately, the court ruled against van Alstyne, but the case effectively ended the consensus that *Cannabis* was monotypic in the United States. The work of Schultes and Anderson also gave rise to a kind of secondary folk taxonomy popularized by consumers of drug-type cannabis. This vernacular persists to this day and is especially evident whenever one enters a cannabis dispensary. Though its use has become widespread, it should not be considered a scientific approach to the classification of *Cannabis*.

3.5 Vernacular Taxonomy—Sativa, Indica, and Ruderalis

Similar to the folk terminology that distinguishes hemp from marijuana, the vernacular taxonomy adopted by American cannabis culture relies on perceivable differences between "Sativa" and "Indica" rather than a formal taxonomical schema (this schema also includes "Ruderalis"). No research has indicated that this is a valid classification system and the amount of crossbreeding between these varieties has undoubtably reduced the population of "pure" examples of either Sativa or Indica significantly. This taxonomy seems to be based more on the subjective experience following consumption. Sativa provides users with a kind of intoxication that is more associated with socialization; Indica is more frequently associated with relaxation.[3] While it is certainly possible that specific chemovars may produce specific effects due to unique concentrations of cannabinoids, terpenes, and other compounds, no evidence beyond the purely anecdotal has arisen to provide objective support for the Sativa/Indica divide.

Though many researchers will note that these distinctions are highly dubious, this vernacular taxonomy is frequently regarded as gospel among cannabis users.[8] It is also an important distinction because many growers view cannabis through this lens when working with specific cultivars. Plants are chosen for breeding based on their characteristics and profiles as understood within this taxonomy. Perhaps most importantly, many dispensaries organize their stores and products by making use of this terminology. In order to effectively help patients navigate through these labyrinths, one should be familiar with the terminology they employ.

Within this vernacular, Sativa refers to taller plants that (allegedly) originated in Southern or Southeast Asia. They favor warmer and more humid climates and have longer growing seasons. In appearance, they are taller and possess long, narrow leaves. Prior to the 1970s, this was almost solely the kind of cannabis consumed for recreational purposes in the United States, as it was imported from countries where it had been grown for centuries—particularly Southeast Asia nations like Thailand and Vietnam, South Africa, East Africa, Colombia, and Mexico.[5] Many of the names of these cultivars (mistakenly referred to as "strains")—Acapulco Gold, Maui Wowie, Kali Mist, etc.—note their purportedly tropical origins.

As noted above, Sativa is more associated with producing the kind of intoxication that one can describe as social. It is said to make users more focused, alert, and creative. Sativa is often said to produce a "head-high," though it is also said to provide significant pain relief.[3]

In the early 1970s, a germplasm that would go on to become the base for Indica plants in the United States was smuggled out of Afghanistan and into this country.[9] It has adapted to drier and cooler climates akin to the western and northern foothills of the Himalayas. Consequently, it is squatter, denser, and has a shorter growing season than Sativa.[3] There are some cultivars of Indica that are believed to closely resemble landraces that have been grown in the Hindu Kush or Pamir highlands for millennia. Consequently, many cultivars of Indica are named for geographical regions in Central Asia. These include Afghani, Afgoo, and Hindu Kush. In fact, the word "Kush" is a common indication that the cultivar is an Indica. Some examples include Purple Kush, Blackberry Kush, Blueberry Kush, Bubba Kush, and Kosher Kush.

Indica cultivars are said to produce an almost narcotic effect that is characterized as a "body-high." It is meant to promote relaxation and an overall sense of calm.[3] Consequently, Indica has often been recommended for individuals who are suffering from chronic pain or undergoing chemotherapy.

Ruderalis is also found within this schema. Of more importance to breeders than consumers, Ruderalis has become a catchall for wild-type varieties. Most are low in THC, but there are features of Ruderalis plants that are of special importance to breeders. Some utilize cultivars' short stature to make plants that only reach two feet in height the time of harvest. Depending on circumstances, this characteristic may be of use for indoor growers. More importantly, many Ruderalis plants autoflower meaning they enter their flowering stage relatively quickly.[10]

For consumers, Ruderalis cultivars are rare. They are only infrequently found in dispensaries. They are used almost solely to impart specific characteristics to hybrid cultivars grown by breeders.

3.6 Contemporary Classification Schema

More recently, the work of Karl Hillig has altered Smalls' classification system by claiming that *sativa* and *indica* are different species based on chemotaxonomic study.[11] For *C. sativa*, there are two biotypes, a domesticated phase that was described by Linnaeus as *C. sativa* and a wild-type phase that was described by Vavilov as *C. sativa* var. *spontanea*. For *C. indica*, there are four biotypes. The first is narrow-leaflet drug (NDL), which corresponds to *sativa* in the parlance of cannabis culture and the *C. indica* described by Lamarck. The second is wide-leaflet drug (WDL), which corresponds to the *indica* that was smuggled into the United States in the early 1970s and the *afghanica* described by Vavilov. Third is a wild-type that corresponds with Small's *Cannabis sativa* subsp. *indica* var. *kafiristanica*. Finally, there is the broad-leaflet fiber (BLF) type that was commonly cultivated in East Asia. Despite its low THC content, it has more in common with other *C. indica* biotypes than with the European *C. sativa*.[12] Hellig has also proposed that *C. ruderalis* is its own species.[5]

There are other, far more confusing discussions about the proper names of these variants that we will avoid. Suffice to say, botanists cannot agree on the subject of the classification of *Cannabis*. However, some researchers have begun to look at the genetic disparities of samples within the *Cannabis* group to assess whether *C. sativa* and *C. indica* should be segregated at the level of species, subspecies, variety, or form.

What they found seems to corroborate Smalls' findings. All variants within cannabis appear to be only slightly disparate. Research conducted in 2007 by Simon Gilmore, Rod Peakall, and James Robertson found very little sequence variation among 188 samples from 76 separate populations that included drug-type, fiber-type, and purportedly wild chemotypes. According to their paper, there were six haplotypes of *Cannabis*, but there was not enough genetic variation to make any of these variants unique species.[13] A paper in 2014 published by John McPartland and Geoffrey Guy found the mean divergence among samples of *C. sativa* and *C. indica* to be 0.41%. For comparison, the mean divergence of five varieties of tea was found to be 0.43%, whereas mean divergence among different species (among them were two species of hop, *H. lupulus* and *Humulus japonicus*) was found to be 3.0%.[14] Finally, researchers who have studied the fixation index (a measurement of how easily groups can interbreed that runs from 0 [can freely interbreed] to 1 [cannot interbreed]) between ostensibly disparate groups of *Cannabis* have found that virtually any group can interbreed with any other relatively easily. The two most genetically disparate groupings tested, fiber-type and drug-type groups, are about as different genetically as human populations from Europe and human populations from East Asia.[5]

The debate will likely continue with some parties claiming that all plants within the group *Cannabis* are members of the species *C. sativa* and other parties claiming that there is a distinction between *C. sativa* and *C. indica* (and perhaps *C. ruderalis*) that warrants the separation of the group into unique species. As clinicians and not botanists, we have sought only to provide the details as to the sides of the debate.

For our purposes going forward, we will break up *Cannabis* into three groups: fiber-type, NLD type, and WLD type. We have excluded nondomesticated variants (often referred to as *ditchweed*) because most patients will never encounter these kinds of plants or use them to treat any condition.

REFERENCES

[1]Li HL. An archaeological and historical account of cannabis in China. *Econ Bot*. 1974;28(4):437-448. doi: 10.1007/BF02862859.

[2]Dioscorides P. *De Materia Medica*. The World Digital Library [website]. https://www.wdl. org/en/item/10632/. Accessed June 4, 2019.

[3]Erkelens JL, Hazekamp A. That which we call *Indica*, by any other name would smell as sweet. *Cannabinoids*. 2014;9(1):9-15. https://www.cannabis-med.org/data/pdf/en_2014_01_2_0.pdf. Accessed October 10, 2019.

[4]Erkelens JL, Hazekamp A. That which we call *Indica*, by any other name would smell as sweet. *Cannabinoids*. 2014;9(1):11. https://www.cannabis-med.org/data/pdf/en_2014_01_2_0. pdf. Accessed October 10, 2019.

[5]McPartland J, Guy GW. Models of cannabis taxonomy, cultural bias, and conflicts between scientific and vernacular names. *Bot Rev*. 2017;83:327-381. doi: 10.1007/s12229-017-9187-0.

[6]Booth M. *Cannabis: A History*. New York, NY: Picador; 2003:109-113.

[7]Booth M. *Cannabis: A History*. New York, NY: Picador; 2003:114.

[8]Piomelli D, Russo EB. The *Cannabis sativa* versus *Cannabis indica* debate: an interview with Ethan Russo, MD. *Cannabis Cannabinoid Res*. 2016;1(1):44-46. doi: 10.1089/can.2015.290003.ebr. eCollection 2016.

[9]Zeman J. *Murder Mountain* [Netflix]. Los Angeles, CA: Lightbox; 2018.

[10]Potter DJ. Cannabis horticulture. In: Pertwee RG, ed. *Handbook on Cannabis*. New York, NY: Oxford University Press; 2013:65-88.

[11]Russo EB. History of cannabis and its preparation in saga, science, and sobriquet. *Chem Biodivers*. 2007;4(8):1614-1648. doi: 10.1002/cbdv.200790144.

[12]Brand EJ, Zhao Z. Cannabis in Chinese medicine: are some traditional indications referenced in ancient literature related to cannabinoids? *Front Pharmacol*. 2017;8:108. doi: 10.3389/fphar.2017.00108.

[13]Gilmore S, Peakall R, Robertson J. Organelle DNA haplotypes reflect crop-use characteristics and geographical origins of *Cannabis sativa*. *Forensic Sci Int*. 2007;172:179-190. doi: 10.1016/j.forsciint.2006.10.025

[14]McPartland JM, Guy GW. A question of rank: using DNA barcodes to classify *Cannabis sativa* and *Cannabis indica*. In: *Proceedings of the 24th Annual Symposium on the Cannabinoids*. Research Triangle Park, NC: International Cannabinoid Research Society; 2014:54. http://www.icrs.co/SYMPOSIUM.2014/ICRS2014.PROGRAMME.pdf. Accessed October 10, 2019.

4

Constituents of Cannabis

4.1 Overview

There are over 500 chemical compounds found within cannabis of which ~140 are *phytocannabinoids*. Evidence suggests that phytocannabinoids are unique to cannabis. Phytocannabinoids are distinct from *endocannabinoids* (such as anandamide and 2-arachidonylglycerol [2-AG]), which occur naturally in the body and interact with receptors within the body's endocannabinoid system (ECS). A detailed description of the ECS follows in Chapter 6 (The Endocannabinoid System).

Almost all noncannabinoid constituents found in cannabis are common throughout the plant world. Such compounds include terpenoids, flavonoids, and other phenolic compounds. A few interact directly with the ECS. Many affect the ECS indirectly.[1] More importantly, when consumed in conjunction with phytocannabinoids, they appear to be capable not only of altering the intoxicating effects of psychotropic phytocannabinoids but also of improving their therapeutic qualities. Many terpenic compounds have been shown to have additional synergistic qualities when consumed in conjunction with phytocannabinoids. This is known as the *entourage effect*.[2] Far more will be said on this subject in Chapter 8 (The Pharmacodynamics of Cannabis).

Interest in the potential medicinal properties these compounds may possess when consumed in conjunction with cannabinoids is increasing. Unfortunately, research remains in its infancy, and very little is known about how these terpenic compounds interact with even some of the better-known phytocannabinoids.

4.2 Phytocannabinoids

Phytocannabinoids fall under a class of compounds that possess C_{19}, C_{21}, or C_{22} terpenophenolic skeletons and tend to show high binding affinities with the G protein–coupled receptors (CB_1 and CB_2) found within the body's ECS. Within individual classes of phytocannabinoids, one finds two subclasses: pentyl phytocannabinoids (phytocannabinoids with side chains containing 5 carbon atoms) and propyl phytocannabinoids (phytocannabinoids with side chains containing 3 carbon atoms). In the case of the former, olivetolic acid is the precursor that leads to the biosynthesis of cannabigerolic acid (CBGA), which is the precursor to other pentyl cannabinoids. In the case of the latter, divarinic acid is the precursor that leads to the biosynthesis of tetrahydrocannabivarin (THCV), which is the precursor to the remaining propyl phytocannabinoids.

The two most abundant phytocannabinoids at the time of harvest, cannabidiolic acid (CBDA) and Δ-9-tetrahydrocannabinolic acid A (THCA-A), are both pentyl cannabinoids. They are converted into cannabidiol (CBD) and Δ-9-tetrahydrocannabinol (THC), respectively, through the process of decarboxylation.[3] A minimal amount of decarboxylation occurs naturally following the curing process of cannabis, but the efficient production of the most sought after phytocannabinoids, whether CBG, CBD, or THC, requires the application of an artificial heat source.

Approximately 140 phytocannabinoids have been isolated at this time with research ongoing. Approximately 20 of these phytocannabinoids have been so recently discovered that there is only anecdotal news of their existence. A listing of the 120 confirmed phytocannabinoids can be found in Table 4.1. The molecular structures of these 120 phytocannabinoids can be found at the end of this chapter.

4.2.1 Cannabigerol Class

The cannabigerol (CBG) class of phytocannabinoids consists of both pentyl and propyl phytocannabinoids, and they are the first biogenic phytocannabinoids the cannabis plant produces. These phytocannabinoids have shown considerable antibacterial activity on gram-positive bacteria.[4] More research is needed to assess additional applications.

Cannabigerolic Acid

CBGA is formed through the synthesis of olivetolic acid and geranyl pyrophosphate, and was first isolated in 1965 by Raphael Mechoulam and Yechiel Gaoni.[5] It is the first biogenic pentyl phytocannabinoid and is converted into other phytocannabinoids as the plant matures, most notably those of the cannabichromene, cannabidiol, and Δ-9-tetrahydrocannabinol classes. Very little research has been conducted on CBGA to assess its potential pharmacological applications.

Cannabigerol

CBG was first isolated in 1964 by Mechoulam and Gaoni. It is formed through the decarboxylation of CBGA and is only found in trace amounts in many chemotypes of cannabis, though some fiber-type plants do produce more significant concentrations. CBG is nonpsychoactive and has been shown to be a poor agonist of

(*text continues on page 104*)

TABLE 4.1 Phytocannabinoids

Figure	Compound Name	Compound Class	Abbreviation
	Cannabigerol	Cannabigerol	CBG [(E)-CBG-C$_5$]
	Cannabigerolic acid	Cannabigerol	CBGA [(E)-CBGA-C$_5$]

CBGM [(*E*)-CBGM-C₅]	Cannabigerol	Cannabigerol monomethyl ether	
CBGAM [(*E*)-CBGAM-C₅]	Cannabigerol	Cannabigerolic acid monomethyl ether	
CBGV [(*E*)-CBGV-C₃]	Cannabigerol	Cannabigerovarin	

(Continued)

TABLE 4.1 Continued

Figure	Compound Name	Compound Class	Abbreviation
	Cannabigerovarinic acid A	Cannabigerol	CBGVA [(E)-CBGVA-C$_3$]
	Cannabinerolic acid A	Cannabigerol	(Z)-CBGVA-C$_5$
	Camagerol	Cannabigerol	N/A
	γ-eudesmyl-cannabigerolate	Cannabigerol	N/A

(Continued)

α-cadinyl-cannabigerolate Cannabigerol N/A

Sesquicannabigerol Cannabigerol N/A

TABLE 4.1 Continued

Figure	Compound Name	Compound Class	Abbreviation
	5-acetyl-4-hydroxy-cannabigerol	Cannabigerol	N/A
	(±)-6,7-*trans*-epoxycannabigerol	Cannabigerol	N/A
	(±)-6,7-*cis*-epoxycannabigerol	Cannabigerol	N/A
	(±)-6,7-*trans*-epoxycannabigerolic acid	Cannabigerol	N/A
	(±)-6,7-*cis*-epoxycannabigerolic acid	Cannabigerol	N/A
	(±)-Cannabichromene	Cannabichromene	CBC [CBC-C₅]

(±)-Cannabichromenic acid	Cannabichromene	CBCA [CBCA-C₅]
(±)-Cannabivarichromene	Cannabichromene	CBCV [CBCV-C₃]
(±)-Cannabivarichromenic acid	Cannabichromene	CBCVA [CBCVA-C₃]
(+)-Cannabichromevarin	Cannabichromene	CBCV [CBCV-C₃]

(Continued)

TABLE 4.1 Continued

Figure	Compound Name	Compound Class	Abbreviation
	2-methyl-2-(4-methyl-2-pentyl)-7-propyl-2H-1-benzopyran-5-ol	Cannabichromene	N/A
	(±)-4-acetoxycannabichromene	Cannabichromene	N/A
	(±)-3"-hydroxy-$\Delta^{(4'',5'')}$-cannabichromene	Cannabichromene	N/A
	(−)-7-hydroxycannabichromene	Cannabichromene	N/A

CBD [CBD-C₅]

Cannabidiol

Cannabidiol

CBDA [CBDA-C₅]

Cannabidiol

Cannabidiolic acid

(Continued)

TABLE 4.1 Continued

Figure	Compound Name	Compound Class	Abbreviation
	Cannabidiol monomethyl ether	Cannabidiol	CBDM [CBDM-C$_5$]
	Cannabidiol-C$_4$	Cannabidiol	CBD-C$_4$

CBD-C4

CBDV [CBDV-C₃]

Cannabidiol

Cannabidivarin

CBDVA [CBDVA-C₃]

Cannabidiol

Cannabidivarinic acid

(Continued)

TABLE 4.1 Continued

Figure	Compound Name	Compound Class	Abbreviation
	Cannabidiorcol	Cannabidiol	CBD-C$_1$
	(−)-Δ^9-*trans*-tetrahydrocannabinol	Δ^9-Tetrahydrocannabinol	THC [Δ^9-THC-C$_5$]
	(−)-Δ^9-*trans*-tetrahydrocannabinolic acid A	Δ^9-Tetrahydrocannabinol	THCA-A [Δ^9-THCA-C$_5$ A]

(−)-Δ⁹-*trans*-
tetrahydrocannabinolic acid B

Δ^9-Tetrahydrocannabinol   THCA-B
[Δ^9-THCA-C$_5$ B]

(−)-Δ⁹-*trans*-
tetrahydrocannabinol-C₄

Δ^9-Tetrahydrocannabinol   THC-C$_4$ [Δ^9-THC-C$_4$]

(−)-Δ⁹-*trans*-
tetrahydrocannabinolic acid
A-C₄

Δ^9-Tetrahydrocannabinol   THCA-A-C$_4$
[Δ^9-THCA-C$_4$]

(Continued)

TABLE 4.1 Continued

Figure	Compound Name	Compound Class	Abbreviation
	(−)-Δ^9-trans-tetrahydrocannabivarin	Δ^9-Tetrahydrocannabinol	THCV [Δ^9-THCV-C$_3$]
	(−)-Δ^9-trans-tetrahydrocannabivarinic acid	Δ^9-Tetrahydrocannabinol	THCVA [Δ^9-THCVA-C$_3$]
	(−)-Δ^9-trans-tetrahydrocannabiorcol	Δ^9-Tetrahydrocannabinol	THC-C1 [Δ^9-THC-C$_1$]

(−)-Δ⁹-*trans*-
tetrahydrocannabiorcolic acid

Δ^9-Tetrahydrocannabinol   THCA-C1
[Δ^9-THCA-C$_1$]

β-fenchyl-Δ²-*trans*-
tetrahydrocannabinolate

Δ^9-Tetrahydrocannabinol   N/A

α-fenchyl-Δ³-*trans*-
tetrahydrocannabinolate

Δ^9-Tetrahydrocannabinol   N/A

(Continued)

TABLE 4.1 Continued

Figure	Compound Name	Compound Class	Abbreviation
	epi-bornyl-Δ^9-*trans*-tetrahydrocannabinolate	Δ^9-Tetrahydrocannabinol	N/A
	bornyl-Δ^9-*trans*-tetrahydrocannabinolate	Δ^9-Tetrahydrocannabinol	N/A
	α-terpenyl-Δ^9-*trans*-tetrahydrocannabinolate	Δ^9-Tetrahydrocannabinol	N/A

4-terpenyl-Δ⁹-*trans*-
tetrahydrocannabinolate

Δ⁹-Tetrahydrocannabinol N/A

α-cadinyl-Δ⁹-*trans*-
tetrahydrocannabinolate

Δ⁹-Tetrahydrocannabinol N/A

γ-eudesmyl-Δ⁹-*trans*-
tetrahydrocannabinolate

Δ⁹-Tetrahydrocannabinol N/A

(Continued)

TABLE 4.1 Continued

Figure	Compound Name	Compound Class	Abbreviation
	Δ^8-tetrahydrocannabinol	Δ^8-Tetrahydrocannabinol	Δ^8-THC [Δ^8-THC-C$_5$]
	Δ^8-tetrahydrocannabinolic acid A	Δ^8-Tetrahydrocannabinol	Δ^8-THCA-A [Δ^8-THCA-C$_5$ A]
	10α-hydroxy-Δ^8-tetrahydrocannabinol	Δ^8-Tetrahydrocannabinol	N/A

Δ^8-Tetrahydrocannabinol N/A

10β-hydroxy-Δ^8-tetrahydrocannabinol

Δ^8-Tetrahydrocannabinol N/A

10α-hydroxy-10-oxo-Δ^8-tetrahydrocannabinol

CBL [CBL-C$_5$]

Cannabicyclol

Cannabicyclol

(Continued)

TABLE 4.1 Continued

Figure	Compound Name	Compound Class	Abbreviation
	Cannabicyclolic acid	Cannabicyclol	CBLA [CBLA-C$_5$]
	Cannabicyclovarin	Cannabicyclol	CBLV [CBLV-C$_3$]
	Cannabielsoin	Cannabielsoin	CBE [CBE-C$_5$]

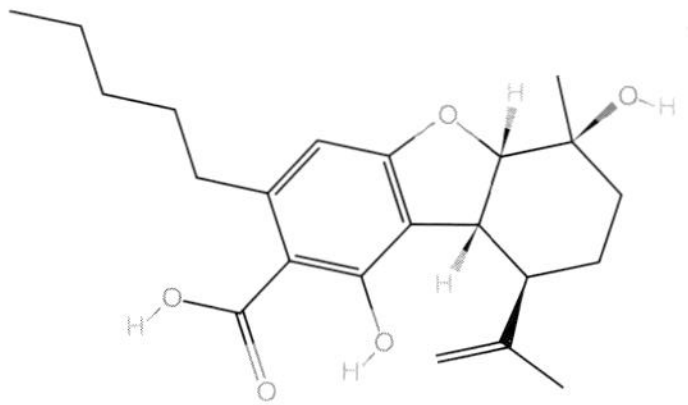

CBEA-A [CBEA-C₅ A]

Cannabielsoin

Cannabielsoic acid A

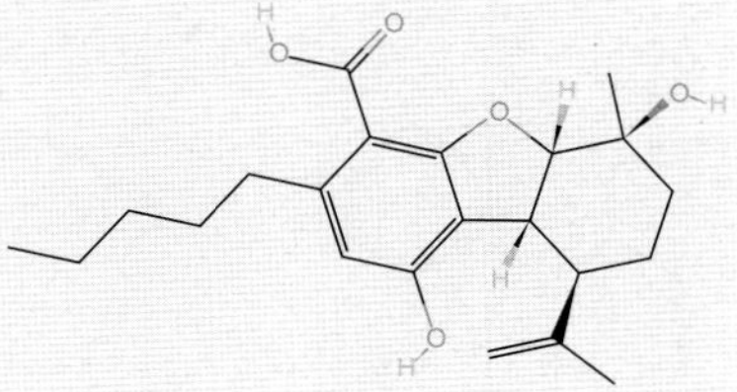

CBEA-B [CBEA-C₅ B]

Cannabielsoin

Cannabielsoic acid B

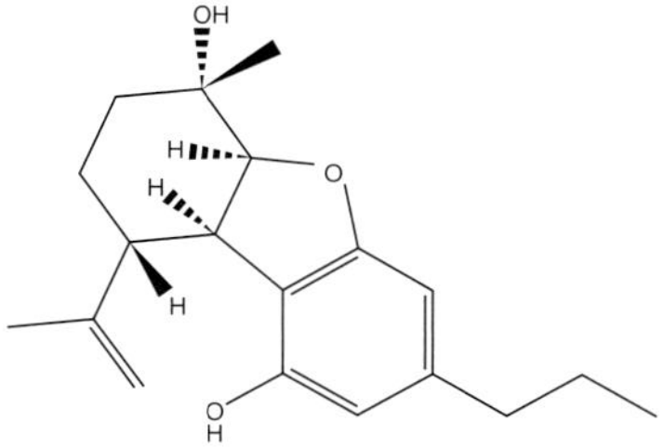

CBE-C₃

Cannabielsoin

Cannabielsoin-C₃

(*Continued*)

TABLE 4.1 Continued

Compound Name	Compound Class	Abbreviation	Figure
Cannabielsoic-C$_3$ acid B	Cannabielsoin	CBEA-C$_3$ B	
Cannabinol	Cannabinol	CBN [CBN-C$_5$]	
Cannabinolic acid	Cannabinol	CBNA [CBNA-C$_5$]	

CBNM-C$_5$ [CBNM-C$_5$]	Cannabinol	Cannabinol methyl ether	
CBN-C$_4$ [CBN-C$_4$]	Cannabinol	Cannabinol-C$_4$	
CBV [CBN-C$_3$ or CBV-C$_3$]	Cannabinol	Cannabivarin	

(Continued)

TABLE 4.1 Continued

Figure	Compound Name	Compound Class	Abbreviation
	Cannabinol-C_2	Cannabinol	CBN-C_2 [CBN-C_2]
	Cannabinol-C_1	Cannabinol	CBN-C_1 [CBN-C_1]
	4-terpenyl cannabinolate	Cannabinol	N/A

8-hydroxy cannabinolic acid A	Cannabinol	N/A
8-hydroxycannabinol	Cannabinol	N/A
1´S-hydroxycannabinol	Cannabinol	N/A

(*Continued*)

TABLE 4.1 Continued

Figure	Compound Name	Compound Class	Abbreviation
	Cannabinodiol	Cannabinodiol	CBND [CBND-C$_5$]
	Cannabinovarin	Cannabinodiol	CBNV [CBNV-C$_5$]
	(−)-*trans*-cannabitriol	Cannabitriol	(−)-*trans*-CBT-C$_5$
	(+)-*trans*-cannabitriol	Cannabitriol	(+)-*trans*-CBT-C$_5$

(±)-*cis*-cannabitriol Cannabitriol (±)-*cis*-CBT-C$_5$

(−)-*trans*-10-ethoxy-9-hydroxy-Δ$^{6a(10a)}$-tetrahydrocannabinol Cannabitriol (−)-*trans*-CBT-OEt-C$_5$

(±)-*trans*-cannabitriol-C$_3$ Cannabitriol (+)-*trans*-CBT-C$_3$

(*Continued*)

TABLE 4.1 Continued

Figure	Compound Name	Compound Class	Abbreviation
	Cannabitriol-C₃ homologue (unknown stereochemistry)	Cannabitriol	CBT-C$_3$-homologue
	(−)-*trans*-10-ethoxy-9-hydroxy-Δ$^{6a(10a)}$-tetra-hydrocannabivarin-C$_3$	Cannabitriol	(−)-*trans*-CBT-OEt-C$_3$
	8,9-dihydroxy-Δ$^{6a(10a)}$-tetrahydrocannabinol	Cannabitriol	8,9-di-OH-CBT-C$_5$
	Cannabidiolic acid tetrahydrocannabitriol ester	Cannabitriol	CBDA-C$_5$-9-OH-CBT-C$_5$-ester

DCBF-C$_5$	Miscellaneous	Dehydrocannabifuran	
CBF-C$_5$	Miscellaneous	Cannabifuran	
OTHC	Miscellaneous	10-oxo-Δ6a(10a)-tetrahydrocannabinol	

(Continued)

TABLE 4.1 Continued

Figure	Compound Name	Compound Class	Abbreviation
	8-hydroxy-isohexa-hydrocannabivarin	Miscellaneous	OH-iso-HHCV-C_3
	Cannabichromanone-C_5	Miscellaneous	CBCN-C_5
	Cannabichromanone-C_3	Miscellaneous	CBCN-C_3
	Cannabicitran	Miscellaneous	N/A

cis-Δ⁹-THC

Miscellaneous

(−)-Δ⁹-*cis*-(6a*S*, 10a*R*)-tetrahydrocannabinol

CBCON-C₅

Miscellaneous

Cannabicoumaronone-C₅

CBR

Miscellaneous

Cannabiripsol

(Continued)

TABLE 4.1 Continued

Figure	Compound Name	Compound Class	Abbreviation
	Cannabitetrol	Miscellaneous	CBTT
	(±)-Δ^7-*cis*-isotetra-hydrocannabivarin-C$_3$	Miscellaneous	*cis*-iso-Δ^7-THCV
	(−)-Δ^7-*trans*-(1R,3R,6R)-isotetrahydrocannabivarin-C$_3$	Miscellaneous	*trans*-iso-Δ^7-THCV

(−)-Δ^7-*trans*-(1R,3R,6R)-isotetrahydrocannabinol-C$_5$	Miscellaneous	*trans*-iso-Δ^7-THC
Cannabichromanone B	Miscellaneous	N/A
Cannabichromanone C	Miscellaneous	N/A
Cannabichromanone D	Miscellaneous	N/A
(−)-(7R)-cannabicoumarononic acid	Miscellaneous	N/A

(*Continued*)

TABLE 4.1 Continued

Figure	Compound Name	Compound Class	Abbreviation
	4-acetoxy-2-geranyl-5-hydroxy-3-*n*-pentylphenol	Miscellaneous	N/A
	2-geranyl-5-hydroxy-3-*n*-pentyl-1,4-benzoquinone	Miscellaneous	N/A
	5-acetoxy-6-geranyl-3-*n*-pentyl-1,4-benzoquinone	Miscellaneous	N/A

(Continued)

Cannabimovone	Miscellaneous	CBM
Cannabioxepane	Miscellaneous	CBX
10α-hydroxy-Δ^{9,11}-hexahydrocannabinol	Miscellaneous	N/A

TABLE 4.1 Continued

Figure	Compound Name	Compound Class	Abbreviation
	9β,10β-epoxyhexa-hydrocannabinol	Miscellaneous	N/A
	9α-hydroxyhexa-hydrocannabinol	Miscellaneous	N/A
	7-oxo-9α-hydroxyhexa-hydrocannabinol	Miscellaneous	N/A

	10α-hydroxyhexa-hydrocannabinol	Miscellaneous	N/A
	10aα-hydroxyhexa-hydrocannabinol	Miscellaneous	N/A
	9α-hydroxy-10-oxo-$\Delta^{6a,10a}$-tetrahydrocannabinol	Miscellaneous	N/A

CB_1 receptors and a partial agonist of CB_2 receptors.[6] Research has suggested that CBG may be used to treat inflammatory bowel disease.[7]

Additional Cannabigerolic Compounds

Other phytocannabinoids of the CBG class have been isolated, but their potential properties have not been adequately studied at this time. This list includes *cannabigerolic acid monomethyl ether* (CBGAM), *cannabigerol monomethyl ether* (CBGM), as well as the propyl homologues *cannabigerovarinic acid* (CBGVA) and *cannabigerovarin* (CBGV).

4.2.2 Cannabichromene Class

The cannabichromene (CBC) class of phytocannabinoids consists of both pentyl and propyl compounds. Pentyl phytocannabinoids of the CBC class are produced by the biosynthesis of CBGA. Propyl phytocannabinoids of the CBC class are produced by the biosynthesis of CBGVA.

Cannabichromenic Acid

Cannabichromenic acid (CBCA) is found in high concentrations among young plants and declines with maturation and was first isolated by a team led by Yukihiro Shoyama in the late 1960s.[5] It is more prevalent in fiber-type plants than drug-type plants.[8] Additional research into the pharmacological properties of CBCA is necessary to establish its potential uses.

Cannabichromene

The decarboxylation of CBCA produces CBC, which was discovered in 1966 by two independent research teams—Claussen et al. and Mechoulam and Gaoni.[4] CBC is the third most prevalent phytocannabinoid (behind THC and CBD). It is nonintoxicating, as it does not have an affinity for CB_1 or CB_2 receptors, but it has been shown to indirectly interact with the ECS and to enhance the effects of other major cannabinoids like THC and CBD through the entourage effect.[8] Studies suggest it may hold anti-inflammatory and analgesic properties.[9,10]

Additional Cannabichromenic Compounds

Two propyl analogues of CBCA and CBC, *cannabichromevarinic acid* (CBCVA) and *cannabichromevarin* (CBCV), have been isolated, but their potential properties have not been adequately studied at this time.

4.2.3 Cannabidiol Class

The CBD class of phytocannabinoids consists of both pentyl and propyl compounds. Pentyl phytocannabinoids of the CBD class are produced by the biosynthesis of CBGA. Propyl phytocannabinoids of the CBD class are produced by the biosynthesis of CBGVA.

Cannabidiolic Acid

CBDA was the first cannabinoid acid to be isolated, in 1955. It is the most abundant phytocannabinoid acid found in fiber-type plants and is typically the second-most abundant phytocannabinoid found in drug-type plants.[11] It is the acidic precursor to CBD, which is formed when CBDA is exposed to heat through decarboxylation. It is a nonintoxicating phytocannabinoid that does not appear to have an affinity for either CB_1 or CB_2 receptors, though studies have found several potential uses for CBDA, as it may treat inflammation, nausea, and psychosis. One study found it to be an effective inhibitor of breast cancer migration.[12]

Cannabidiol

CBD was isolated in 1940 and is produced following the decarboxylation of CBDA.[11] Following decarboxylation, it is the most abundant phytocannabinoid in fiber-type plants and typically the second-most abundant phytocannabinoid in drug-type plants. CBD is a nonintoxicating phytocannabinoid that indirectly affects CB_1 and CB_2 receptors but does not have a high affinity for either.[13] CBD has a host of potential medicinal uses that may possess antianxiety, antibacterial, anticonvulsant, antifungal, anti-inflammatory, antinausea, antipsychotic, antispasmodic, and immunomodulatory properties. It may also be able to treat some disorders that affect the central nervous system and could mitigate some of the unwanted side effects of cannabis with high levels of THC.[8]

Cannabidivarin

CBDV was first isolated in 1969 and is the propyl analogue of CBD and the decarboxylated form of cannabidivarinic acid (CBDVA).[14] CBDV is nonintoxicating, though it does have a weak affinity for CB_1 and CB_2 receptors and may be an effective anticonvulsant and antiepileptic.[15] It is not found in high concentrations in most cultivars, though some landraces in India, Pakistan, and Mexico produce significant amounts of CBDV. GW Pharmaceuticals is conducting phase 2 trials for a drug containing CBDV that it hopes will treat adult epilepsy.

Additional Cannabidiolic Compounds

Research is wanting on the remaining cannabidiolic compounds that have been isolated. These compounds include *cannabidiol monomethyl ether* (CBDM), *cannabidiol-C$_4$* (CBD-C$_4$), *cannabidiorcol* (CBD-C$_1$), and *cannabidivarinic acid* (CBDVA). Consequently, not enough information is available to describe their potential medicinal properties.

4.2.4 Δ-9-Tetrahydrocannabinol Class

The Δ-9-tetrahydrocannabinol class of phytocannabinoids consists of both pentyl and propyl compounds. Pentyl phytocannabinoids of this class are produced by the biosynthesis of CBGA. Propyl phytocannabinoids of this class are produced by the biosynthesis of CBGVA. Some of the phytocannabinoids found in this class produce an intoxicating effect.

Δ-9-Tetrahydrocannabinolic Acid

Δ-9-tetrahydrocannabinolic acid (THCA) is found in abundance among drug-type plants and to a far lesser extent in fiber-type plants that have yet to undergo decarboxylation, after which point it becomes psychoactive Δ-9-tetrahydrocannabinolic (THC). There are two isomers of THCA, THCA-A and THCA-B, both of which are nonintoxicating and appear to have little affinity for CB$_1$ and CB$_2$ receptors.[16] THCA-A is far more common than THCA-B, though THCA-B is more stable.[16] Research has indicated that THCA has anti-inflammatory properties and may be effective at treating IBD when used in conjunction with other phytocannabinoids.[17]

Δ-9-Tetrahydrocannabinol

Δ-9-tetrahydrocannabinol (THC) was first isolated in 1964 by Mechoulam and Gaoni. It is produced following the decarboxylation of THCA and is the primary psychoactive phytocannabinoid in cannabis. As such, drug-type plants have been bred to contain extremely high concentrations of THC (sometimes exceeding 30%), while fiber-type plants tend to contain very low concentrations of THC. Broad-leaflet fiber-type (BLF) plants, which are commonly cultivated in East Asia, have a notably higher THC content than do their European counterparts, but still do not produce a significant amount of THC when compared to drug-type plants.[18] THC binds to both CB$_1$ and CB$_2$ receptors and has been shown to have a wide range of potential applications, particularly as an antiemetic, anti-inflammatory, and analgesic. THC has also been shown to activate the orphan receptor GPR55, which some have claimed is a third endocannabinoid receptor.[13]

Δ-9-Tetrahydrocannabivarinic acid

Δ-9-tetrahydrocannabivarinic acid (THCVA) is the propyl homologue of THCA that is not found in high concentrations in most cultivars of cannabis available in the United States, though some have been specially bred to contain high concentrations of propyl phytocannabinoids, including THCVA, to allow for the study of these compounds. There are two isomers of THCVA, THCVA-A and THCVA-B, both of which are nonintoxicating and appear to interact indirectly with CB_1 and CB_2 receptors.[19]

Δ-9-Tetrahydrocannabivarin

Δ-9-tetrahydrocannabivarin (THCV) was first isolated in 1970 by a team led by Edward Gill and is produced following the decarboxylation of THCVA.[20] Like THCVA, it is not found in high concentrations among cultivars commonly grown in the United States, though, also like THCVA, some have been developed to contain significant concentrations of propyl phytocannabinoids, including THCV. THCV is a nonintoxicating compound that has been shown to be a high-affinity CB_1 receptor ligand and can serve as both a CB_1 antagonist and a CB_1 agonist depending on dosage, as well as a high-affinity CB_2 receptor ligand and partial CB_2 receptor agonist.[13] THCV may also be a partial agonist of orphan receptor GPR55.[13]

Additional Δ-9-Tetrahydrocannabinolic Compounds

There are multiple homologues of the phytocannabinoids found within the Δ-9-tetrahydrocannabinol class. These include *Δ-9-tetrahydrocannabiorcolic acid-C₁* (THCA-C_1) and *Δ-9-tetrahydrocannabinolic acid-C₄* (THCA-C_4), as well as their decarboxylates, *Δ-9-tetrahydrocannabiorcol-C₁* (THC-C_1) and *Δ-9-tetrahydrocannabinol-C₄* (THC-C_4). Not enough research has been performed on these compounds to determine their potential medicinal values. Additionally, the numerous esters found within this class, including but not limited to α-fenchyl-Δ-9-tetrahydrocannabinolate and α-terpenyl-Δ-9-tetrahydrocannabinolate, have not been sufficiently studied to provide a detailed analysis of their potential values as of this time.[21]

4.2.5 Δ-8-Tetrahydrocannabinol Class

The Δ-8-tetrahydrocannabinol class of phytocannabinoids is limited to Δ-8-tetrahydrocannabinolic acid (Δ^8-THCA) and its decarboxylated relative, Δ-8-tetrahydrocannabinol (Δ^8-THC). Δ^8-THCA and Δ^8-THC are considered artifacts of Δ-9-tetrahydrocannabinolic acid (Δ^9-THCA) and Δ-9-tetrahydrocannabinol (Δ^9-THC), respectively. Δ^8-THCA and Δ^8-THC do not occur in as high concentrations as Δ^9-THCA and Δ^9-THC.[11]

Δ-8-tetrahydrocannabinolic acid

Δ^8-THCA is not found in high concentrations in most cannabis cultivars. Following decarboxylation, it becomes Δ^8-THC. Very little research on this phytocannabinoid has been conducted.

Δ-8-tetrahydrocannabinol

Δ^8-THC is an isomer of its more famous relative, Δ-9-tetrahydrocannabinol, that was first isolated in 1966 by Hively et al. and differs from Δ^9-THC because of the position of a double bond.[5] It does have psychoactive properties, though it is not as powerful as Δ^9-THC in this regard, and is not found in high concentrations in most cultivars of cannabis. Δ^8-THC is a moderate agonist of both CB_1 and CB_2 receptors and shares a similar pharmacological profile to that of Δ^9-THC.[22]

4.2.6 Cannabicyclol Class

The cannabicyclol (CBL) class of phytocannabinoids includes CBL, its corresponding acid (cannabicyclolic acid [CBLA]), and a propylic homologue, cannabicyclovarin (CBLV). This class of phytocannabinoids comprises photochemical artifacts of the CBC class of phytocannabinoids created when heat or ultraviolet light is applied to cannabis.[22]

Cannabicyclolic Acid

CBLA was first isolated by the team led by Yukihiro Shoyama in the early 1970s and is not found in high concentrations in any known cultivar of cannabis.[4] CBLA has not been studied enough to provide a detailed analysis of its potential values as of this time.

Cannabicyclol

CBL was first isolated in 1967, but little research has been performed on it because CBL is more difficult to decarboxylate than other phytocannabinoids and is not produced in high qualities in any known cultivars of cannabis.[5] As it is an artifact of CBC, it is found in chemotypes with relatively high concentrations of CBC. No pharmacological evaluation for CBL has been conducted at this time.[22]

Cannabicyclovarin

Like the other phytocannabinoids in this class, little is known about CBLV. It was isolated in the early 1980s by a team led by Yukihiro Shoyama.[4]

4.2.7 Cannabielsoin Class

The cannabielsoin class of phytocannabinoids includes five compounds: cannabielsoic acid A, cannabielsoic acid B, cannabielsoin, cannabielsoin-C_3, and cannabielsoic-C_3 acid B. Like those found in the CBL class, phytocannabinoids in the cannabielsoin class are photochemical artifacts of the CBD class of phytocannabinoids. They occur in extremely low concentrations in most cultivars of cannabis, if at all. Consequently, it is unclear if this class of compounds has pharmacological applications.[4]

Cannabielsoic-C_5 Acid A (CBEA-C_5 A), Cannabielsoic-C_5 Acid B (CBEA-C_5 B), and Cannabielsoic-C_3 Acid B (CBEA-C_3 B)

The isomers cannabielsoic-C_5 acid A (CBEA-C_5 A) and cannabielsoic-C_5 acid B (CBEA-C_5 B) are both produced by the photo-oxidation of CBDA, while the propylic homologue cannabielsoic-C_3 acid B (CBEA-C_3 B) is produced by the photo-oxidation of CBDVA. The two pentylic isomers were first isolated in the 1970s by Raphael Mechoulam and Arnon Shani.[5] Heinfried Grote and Gerhard Spiteller published their paper on the isolation of CBEA-C_3 B in 1978.[23]

Cannabielsoin-C_5

Cannabielsoin-C_5 (CBE-C_5 or CBE) was first detected by a research team headed by C.A. Ludwig Bercht in the early 1970s.[5] Its structure was subsequently established by a research team headed by David B. Uliss, Raj K. Razdan, and Haldean C. Dalzell.[24] CBE is produced by the photo-oxidation of CBD. When administered to rodents, CBE did not appear to have any effect on the central nervous system, and a 5 mg/kg injection in rabbits was shown to reduce intraocular pressure.[25] There are no known publications describing the biological activity of CBE in humans.[25]

Cannabielsoin-C_3

Cannabielsoin-C_3 (CBE-C_3) is produced by the photo-oxidation of CBDV and was first isolated in the late 1970s by Heinfried Grote and Gerhard Spiteller.[23] To date, no research has been conducted on this phytocannabinoid.

4.2.8 Cannabinol Class

Phytocannabinoids of the cannabinol (CBN) class are the aromatized derivatives of Δ-9-tetrahydrocannabinol. As cannabis ages, it increases in its concentration of these types of phytocannabinoids while decreasing in THC.[4]

Cannabinolic Acid

Cannabinolic acid (CBNA) is the aromatized derivative of Δ-9-tetrahydrocannabinolic acid (THCA) and the acidic precursor of CBN. It was first isolated by the team of Mechoulam and Gaoni in the 1960s.[5] Not enough research has been conducted at this time to make any claims about the biological effects of CBNA.

Cannabinol

CBN is the aromatized derivative of Δ-9-tetrahydrocannabiol (THC) and was the first cannabinoid to be isolated—in the 1890s by Wood, Spivey, and Easterfield. It was given the correct structure in 1940 by Adams, Baker, and Wearn.[5] As it is an oxidation artifact of THC, CBN concentration depends on the age and storage conditions of cannabis and is far less prominent in fresh cannabis.[11] CBN is mildly psychoactive and expresses a lower affinity for CB_1 receptors and a threefold higher affinity for CB_2 receptors relative to THC.[26] CBN is also a TRPV2 agonist.[27] It has been noted for its sedative and anxiolytic qualities and appears to play a role in the entourage effect.

Additional Cannabinol Compounds

There are numerous compounds within the CBN class, including cannabinol-C_4 (CBN-C_4), cannabivarin (CBV), cannabinol-C_2 (CBN-C_2), cannabiorcol (CBN-C_1), cannabinol methyl ether (CBNM), 4-terpenyl cannabinolate, 8-hydroxy cannabinolic acid A, 8-hydroxycannabinol, and 1`S-hydroxy-cannabinol, but they have not been sufficiently studied. Little is known of their biological effects at this time.

4.2.9 Cannabinodiol Class

There are two phytocannabinoids within the cannabinodiol class, cannabinodiol (CBND) and its prolylic relative, cannabinodivarin (CBVD). CBND is the aromatized derivative of CBD, while CBVD is the aromatized derivative of CBDV.[5] Robert Lousberg et al. published a paper describing the first isolation of CBND in 1977, while Turner et al. published a paper describing the first isolation of

CBVD in 1980.[5] Very little research has been done on the biological effects of CBND and CBVD.

4.2.10 Cannabitriol Class

Though there are nine cannabitriol-type phytocannabinoids, and though cannabitriol (CBT) was first isolated in 1966 by Obata and Ishikawa in 1966, very little is known of CBT (which exists as both isomers and racemates) or any other phytocannabinoid from within this class.[5]

4.2.11 Miscellaneous Phytocannabinoids

Finally, there several phytocannabinoids of unusual structure that do not fall into any of the above categories. Not enough research has been done on any of these phytocannabinoids to understand their biological effects.

4.3 Terpenes and Terpenoids

Terpenes and terpenoids are organic hydrocarbons. The terms "terpene" and "terpenoid" are often used interchangeably, though there is a distinction between the two. Terpenes become terpenoids following oxidation, which typically occurs when the cannabis plant is cured and dried.[28]

There are hundreds of terpenes and terpenoids throughout the plant kingdom, and ~200 individual terpene and terpenoid compounds have been found in various chemotypes of cannabis.[28] This includes monoterpenes with C_{10} skeletons, sesquiterpenes with C_{15} skeletons, diterpenes with C_{20} skeletons, and triterpenes with C_{30} skeletons. Terpene and terpenoid content depend largely upon cultivar and may change even from one chemotype to another.

The essential oils of these terpenes are obtained through steam distillation or vaporization and tend to degrade quickly during the drying process, though they do not seem to disappear entirely.[11] Ross and ElSohly reported that fresh cannabis from an Afghani landrace yielded 0.29% essential oils at harvest and only 0.20% and 0.13% after being dried and stored for a period of 1 week and 3 months, respectively. This phenomenon is particularly discernible among monoterpenes, which are the most common types of terpenes when cannabis is fresh. Concentrations of sesquiterpenoids at harvest are typically lower than those of monoterpenes by a wide margin, but higher than those of diterpenoids and triterpenoids, which appear in trace quantities. As the cannabis ages and monoterpenes are lost at a far greater rate than sesquiterpenes, diterpenes, or triterpenes, the ratio of monoterpenes to the other terpenes becomes significantly lower. Ross and ElSohly found that monoterpenes accounted for 92.48% of volatile oils in the Afghani landrace at the time of harvest (sesquiterpenoids accounted for 6.84% and all other terpenic compounds accounted for 0.68%). After 3 months, monoterpenes accounted for 62.02% of volatile oils, sesquiterpenoids accounted for 35.63%, and all other terpenic compounds accounted for 2.35%.[29]

What follows is a brief summary about some of the most common terpenes and terpenoids found in cannabis. How these compounds interact with the ECS will be explored at greater length in Chapter 6 (The Endocannabinoid System).

Myrcene

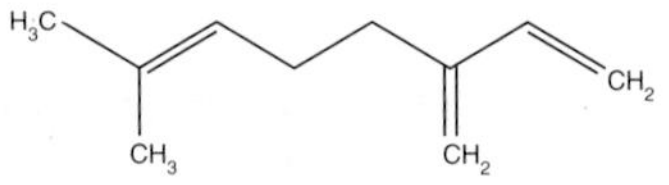

Figure 4.1 Myrcene ($C_{10}H_{16}$).

Myrcene (or β-myrcene) is the most abundant terpene in cannabis (Fig. 4.1). Both are monoterpenes that have been shown to produce a sedative effect when paired with CBD and THC that is familiarly known as "couch lock." Myrcene also has anti-inflammatory properties and was shown to be both a muscle relaxant and an analgesic in murine testing.[2] It is commonly found in mangos, hops, lemongrass, and cardamom.

Limonene

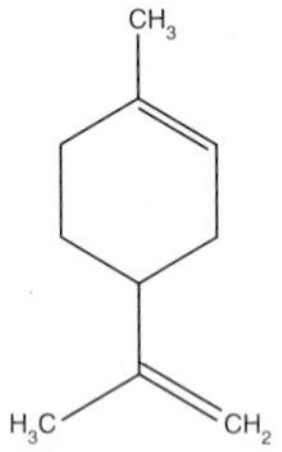

Figure 4.2 Limonene ($C_{10}H_{16}$).

Limonene is a monoterpene that is one of the most abundant terpenes in the plant kingdom and is frequently found in most cannabis cultivars (Fig. 4.2). As the name suggests, it possesses a strong citric scent and flavor. Limonene has been shown to be an anxiolytic, to cause apoptosis in breast cancer cells, and to inhibit the pathogen responsible for acne.[2] It may also improve one's mood.[30] Anecdotal evidence suggests that this latter feature of limonene is enhanced by the entourage effect.

Linalool

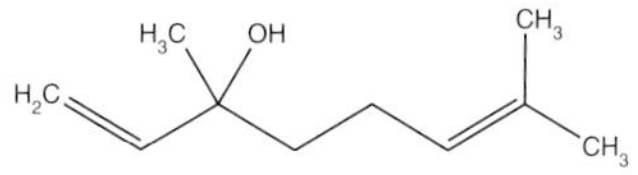

Linalool is a monoterpene regularly found in many cultivars of cannabis, as well as in lavender (Fig. 4.3). Research indicates it is the agent responsible for lavender's anxiolytic properties and capacity to treat skin burns without scarring.[2] Linalool has also been shown to be an anticonvulsant in rats and decreased K^+-stimulated glutamate release and uptake in murine synaptosomes.[31,32] Cultivars of cannabis high in linalool are said to help patients with pain management and anxiety.

Figure 4.3 Linalool ($C_{10}H_{18}O$).

Pinene (α-Pinene and β-Pinene)

There are two isomers of the monoterpene pinene, α-pinene and β-pinene (Fig. 4.4). α-Pinene is the most common terpene in nature and, as to be expected, is typically found in higher concentrations in cannabis than β-pinene. Anecdotal evidence suggests that α-pinene may reduce unwanted side effect of THC intoxication.[2] Both terpenoids have shown antimicrobial properties, and were able to produce a bactericidal effect in methicillin-resistant *Staphylococcus albicans* (MRSA).[33] Both isomers have also been shown to improve memory, suppress the pathogen responsible for acne, and serve as bronchodilators.[2]

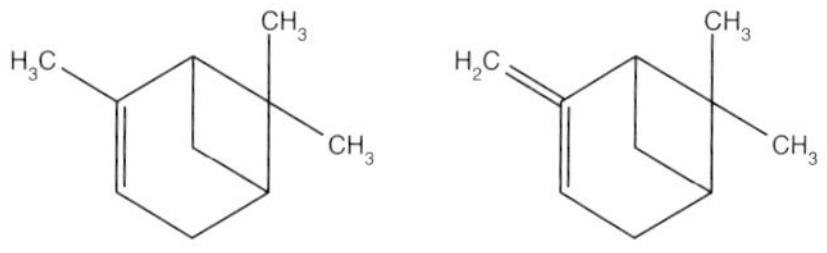

Figure 4.4 *Left.* α-Pinene ($C_{10}H_{16}$). *Right.* β-Pinene ($C_{10}H_{16}$).

β-Caryophyllene

β-Caryophyllene is generally the most common sesquiterpene in cannabis (Fig. 4.5). It is also found in black pepper, cloves, basil, and cinnamon. Of particular importance is the ability of β-caryophyllene to bind with the body's CB_2 receptor as a full agonist, thereby making it *the only terpene that has been shown to bind to either cannabinoid receptor*.[34] Consequently, anecdotal evidence suggests that cultivars with high concentrations of β-caryophyllene and CBD can help patients manage symptoms associated with autoimmune disorders such as arthritis and multiple sclerosis.

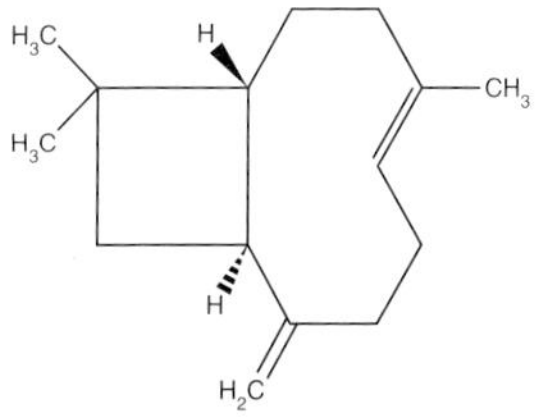

Figure 4.5 β-Caryophyllene ($C_{15}H_{24}$).

Humulene (α-Humulene, α-Caryophyllene)

Humulene (also known as α-humulene and α-caryophyllene) is a sesquiterpene and an isomer of β-caryophyllene that is typically found in hops, as well as cannabis (Fig. 4.6). Humulene has demonstrated anti-inflammatory and pharmacokinetic properties.[35,36] Humulene may also be an appetite suppressant.

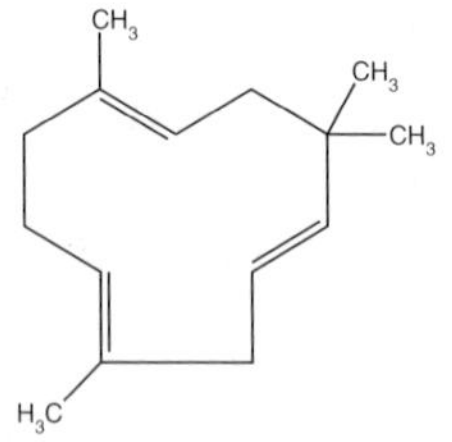

Figure 4.6 α-Humulene or α-Caryophyllene ($C_{15}H_{24}$).

Nerolidol

Nerolidol is a sesquiterpene found in the peels of many citrus fruits, though it does not frequently occur in high concentrations in cannabis (Fig. 4.7). It has been shown to be an antimalarial and a skin penetrant.[2] The latter attribute may enhance transdermal medications without impacting drug solubility.[37]

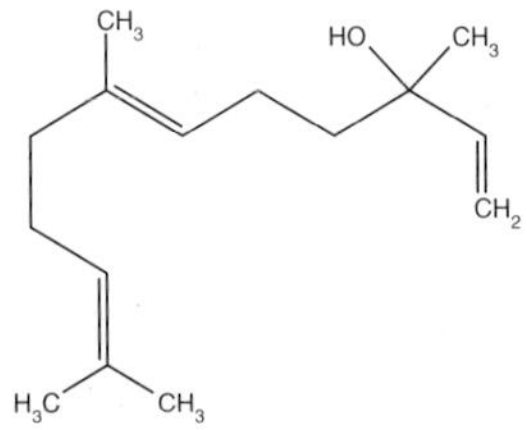

Figure 4.7 Nerolidol ($C_{15}H_{26}O$).

Geraniol

Geraniol is a monoterpene alcohol commonly found in geraniums, roses, and lemons (Fig. 4.8). It is also commonly used in the flavor and fragrance industries. Most notably, it is one of the main ingredients in citronella oil, as it is considered a natural mosquito repellent. Research has found that geraniol is an effective antimicrobial, antioxidant, and anti-inflammatory, as well as a powerful a skin penetrant.[38] Cannabis cultivars with high concentrations of geraniol may be beneficial to patients with diabetic neuropathy, as it has shown to provide therapeutic relief for this kind of pain in murine subjects.[39]

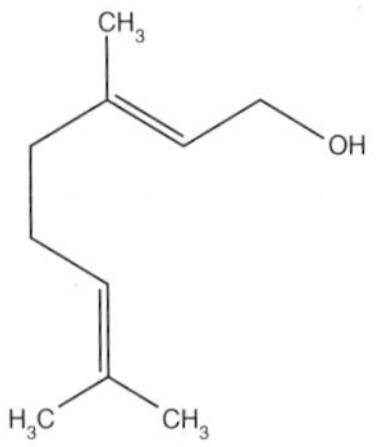

Figure 4.8 Geraniol ($C_{10}H_{18}O$).

Borneol

Borneol is a bicyclic monoterpene alcohol that is found in other species such as camphor, mint, and rosemary (Fig. 4.9). It has been shown to possess anti-inflammatory

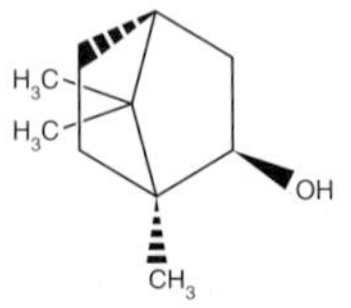

Figure 4.9 Borneol ($C_{10}H_{18}O$).

and anesthetic properties via antinociceptive activity.[40] Borneol has also demonstrated that it could be a drug potentiator, as studies indicated it enhanced the effects of selenocystine on human hepatocellular carcinoma cells.[41]

Δ-3-Carene

Δ-3-carene is a bicyclic monoterpene that is found in many cultivars of cannabis (Fig. 4.10). It is a constituent of turpentine and is a mild irritant.[42] Δ-3-carene in lower concentrations has been linked to the stimulation of bone growth in murine subjects.[43]

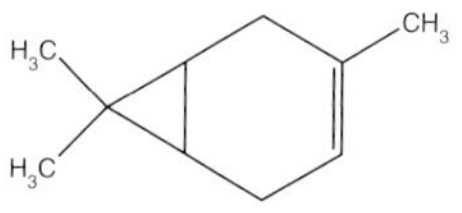

Figure 4.10 Δ-3-Carene ($C_{10}H_{16}$).

Terpinolene

Terpinolene is a monoterpene commonly found in many cultivars of cannabis, as well as species as varied as lilacs, nutmeg, and apples (Fig. 4.11). Terpinolene has been found to have antioxidant properties, and a separate study found that it produced a sedative effect in mice.[44,45] Consequently, cannabis cultivars that are high in terpinolene may enhance the sedative effects of phytocannabinoids.

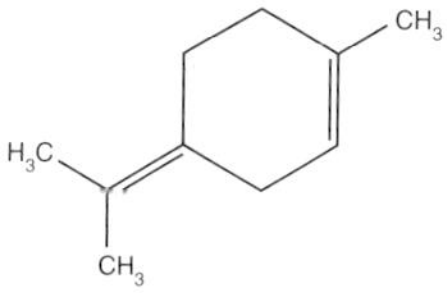

Figure 4.11 Terpinolene ($C_{10}H_{16}$).

α-Bisabolene

α-Bisabolene is a sesquiterpene that is typically found in many cannabis cultivars, but typically in low concentrations (Fig. 4.12). It is also a component of the essential oil of opoponax (sweet myrrh). It has been shown to exhibit cytotoxicity in breast cancer cell lines in murine subjects.[46]

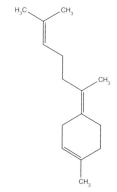

Figure 4.12 α-Bisabolene ($C_{15}H_{24}$).

4.4 Flavonoids

There are at least 23 flavonoids that commonly exist in cannabis, most of which are C-/O- and O-glycosides. The O-glycosides cannflavin A (Fig. 4.13) and cannflavin B (Fig. 4.14) are methylated isoprenoid flavones unique to cannabis that are produced as early

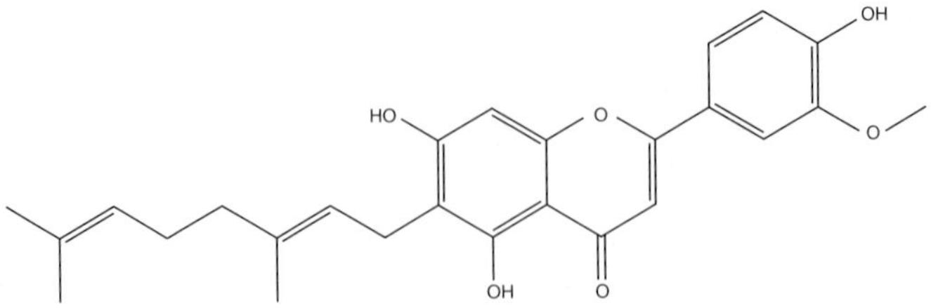

Figure 4.13 Cannflavin A ($C_{26}H_{28}O_6$).

as when the cannabis plant first sprouts. They have been shown to have anti-inflammatory properties.[47]

Cannflavin A and cannflavin B are not the only flavonoids that can produce beneficial biological activities. Additional flavonoids that are not unique to cannabis have been shown to possess anti-inflammatory, anticancer, neuroprotective, anxiolytic, and osteogenic properties.[48]

4.5 Additional Compounds

The following types compounds have also been found in cannabis and can vary in concentrations depending on upon cultivar[4].

- Nitrogenous compounds: 27
- Amino acids: 18
- Proteins: 3
- Glycoproteins: 2
- Enzymes: 6
- Sugars and related compounds: 34
- Hydrocarbons: 50
- Simple alcohols: 7
- Simple aldehydes: 12
- Simple ketones: 13
- Simple acids: 20
- Simple esters: 12
- Fatty acids: 23
- Lactones: 1
- Steroids: 11
- Noncannabinoid phenols: 25
- Vitamin K

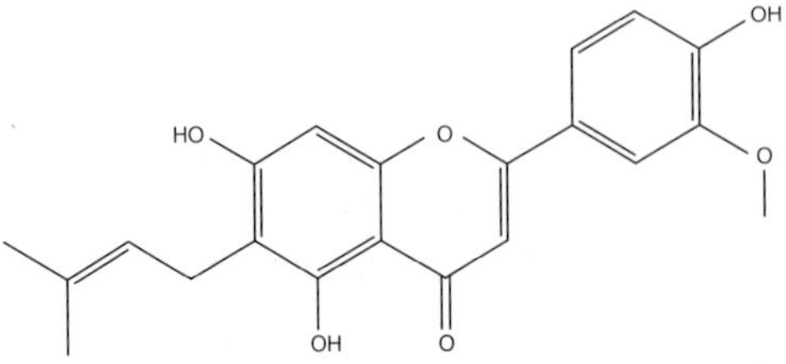

Figure 4.14 Cannflavin B ($C_{21}H_{20}O_6$).

REFERENCES

[1]Gertsch J, Pertwee RG, Di Marzo V. Phytocannabinoids beyond the Cannabis plant – do they exist? *Br J Pharmacol.* 2010;160(3):523-529. doi: 10.1111/j.1476-5381.2010.00745.x.

[2]Russo EB. Taming THC: potential cannabis synergy and phytocannabinoid-terpenoid entourage effects. *Br J Pharmacol.* 2011;163(7):1344-1364. doi: 10.1111/j.1476-5381.2011.01238.x.

[3]Russo EB. History of cannabis and its preparation in saga, science, and sobriquet. *Chem Biodivers.* 2007;4(8):1614-1648. doi: 10.1002/cbdv.200790144.

[4]ElSohly MA, Slade D. Chemical constituents of marijuana: the complex mixture of natural cannabinoids. *Life Sciences.* 2005;78:539-548. doi: 10.1016/j.lfs.2005.09.011.

[5]ElSohly M, Gul W. Constituents of Cannabis sativa. In: Pertwee RG, ed. *Handbook on Cannabis.* New York, NY: Oxford University Press; 2014:3-22.

[6]Navarro G, Varani K, Reyes-Resina I, et al. Cannabigerol action at cannabinoid CB1 and CB2 receptors at CB1-CB2 heteroreceptor complexes. *Front Pharmacol.* 2018;632(9). doi: 10.3389/fphar.2018.00632.

[7]Borrelli F, Fasolino I, Romano B, et al. Beneficial effect of the non-psychotropic plant cannabinoid cannabigerol on experimental inflammatory bowel disease. *Biochem Pharmacol.* 2013;85:1306-1316. doi: 10.1016/j.bcp.2013.01.017.

[8]Andre CM, Hausman JF, Guerriero G. Cannabis sativa: the plant of the thousand and one molecules. *Front Plant Sci.* 2016;7:19. doi: 10.3389/fpls.2016.00019.

[9]Izzo AA, Capasso R, Aviello G, et al. Inhibitory effect of cannabichromene, a major non-psychotropic cannabinoid extracted from Cannabis sativa, on inflammation-induced hypermotility in mice. *Br J Pharmacol.* 2012;166:1444-1460. doi: 10.1111/j.1476-5381.2012.01879.x.

[10]Maione S, Piscitelli F, Gatta L, et al. Non-psychoactive cannabinoids modulate the descending pathway of antinociception in anaesthetized rats through several mechanisms of action. *Br J Pharmacol.* 2011;162:584-596. doi: 10.1111/j.1476-5381.2010.01063.x.

[11]Brenneisen R. Chemistry and analysis of phytocannabinoids and other Cannabis constituents. In: ElSohly MA, ed. *Marijuana and the Cannabinoids.* Totowa, NJ: Humana Press Inc; 2007:17-49.

[12]Takeda S, Okajima S, Miyoshi H. Cannabidiolic acid, a major cannabinoid in fiber-type cannabis, is an inhibitor of MDA-MB-231 breast cancer cell migration. *Toxicol Lett.* 2012;214(3):314-319. doi: 10.1016/j.toxlet.2012.08.029.

[13]Pertwee RG. The diverse CB1 and CB2 receptor pharmacology of three plant cannabinoids: Δ9-tetrahydrocannabidol, cannabidiol, and Δ9-tetrahydrocannabivarn. *Br J Pharmacol.* 2007;153(2):199-215. doi: 10.1038/sj.bjp.0707442.

[14]Amada N, Yamasaki Y, Williams CM, Whalley BJ. Cannabidivarin (CBDV) suppresses pentylenetetrazole (PTZ)-induced increases in epilepsy-related gene expression. *Peer J.* 2013;1:e214. doi: 10.7717/peerj.214.

[15]Morales P, Reggio PH, Jagerovic N. An overview of medicinal chemistry of synthetic and natural derivatives of cannabidiol. *Front Pharmacol.* 2017;8:422. doi: 10.3389/fphar.2017.00422.

[16]McPartland JM, MacDonald C, Young M, Grant PS, Furkert DP, Glass M. Affinity and efficacy studies of tetrahydrocannabinolic acid A at cannabinoid receptor types one and two. *Cannabis Cannabinoid Res.* 2017;2(1):87-95. doi: 10.1089/can.2016.0032.

[17]Nallathambi R, Mazuz M, Ion A, et al. Anti-inflammatory activity in colon models is derived from Δ-9-tetrahydrocannabinolic acid that interacts with additional compounds in Cannabis extracts. *Cannabis Cannabinoid Res.* 2017;2(1):167-182. doi: 10.1089/can.2017.0027.

[18]Brand EJ, Zhao Z. Cannabis in Chinese medicine: are some traditional indications referenced in ancient literature related to cannabinoids? *Front Pharmacol.* 2017;8:108. doi: 10.3389/fphar.2017.00108.

[19]Soderstrom K, Soliman E, Van Dross R. Cannabinoids modulate neuronal activity and cancer by CB1 and CB2 receptor-independent mechanisms. *Front Pharmacol*. 2017;8:720. doi: 10.3389/fphar.2017.00720.

[20]Pertwee RG. Cannabinoid pharmacology: the first 66 years. *Br J Pharmacol*. 2006;147:S163-S171. doi: 10.1038/sj.bjp.0706406.

[21]Ahmed SA, Ross SA, Slade D, Radwan MM, Zulfigar F, ElSohly MA. Cannabinoid ester constituents from high-potency Cannabis sativa. *J Nat Prod*. 2008;71(4):536-542. doi: 10.1021/np070454a.

[22]Morales P, Hurst DP, Reggio PH. Molecular targets of the phytocannabinoids—a complex picture. *Prog Chem Org Nat Prod*. 2017;103:103–131. doi: 10.1007/978-3-319-45541-9_4.

[23]Grote H, Spiteller G. New cannabinoids II. *J Chromatogr A*. 1978;154(1):13-23. doi: 10.1016/S0021-9673(00)88475-7.

[24]Uliss DB, Razdan RK, Dalzell HC. Stereospecific intramolecular epoxide cleavage by phenolate anion. Synthesis of novel and biologically active cannabinoids. *J Am Chem Soc*. 1974;96(23):7372-7374. doi: 10.1021/ja00830a045.

[25]Ujváry I, Hanuš L. Human metabolites of cannabidiol: a review on their formation, biological activity, and relevance in therapy. *Cannabis Cannabinoid Res*. 2016;1(1):90-101. doi: 10.1089/can.2015.0012.

[26]Hanuš LO, Meyer SM, Muñoz E, Taglialatela-Scafati O, Appendino G. Phytocannabinoids: a unified critical inventory. *Nat Prod Rep*. 2016;33:1357-1392. doi: 10.1039/C6NP00074F.

[27]Qin N, Neeper MP, Liu Y, Hutchinson TL, Lubin ML, Flores CM. TRPV2 is activated by cannabidiol and mediates CGRP release in cultured rat dorsal root ganglion neurons. *J Neurosci*. 2008;28(24):6231-6238. doi: 10.1523/JNEUROSCI.0504-08.2008.

[28]What are terpenes & terpenoids? Why do they matter. Terpenes and Testing Magazine website. Available at https://terpenesandtesting.com/category/science/terpenes-terpenoids-difference/. Accessed June 4, 2019.

[29]Ross SA, ElSohly MA. The volatile oil composition of fresh and air-dried buds of Cannabis sativa. *J Nat Prod*. 1996;59(1):49-51. doi: 10.1021/np960004a.

[30]Hoenen M, Müller K, Pause BM, Lübke KT. Fancy citrus, feel good: positive judgment of citrus odor, but not the odor itself, is associated with elevated mood during experienced helplessness. *Front Psychol*. 2016;7:74. doi: 10.3389/fpsyg.2016.00074.

[31]Elisabetsky E, Marschner J, Souza Do. Effects of linalool on glutamatergic system in the rat cerebral cortex. *Neurochem Res*. 1995;20(4):461-465. doi: 10/.1007/BF00973103.

[32]Batista PA, Werner MF, Oliveira EC, et al. Evidence for the involvement of ionotropic glutamatergic receptors on the antinociceptive effect of (−)-linalool in mice. *Neurosci Lett*. 2008;440(3):299-303. doi: 10.1016/j.neulet.2008.05.092.

[33]da Silva AC, Lopes PM, de Azevedo MM, Costa DC, Alviano CS, Alviano DS. Biological activities of α-pinene and ß-pinene enantiomers. *Molecules*. 2012;17(6):6305-6316. doi: 10.3390/molecules17066305.

[34]Gertsch J, Leonti M, Raduner S, et al. Beta-caryophyllene is a dietary cannabinoid. *Proc Natl Acad Sci U S A*. 2008;105(26):9099-9104. doi: 10.1073/pnas.0803601105.

[35]Fernandes ES, Passos GF, Medeiros R, et al. Anti-inflammatory effects of compounds alpha-humulene and (−)-trans-caryophyllene isolated from the essential oil of Cordia verbenacea. *Eur J Pharmacol*. 2007;569(3):228-236. doi: 10.1016/j.ephar.2007.04.059.

[36]Chaves JS, Leal PC, Pianowisky L, Calixto JB. Pharmacokinetics and tissue distribution of the sesquiterpene alpha-humulene in mice. *Planta Med*. 2008;74(14):1678-1683. doi: 10.1055/s-0028-1088307.

[37]Nokhodchi A, Sharabiani K, Rashidi MR, Ghafourian T. The effect of terpene concentrations on the skin penetration of diclofenac sodium. *Int J Pharm*. 2007;335(1-2):97-105. doi: 10.1016/j.jpharm.2006.10.041.

[38]Chen W, Viljoen AM. Geraniol—a review of a commercially important fragrance material. *S Afr J Bot.* 2010;76(4):643-651. doi: 10.1016/j.sajb.2010.05.008.

[39]Prasad SN, Muralidhara. Protective effects of geraniol (a monoterpene) in a diabetic neuropathy rat model: Attenuation of behavioral impairments and biochemical perturbations. *J Neurosci Res.* 2014;92(9):1205-1216. doi: 10.1002/jnr.23393.

[40]Almeida JR, Souza GR, Silva JC, et al. Borneol, a bicyclic monoterpene alcohol, reduces nociceptive behavior and inflammatory response in mice. *ScientificWorldJournal.* 2013;808460. doi: 10.1155/2013/808460.

[41]Su J, Lai H, Chen J, et al. Natural borneol, a monoterpenoid compound, potentiates selenocystine-induced apoptosis in human hepatocellular carcinoma cells by enhancement of cellular uptake and activation of ROS-mediated DNA damage. *PLoS One.* 2013;8(5):e63502. doi: 10.1371/journal.pone.0063502.

[42]Kasanen JP, Pasanen AL, Pasanen P, Liesivuori J, Kosma VM, Alarie Y. Evaluation of sensory irritation of delta-3-carene and turpentine, and acceptable levels of monoterpenes in occupational and indoor environment. *J Toxicol Environ Health A.* 1999;57(2):89-114. doi: 10.1080/009841099157809.

[43]Jeong JG, Kim YS, Min YK, Kim SH. Low concentration of 3-carene stimulates the differentiation of mouse osteoblastic MC3T3-F1 subclone 4 cells. *Phytother Res.* 2008;22:18-22. doi: 10.1002/ptr.2247.

[44]Grassman J, Hippeli S, Spitzenberger R, Elstner EF. The monoterpene terpinolene from the oil Pinus mugo L. in concert with alpha-tocopherol and beta-carotene effectively prevents oxidation of LDL. *Phytomedicine.* 2005;12(6-7):416-423. doi: 10.1016/j.phymed.2003.10.005.

[45]Ito K, Ito M. The sedative effect of inhaled terpinolene in mice and its structure-activity relationships. *J Nat Med.* 2013;67(4):833-937. doi: 10.1007/s11418-012-0732-1.

[46]Yeo SK, Ali AY, Hayward OA, et al. ß-Bisabolene, a sesquiterpene from the essential oil extract of opoponax (Commiphora guidottii), exhibits cytotoxicity in breast cancer cell lines. *Phytother Res.* 2015;30(3):418-425. doi: 10.1002/ptr.5543.

[47]Werz O, Seegers J, Schaible AM, et al. Cannaflavins from hemp sprouts, a novel cannabinoid-free hemp food product, target microsomal prostaglandin E2 synthase-1 and 5-lipoxygenase. *PharmaNutrition.* 2014;2(3):53-60. doi: 10.1016/j.phanu.2014.05.001.

5

U.S. Cannabis Regulations From Past to Present

5.1 Overview

This chapter discusses the rules and regulations on the use and distribution of cannabis in the United States. It brings to light important historical information dating back to the 19-century tinged with racial insensitivity but is relevant to our discussion since these cultural undertones led to the adoption of laws concerning cannabis use. These regulations were often based on inaccurate scientific data and instead were influenced by immigration policies and cultural nuances of the time. The chapter addresses the misrepresentation that shaped the thinking of the general public, as well as scientific community at the time, and haltered the clinical research and use of cannabis in the 20th century.

Despite the widespread availability of unregulated cannabis in pharmacies during the 19th and early 20th centuries, its recreational usage remained somewhat uncommon in the United States and Europe prior to World War I. Cannabis use did not significantly increase in Europe during the interwar years but did become more prevalent in the United States during this time. Many working-class Mexicans had begun smoking cannabis in the form of marijuana cigarettes during the late 19th century, and some brought the habit with them when they came to the United States to escape Mexico's civil war, but it would be incorrect to say that recreational cannabis was unheard of in the United States prior to this time or that it was introduced to the United States by Mexican immigrants.

By the 1920s, marijuana had become a significant part of Jazz Age culture, particularly among musicians and residents of working-class communities in urban areas in the South, where there were significant Mexican populations. Because of its popularity among the marginalized communities, as well as the ignorance of middle class and more affluent members of the general population with regard to the effects of cannabis, it came to be regarded as a menace equal to or greater than opium and its derivatives—that is, heroin.

Concurrently, interest in cannabis among medical professionals began to wane. Medicinal use had been common throughout the late-19th and early-20th centuries, but its use had declined because it was difficult to standardize doses and it did not take immediate effect when consumed orally. Additionally, it could not be injected intravenously because cannabinoids are not soluble in water, and many of the conditions for which it was prescribed were being treated by new, synthetic medicines. Cannabis was, ironically, considered something of an old-fashioned remedy by the time the people of Main Street America were panicking about the dangers of marijuana in the 1920s and 1930s. It seems as though these individuals did not understand that the two, cannabis and marijuana, were the same plant. Decline in interest from the medical community, in conjunction with public pressure that was largely fueled by racially motivated tales of marijuana-driven mayhem, led to increased prohibition at the state level in the 1920s and 1930s. In 1937, Congress passed the Marihuana Tax Act,* thereby making its legal use as a medicine prohibitively

---

*The words "marijuana" and "marihuana" have the same meaning. The latter and less common spelling fell out of use gradually and is now considered obsolete, but it still appears in some federal documents. Both "marijuana" and "marihuana" were often favored over "cannabis" by those who sought to prohibit its use and believed that making the drug sound more foreign would make it seem more dangerous. Cannabis eventually came to be referred to as "marijuana" even by proponents of its use, though many now consider both "marijuana" and "marihuana" to be problematic. "Cannabis" is the preferred nomenclature.

expensive and it was dropped from the U.S. Pharmacopeia in 1941.

Even before the passage of the Marihuana Tax Act, the United States had taken the lead on disrupting the illicit cannabis trade on an international level. Most within the international community followed a similar policy, though cannabis continued to be produced in India, Pakistan, Afghanistan, Syria, Lebanon, and Morocco, among other countries. Recreational usage ballooned from the 1940s through the 1960s, particularly among working-class and countercultural communities. Eventually, members of the predominately white counterculture movements of the 1950s and 1960s—the Beats and the hippies, respectively— helped to turn cannabis into a symbol of defiance against the established order. The established order, often personified by former President Richard Nixon, responded by classifying cannabis as a Schedule I drug under the Controlled Substances Act (CSA) of 1970, thereby putting a tight stranglehold on cannabis research.

The effects of the CSA put a hold on cannabis research, but it did not end it entirely and interest in cannabis as a medicinal drug was renewed in the 1970s as more researchers and patients began to examine alternatives to conventional medicine. Though initially a fringe movement, anecdotal evidence and limited scientific analysis began to reveal that medicinal cannabis was an effective treatment for glaucoma and certain types of neuropathy, and that it had the ability to stimulate the appetites of individuals suffering from wasting diseases or the effects of cancer treatments, particularly chemotherapy. The effort to legalize medicinal cannabis gradually gained traction throughout the early 1990s, especially in western states like California, Arizona, and New Mexico. It culminated in California's decision to allow for the use of medicinal cannabis in 1996. Since that time, numerous states have followed suit even though the federal government continued to label all forms of cannabis as Schedule I drugs until December 2018, when Congress enacted legislation to legally differentiate between hemp and marijuana, thereby allowing states to implement plans allowing people to grow hemp for industrial purposes or for the sake of producing extracts that contain high amounts of cannabidiol (CBD), a nonintoxicating phytocannabinoid that has recently become popular among consumers for its wide range of purported therapeutic effects.

5.2 America's First Opiate Crisis

This section addresses the impact of opium crises and subsequent legislation to regulate its use. To better understand the laws governing cannabis, it is important to discuss the history of the opium crises that emerged in the 19th century since they are direct consequences of the laws that were later enacted to regulate drugs in the early 20th century.

Like cannabis, opium has been used medicinally for millennia, though it is unclear when and where humans first began using it. The Sumerians, who inhabited modern Iraq as long ago as 4500 Before Common Era (BCE), were cultivating poppies for opium as early as the third millennium BCE, and they referred to the drug as *gil*, meaning "joy," and the poppy as *hul gil*, which translates into "plant of joy."[1] By the second millennium BCE, it was being used by cultures in the Near East, Northern Africa, and in parts of Europe.[2] Evidence also indicates that the Chinese doctor Hua To, who lived during the Three Kingdoms (220-264 Common Era [CE]), used a mixture of opium and cannabis when preparing patients for surgery.[3]

While used medicinally in the ancient world to treat a wide variety of conditions (as well as a popular poison), evidence suggests that it was also used as a euphoriant and what could today be described as a recreational drug. It is difficult to assess how widespread usage or abuse was, but there is evidence that Galen (129-210 CE), the last of the great Greek physicians, was familiar with both the toxic effects of opium and the concept of tolerance.[4] European physicians writing more than 1000 years later, after opium had been reintroduced to the continent by Arab traders, also recognized the problems of addiction and tolerance.[1] Chinese writers were familiar with opium's deadly potential, too. Zhu Zhenheng, a physician writing in the 14th century, claimed that a paste made from opium was a useful treatment for diarrhea and dysentery, but noted that one should be cautious with the medicine, "for it kills like a knife."[5]

Prior to the 16th century, opium was consumed orally, and use was restricted to the wealthy elite throughout Europe and Asia. This began to change as European traders spread the habit of tobacco smoking throughout the world. The practice became increasingly common in the late 16th and early 17th centuries, and many cultures began to experiment with smoking other substances.

As mentioned in Chapter 2 (The History of Cannabis), it was at this time that the habit of smoking preparations of cannabis became common throughout India and much of the Muslim world. Smoking opium, meanwhile, became common in Southeast Asia, particularly in China, where it was initially mixed with either betel leaves or tobacco and called *madak*.[6]

By the end of the 18th century, opium smoking in China had become extremely widespread, and the importation of the drug had become a lucrative operation for European merchants. The British East India Company, who procured opium from the poppy fields of India, came to dominate this trade even after the Jiaqing Emperor prohibited the importation of opium into China in 1799.[7] Consequently, what had been a legal, albeit frowned-upon trade became a smuggling operation carried out furtively by the East India Company.[8]

Opium smoking continued to be a major problem in China, not only because of its costs in human misery but because it drained the empire's silver reserves. Between 1793 and 1820, China's silver reserves plummeted by roughly 85%—from 70 million taels (~5.83 million pounds) to 10 million taels.[9] It is estimated that there were as many as 3 million people in China addicted to opium as of 1830, with addiction rates reaching close to 90% in some coastal provinces.[9] More than 10% of the revenue that the British drew from India came from the illicit opium trade.[9] When the ambitious high commissioner in Guangzhou (then known as Canton) attempted to disrupt the supply of British opium into China, the result was the First Opium War, which lasted from 1840 to 1842. It ended in a British victory, as well as continuation of the illicit opium trade. The Second Opium War, waged between 1856 and 1860, resulted in another Chinese defeat and the legalization of the opium trade in China.

As a consequence of the opium wars, widespread opium addiction, rebellions, and several other factors, China became less stable, thereby making life difficult for many peasants and members of the nascent working class. To escape these conditions, many emigrated to regions within Asia or to Oceana, where there was a significant demand for labor. Beginning in the 1840s, an increasing number of Chinese workers also began coming to the West Coast of the United States, oftentimes in a form of indentured servitude, where they found jobs working in the mines or on the railroads. The work was arduous and physically taxing, and one of the ways they coped with these demanding jobs was by smoking opium.[10]

While the habit of smoking opium was something of a novelty in the United States when Chinese immigrants started to arrive in the 1840s, the drug was anything but new to Americans of European decent. It had been widely used in Europe for several hundred years and its use had continued among Europeans who came to North America. During colonial times, it was used medicinally by doctors, as well as laymen, and handbooks regularly provided recipes for opium-based concoctions like laudanum (a tincture typically containing ~10% powdered opium by weight) and paregoric (a tincture containing ~4% powdered opium by weight).[11] Opium could be readily procured at the general store or one could grow it in a private medicinal garden, a practice that was common throughout the 13 Colonies before, during, and after the Revolutionary War. Thomas Jefferson, the author of the Declaration of Independence and the third President of the United States, grew poppies in his medicinal garden at Monticello, and they continued to bloom there year after year until the Drug Enforcement Agency had them yanked from the grounds in 1991.[12]

Opium was not only being used for medicinal purposes. The physician James Thacher, in his 1810 *materia medica* on species native to North America and European transplants, rather ornately lamented the growing trend of using opium for its intoxicating effects. "It is a melancholy consideration, that the excellent, kind assuager of our bodily pains and mental distress, is frequently resorted to for the horrid purpose of self-destruction," he wrote.[13] Author Thomas de Quincy's 1821 *Confessions of an English Opium Eater*, which was published in installments throughout 1821 in *London Magazine*, paints a far more vivid picture of this era of recreational opium abuse. The work makes clear that opium was being used as a recreational drug, but the problem was not considered a public health crisis.

Still, physicians were often cautious about giving full-throated support to the virtues of opium and opiates. Friedrich Wilhelm Adam Sertürner, who discovered morphine[†] in either 1804 or 1805, later wrote, "I consider it my duty to attract attention to the terrible effects of this new substance in order that calamity may be averted."[14] In 1838, a writer for the *Boston Medical and Surgical Journal* recognized that opium was addictive, that long-term usage could lead to tolerance and problems with abuse, and that those who became severely addicted to the substance in youth rarely

---

[†]Sertürner's discovery of morphine was also the first discovery of an alkaloid.

lived to the age of forty. The author added, "By degrees, as the habit becomes more confirmed, his strength continues decreasing, the craving for the stimulus becomes even greater, and to produce the desired effect, the dose must be constantly augmented."[15]

Despite these warnings, opiate use continued to increase both as a therapeutic agent and as a recreational drug, largely due to the proliferation of morphine and subsequently to the development of the hypodermic needle in the 1850s. During the U.S. Civil War, medics regularly used morphine to prevent dysentery and to relieve the pain of those wounded in battle. As a result, many veterans inadvertently became addicted to morphine and opiate addiction became known as the "army disease."[16]

Concurrently, opium imports into the United States steadily began to climb, from 24 000 lb in 1840 to 110 470 lb in 1865, before skyrocketing to 416 864 lb in 1872. For the rest of the century, opium imports remained between 400 000 and 500 000 lb per year with rare exception.[17]

As these data suggest, opiate use after the war was widespread, and it was not only restricted to former soldiers and Chinese immigrants but affected Americans of all backgrounds. Physicians lacked an understanding of the complexity and dangers of addiction, which led many to prescribe opiates not only for pain relief (for which there were no alternatives at the time) but even minor problems. For example, one North Carolina doctor as late as 1880 claimed to have given a patient between 2500 and 3000 morphine injections over the course of 18 months and seemed convinced that no signs of "the opium habit" had developed—probably because the patient never went more than a few hours without a dose and, consequently, never experienced the onset of withdrawal symptoms.[18] Male doctors appear to have been particularly prone to overprescribing opiates to women who were suffering from menstrual cramps, morning sickness, and neurasthenia.[19]

Patients were not required to see a physician to procure opiates, and there were virtually no restrictions preventing the public from self-medicating. One could easily procure opium, morphine, laudanum, or paregoric in the United States or the United Kingdom even after the passage of the Poisons and Pharmacy Act of 1868, which restricted the sale of opium in Britain to registered chemists.[20] Opiates were also found in patent medicines, which were premade formulae designed to invigorate the senses of adults, quell the tantrums of teething children, and even cure alcoholism. Between 1840 and 1870, patent medicine sales increased more than 7 times faster than the rate of population growth.[21] The popularity of these tonics is part of the reason why only one-fifth of the opium imported into the United States in the 1870s was believed to be used in a medicinally legitimate manner.[22] Opiates, whether in the form of morphine or laudanum or a patent medicine whose contents were an utter mystery to consumers, were as freely accessible as aspirin is today.[23]

Those who developed a dependency to opiate-based drugs and tonics were not social pariahs or individuals on the lower rungs of the existing social order, nor was casual opiate consumption something in which only libertines participated. Consuming patent medicines that contained opiates was particularly common among middle-class women and society ladies. They were used as analgesics or for recreational purposes—the latter usage being common because respectable women were not supposed to drink alcohol. Such social mores remained in place even into the 1890s, a point that is illustrated by a physician writing in Philadelphia's *Medical and Surgical Reporter* in 1895. "The female sex does not often, in the country and small towns, become addicted to the use of alcohol, while opium claims more of them as its devotees than of the male sex," he wrote. "The latter attracts men and women; the former, as a rule, men only."[24]

As opium use continued to increase into the 1870s and 1880s, concern about the prevalence of addiction grew, too. Though a highly effective analgesic and a necessary part of any physician's toolkit, many within the medical community and beyond recognized that opiates were extremely addictive and that their use should be restricted. The public also began to recognize the dangers of opiate addiction at this time.

Despite the growing evidence of opium's addictive qualities, however, there continued to be a belief in some circles that opium use was preferable to drinking alcohol, particularly for women, and even some prominent temperance activists were habituated, as the stigma against opiates was less severe than that of alcohol.[25] This was a common opinion that was openly expressed by some physicians and members of the public.[26] In a *New York Times* article about the dangers of opiate addiction published in 1878, one writer claimed that, "Far from disordering the mental faculties as wine and spirituous liquors do, opium, in its immediate effect, strengthens the mind, composes what has been agitated, and communicates calmness and serenity to all the faculties."

been in previous decades, and this avoided another large wave of physician-inspired addiction. Still, word of its euphoric effects quickly spread and, by the early 1910s, heroin had become a popular street drug in major urban centers around the country.[40]

Throughout the second half of the 19th century and the early 20th century, the public's attitude toward people struggling with addiction, whether to opiates or alcohol, was varied. In some cases, individuals had sympathy for those who had become addicted to opiates, particularly if the addiction was inadvertent, as was the case with many veterans from the Civil War or women who had developed a dependency either due to overprescription or the use of patent medicines that contained opiates. Not everyone was so understanding, and many considered both alcoholism and opiate addiction to be a moral failure or weakness on the part of the individual. Those of this opinion perceived addiction as an indulgence and a character flaw that could be overcome by willpower, and not a disease.

The fact that these two sentiments were always present in the public debate about addiction is clear from historical evidence, but they waxed and waned in popularity over time. Prior to 1900, those who were sympathetic to addicted individuals appear to have outnumbered those who held the sterner position concerning addiction. This changed in the early 20th century, largely because of the rise of heroin abuse and the consequent shift in the image of the typical opiate user.[41] The popular perception of the opiate addict became defined by voluntary heroin use, idleness, and public displays of intoxication, and the image of the "average addict" became a criminal or vagrant and ceased to be a respectable person who developed a physical dependency because they unknowingly consumed a tonic that contained morphine and privately maintained their addiction at home.[42] Consequently, public opinion about the kinds of policies that should be enacted to fight addiction began to change, as well, and many Americans began to favor a hardline and punitive approach to drug users, whether their drug of choice was cocaine, heroin, morphine, or another opiate. This would come to be reflected in the drug laws that were passed in the first half of the 20th century, and it would also shape how the public responded to the growing use of recreational cannabis in the 1920s and 1930s.

U.S. foreign policy regarding opiates also changed at the end of the century and was largely due to the annexation of the Philippines following the Spanish-American War of 1898.[43] Throughout the 19th century, U.S. merchants had actively participated in the opium trade in East Asia, even though the federal government had prohibited the importation of opium into China since 1858, but there was not a strong effort to crack down on those who ignored the ban.[44] Once the Philippines became a U.S. territory, American missionaries reported widespread opium use to diplomats who wanted to create an image of benevolent rule over the former Spanish colony.[45] In 1903, the Philippines Opium Commission was created, and their report led to the prohibition of opium imports into the Philippines, except for medicinal purposes, which went into effect in 1908.[46] A similar law would go into effect in the United States in 1909 following the passage of House bill H.R. 27427, also known as the Smoking Opium Exclusion Act of 1909 or the Opium Exclusion Act of 1909. Both bans took on the appearance of a moral crusade against opium abuse, and such an attitude would eventually become a feature of U.S. foreign policy in East Asia and beyond. The Shanghai International Opium Commission of 1909, organized largely at the behest of the United States and individuals like Dr. Hamilton Wright, would represent the first coordinated effort among numerous nations to combat the opiate problem.[47]

5.3 The Rise of Regulations

Concomitant to the rise in awareness about the dangers of addiction on both the national and international level, the public was also becoming worried about the levity food and drug manufacturers were afforded. The call for more transparency became louder due to the work of crusaders like the scientist Harvey Washington Wiley and the activist Alice Lakey, as well as a group of investigative journalists known as the muckrakers. These journalists regularly published stories and books about the hazards of unregulated industry and corruption among businessmen and within the government. The most famous of the muckrakers' works, *The Jungle*, was published in 1906 by Upton Sinclair. He wrote the book to describe the oppressive labor conditions faced by Chicago's meatpackers, but it instead shocked the public with its vivid descriptions of how the sausage literally gets made.[48] As Sinclair remarked after the book's success, "I aimed at the public's heart and by accident I hit it in the stomach."[49]

The Jungle has enjoyed the most enduring legacy of any book written by a muckraker, but it was not the only book to have caused a stir among the public at the time of publication. Samuel Hopkins Adams accomplished a similar feat when he wrote 11 articles for *Collier's* in 1905 detailing the dangers of allowing patent medicines to remain unregulated.[50] The series, which was subsequently published as a pamphlet entitled *The Great American Fraud* in 1906, was widely read by both physicians and the general public.[51] The average American was shocked when they learned that many of these concoctions contained drugs, alcohol, and even poisons like strychnine and arsenic (Fig. 5.2).[37]

The public outcry aroused by activists and works like *The Jungle* and *The Great American Fraud* pressured Congress to pass the *1906 Safe Food and Drug Act*. The law created the Food and Drug Administration (FDA) and made it unlawful to misbrand any food or drug sold to the public. Furthermore, the law required manufacturers label the quantity or proportion of the following substances found in any medicines: "alcohol, morphine, opium, cocaine, heroin, alpha or beta eucaine, chloroform, *Cannabis indica*, chloral hydrate, or acetanilide, or any derivative or preparation of any such substances contained therein."[52]

The law did not entirely eliminate opiates from patent medicines, but it did expose charlatans who had used opiates to make their tonics addictive, and many promptly went out of business. However, America's drug problem was far from cured. Usage rates were still high and there continued to be few restrictions on the sale of extremely potent and addictive drugs. As mentioned above, heroin could be found in some pharmacies until the 1910s, while other

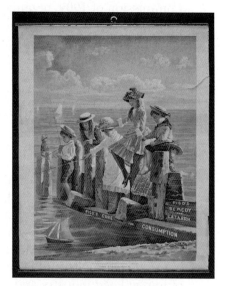

Figure 5.2 Piso's Cure for Consumption, Piso's Remedy for Catarrh. Courtesy of Historic New England. According to Samuel Hopkins Adams' *The Great American Fraud*, Piso's contained alcohol, chloroform, opium, and cannabis.

preparations containing opiates, such as laudanum and paregoric, could be found in grocery stores.[53] Furthermore, the public began to associate drugs with crime. Heroin users, for example, were often depicted as unemployed or underemployed young men who stole to finance their habit.[40] Cocaine also became associated with crime, particularly among African Americans in the South.[54] Public opinion favored the call for additional regulations.

Enacting a ban on the sale of opiates or other drugs for nonmedicinal purposes was not possible at the time. Even the most vehement antidrug crusaders recognized that there were constitutional limitations that would not allow the federal government to police drug use or sales. However, they reasoned that the constitution would allow the federal government to use its ability to impose taxes and require strict record keeping as a mechanism through which restrictions on opiates and other drugs could be put into place.[55] The initial piece of legislation that sought to employ this method, known as the Foster bill, died in 1911. A similar piece of legislation, the Harrison Act, was passed in 1914 without significant opposition.

The Harrison Act required anyone who sold or manufactured opiates, cocaine, or numerous other drugs to register and buy tax stamps through the collector of internal revenue. Violators were fined no more than $2000 (~$50 000 in 2019 dollars) and faced a maximum of 5 years in prison. Attempts to include cannabis in the list of drugs found in the Harrison Act were halted by the pharmaceutical industry.[56] They argued that it was a useful remedy for glaucoma and migraines and that it was used in veterinary practices and to treat corns. Legislation requiring a record of every sale of a corn plaster because it contained an illicit substance seemed ridiculous.[57]

It became clear in the following years that the language of the Harrison Act lacked precision, and it consequently faced numerous challenges in the Supreme Court. Most notably, several doctors and pharmacists argued that the law still allowed them to prescribe small amounts of opiates to individuals who were dependent solely to mitigate withdrawal symptoms. The Supreme Court ultimately ruled against this interpretation of the law in 1919 in two different cases: *U.S. v. Doremus* and *Webb et al v. U.S.*[58]

For official records, the law significantly reduced the number of Americans who were addicted to opiates, though it is difficult to establish how many Americans struggled with dependency in secret following its implementation. As the opiate trade became illicit and was not subject to record keeping, the estimated number of individuals addicted to opiates fluctuated wildly. A committee appointed by the Secretary of the Treasury in 1918 determined that there were ~1 000 000 individuals addicted to opiates.[59] An Army survey, meanwhile, placed their low estimate at 104 300.[60] Later analysis suggests that the number of Americans addicted to opiates in 1915 was ~215 000, and that the number had dropped to 110 000 by 1922.[60]

It is at the very least reasonable to assert that the Harrison Act was effective at reducing the number of individuals addicted to opiates, but the act made life for those who continued using opiates more difficult. It also made doctors far more cautious about prescribing them out of fear that they could run afoul of the law.[61] As addicts could no longer obtain opiates through legitimate means, they instead sought out unscrupulous street peddlers who exploited the situation by both reducing the quality of the drugs they sold (often by adulterating it with other powders like powdered milk) and increasing their price. A lieutenant in the New York City Police Department told the *New York Times* in 1915 that the trade price of heroin was $6.50 for an ounce, but that street sales of the drug were closer to $12 for one-eighth of that amount.[62]

Prohibition progressed on the international level, as well—at least in spirit. The Shanghai Opium Conference of 1909 had recognized that the opium epidemic was a global problem that required global solutions, though these solutions were recommendations rather than binding terms.[63] The next international conference, the Hague Convention of 1912, similarly accomplished little beyond making the suppression of opium smoking "a principle of international law."[64] According to Harry Jacob Anslinger, the future head of the Federal Bureau of Narcotics (FBN) (a precursor to the Drug Enforcement Agency), "Its main defect was that it created no administrative machinery for the implementation of the agreed principles."[65]

As the focus of these first two international conventions was to address the opiate problem, and not all drugs that were at the time designated as narcotics,‡ relatively little was said about cannabis.[66]

---

‡Presently, narcotics refer to psychoactive compounds that induce sleep, and the word has come to be synonymous with opiates and opioids. In the past, a narcotic referred to any kind of illicit drug, even cocaine. Cocaine is still defined as a narcotic by Title 21 section 802 of the United States Code, even if it is technically a non-narcotic stimulant.

It was not until the Second Geneva Convention of 1925 that the international community attempted to come to an agreement about the regulation of the cannabis trade.[66] Due to infighting between the nations in attendance, the only agreement to be forged was a suggested restriction on the export of hashish only, but not all participating nations signed onto an agreement, as Egypt and the United States walked out of the convention before it ended.[67] The situation in the United States had changed dramatically by this time, and the delegation had wanted more to be done in addressing what was perceived to be a growing cannabis epidemic.

5.4 Cannabis and Opium

Though cannabis and opium are very different drugs, the two were often lumped together under the title of narcotics, a term that referred to a drug capable of producing both psychoactive and soporific effects. Additionally, physicians and pharmacists in the 19th century often compared them to one another because they were both used as analgesics.

As has been stated elsewhere, relatively few Americans experimented with cannabis as a recreational drug, though there is evidence that stories about the effects of cannabis had entered into public discourse not long after O'Shaughnessy's study on "Indian hemp" was published in the United States in the early 1840s. One of the more colorful descriptions can be found in the work of Fitz Hugh Ludlow, who published *The Hasheesh Eater* in 1857.

According to Ludlow, few Europeans or Americans of European ancestry were using cannabis recreationally even in the 1850s. He claims that some Europeans may have tried hashish while travelling in the East, but, "The results of the experiment were dignified with no further notice than a page or a chapter in the note-book of his journeyings, and the hasheesh [*sic.*] phenomena, with an exclamation of wonder, were thenceforward dismissed from his own and the public mind."[68] He continues, "Very few even of the permanently domesticated foreign residents in the countries of the East have ever adopted this indulgence as a habit, and of those few I am not aware of any who have communicated their experience to the world, or treated it as a subject possessing scientific interest."[68]

Ludlow, however, did not have to travel to the East to discover hashish. Instead, he found it in Poughkeepsie when he stumbled upon a tincture made from "East Indian hemp" produced by Tilden & Co. in his local pharmacy. Though it did not produce any observable effect the first 2 times he used it, a third and far larger dose clearly did. As he tells his physician during the height of his experience: "I have been taking hasheesh [*sic.*]—*C. indica* [*sic.*], and I fear that I am going to die."[69] Later passages were far more poetic. Much of the prose is reminiscent (though derivative) of the work of De Quincy. Even the title of the book appears to be an homage to De Quincy's 1821 work.

Ludlow was not the only American to experience the intoxicating effects of hashish. Many doctors throughout the second half of the 19th century did so, as well.[70] More importantly, several doctors also provided testimony about the efficacy of cannabis and its similarities to opium.

Dr. Fronmueller of Feurth, Ohio, for example, contributed to the 1860 report of the Ohio State Medical Committee on *C. indica*. "I have used hemp many hundred times to relieve local pains of an inflammatory as well as neuralgic nature," he wrote, "and judging from these experiments, I have to assign to the Indian hemp a place among the so-called hypnotic medicines next to opium."[71] While similar to opium, he noted that, "The whole effect of hemp being less violent, and producing a more natural sleep, without interfering with the actions of the internal organs, it is certainly often preferable to opium, although it is not equal to that drug in strength and reliability."[71]

The 20th edition of *The Dispensatory of the United States of America*, published in 1918, contained similar claims. "Its action upon the nerve centers resembles opium," its authors wrote.[72] However, as Dr. Fronmueller noted 58 years before, "One of the great hindrances to the wider use of this drug is its extreme variability."[72]

Though some drug manufacturers claimed to have developed standardized doses by 1930, it was too little too late.[73] Synthetic pharmaceuticals had made cannabis-based medicines largely obsolete and it was beginning to be considered something of an antiquated treatment option. Furthermore, the opinion that one could use intoxicating drugs, including alcohol, responsibly had become less popular among Americans during the first two decades of the 20th century. The temperance movement had succeeded in pressuring Congress to pass the Volstead Act in 1919, which ushered in the era of Prohibition in 1920, and the horrors of opiate addiction were still fresh in the collective American memory. These fears were given credence and fueled by regular media reports describing crazed drug addicts rampaging through the streets while under the influence of heroin or cocaine.

Allowing cannabis to go unregulated—even if recreational use was minimal and its most common medicinal preparation by this time was as a topical plaster used to treat corns—seemed like a dangerous move. While it was not regulated by the Harrison Act, some state laws (such as New York's Boylan Anti-Drug Act, which was passed in 1914) did define cannabis as a "habit-forming drug" and restricted nonmedicinal sales. In 1914, the *New York Times* applauded an amendment to the Boylan Anti-Drug Act, which added cannabis to the list of "habit-forming drugs" contained in the legislation, and wrote, "Devotees of hashish are now hardly numerous enough here to count, but they are likely to increase as other narcotics become harder to obtain."[74]

That both the readers and writers of the *Times* had little idea as to effects of cannabis is made clear by language from an article that had been published the previous day, wherein the *Times* claimed that cannabis "has practically the same effect as morphine and cocaine, but it was not used in this country to any extent."[75]

5.5 Reefer Madness

As cannabis' figurative star was falling among the medical community in the 1910s and 1920s, recreational use began to increase. Tinctures of hashish or other forms of cannabis had been available in pharmacies since the 19th century, but recreational use of these preparations had not become common, largely because they tended to be unpredictable or extremely strong, and many of those who experimented with them found the experience to be a highly unpleasant and protracted one.[76] The capricious nature of the preparation led the authors of a 1913 article published in the *Journal of the American Pharmaceutical Association* to conclude, "...[N]o two persons can be expected to exhibit the same symptoms as a result of ingesting equal quantities of the same drug, and no person can be depended upon to react in exactly the same manner from the same drug on different occasions."[77]

In Mexico, recreational cannabis use had been on the rise for several decades among farm laborers who rolled the dried flower of the female cannabis plant into cigarettes.[78] They called this preparation of cannabis "marijuana," though the etymology of this word remains a mystery. Unlike oral administration, intoxication is felt almost immediately when cannabis is inhaled, thereby allowing users to better titrate their dosages and to avoid the unpleasant experience of taking far too much (see Chapter 7 [The Pharmacology of Cannabis]) for a more detailed analysis of routes of administration). The widespread availability of marijuana, rather than tinctures of cannabis or hashish, could be one possible reason why recreational cannabis became popular in Mexico during the 19th century, but not in the United States or Europe.

By 1900, cannabis use appears to have been fairly common among poor northern farmworkers, but the practice was frowned upon by the more urbane residents within the country's major cities. As they had no association with cannabis, their only knowledge of its effects came from the press, who printed stories claiming that it was causing crime, mayhem, and suicidal behavior. In 1898, a leading newspaper in Mexico City claimed that, "For years the press has described horrifying crimes, criminal eccentricities and suicides, which place before the court of public opinion individuals whose type oscillates between furious madmen and criminals worthy of being placed before the firing squad, and one after another case demonstrates that the murderer, the rapist, the insubordinate, the presumed suicide, and the scandalous acted under the influence of marijuana."[79]

The northern farmworkers who used cannabis had become increasingly disenfranchised as the owners of massive estates (*haciendas*) rapidly consolidated land and power during the reign of Porfirio Díaz (an era often known as the Porfiriato), which lasted from 1876 to 1911, and the effects were disastrous for small ranchers, farmers, and landowners. T.R. Fehrenbach, the author of *Fire & Blood*, one of the seminal works on Mexican history in the English language, notes that the era saw as many as one million families dispossessed of their land while the country experienced a concomitant surge in population, from 9 to 15 million. Many of these individuals could not be absorbed into the country's cities due to a lack of industrialization, which meant that millions of Mexicans had neither land nor job prospects in their homeland.[80] Facing limited opportunities, many Mexicans migrated to the United States in search of a better life and brought their culture and habits (including the use of marijuana) with them. Little was said of the habit during the 19th century or for much of the first decade of the 20th century.

This changed in the 1910s, largely because immigration to the United States accelerated due to the bloody Revolution, which lasted from ~1910 to 1920 and forced roughly 264 000 Mexicans, both rich and poor, to emigrate to Texas.[81] As more Mexicans fled the violence and poverty ravaging their homeland, racial tensions between rural whites in the Southwest United States and the new arrivals began to flare up. Many of the laborers from Mexico were willing to work for low wages, which threatened the job security of white farmhands and ranchers, and violence did erupt between the two groups. Authorities frequently blamed this violence on the use of cannabis among the Mexican immigrants, and its use soon became vilified in much the same way opium smoking among Chinese immigrants had been demonized in the 1880s.[82]

Reports oftentimes equated the effects and addictive qualities of cocaine or opiates with cannabis and echoed the reports from Mexico several decades beforehand, where it had been claimed that cannabis could cause insanity or violent behavior.[83] In some cases, it was said that those who smoked it developed a "lust for blood" or "superhuman strength," while in others it was said to be fatal.[84] According to a 1905 report from the *Los Angeles Times*, it was said that use led to sudden death because it caused the brains of those who smoked it to "dry up."[85] In 1927, the *New York Times* published a story about a mother and her four children who had accidentally eaten cannabis in Mexico, and that doctors believed that the children would die, while the mother would be left insane for the rest of her life.[86] Additionally, reports indicated that its use was spreading to children and causing juvenile delinquency.[87]

News stories like those noted above led to frenzied calls to ban what had been dubbed either "demon weed" or the more racist "loco weed."[83] By 1927, 17 states had passed legislation prohibiting cannabis, but each of these laws did include exceptions for its medicinal use.

Despite the tales of corrupted youth and the rush to pass laws banning nonmedicinal cannabis, at least one official report from the era suggested that cannabis was not as dangerous as many news reports had made it seem. In 1925, Colonel M. L. Walker, the governor of the American-held Panama Canal Zone, ordered an investigation into the safety of cannabis. The investigation studied the existing literature on cannabis—most notably the British report produced by the Indian Hemp Drugs Commission of 1894 discussed in Chapter 2 (The History of Cannabis)—and conducted experiments on 17 American servicemen who claimed to be acquainted with the effects of the drug. The Panama investigation found no medical evidence to support the claims that cannabis caused insanity, that moderate use led to dependency, or that it had "any appreciable deleterious effect on the individual using it."[88]

largely become an obsolete herb from an industrial standpoint and the public was terrified of the menace of marijuana, which, the press reported, was "...considered more dangerous than cocaine or opium."[101]

Though cannabis had been used medicinally throughout the United States with regularity, it was commonly referred to as either cannabis, hemp, Indian hemp, or *C. indica*. Consequently, many Americans thought that marijuana (or marihuana) was a new and foreign drug. They did not know that the dusty tinctures of *C. indica* that their parents and grandparents used to treat corns contained the same active psychotropic ingredient as found in the dreaded marijuana. The public would have likely been less credulous about the dangers of "killer weed" had the media referred to the drug by the name with which they were more familiar.

There were few voices of opposition when HR6385, which would later become known as the Marihuana Tax Act of 1937, was being considered by Congress, but the bill did receive some significant criticism, particularly from members of the medical community. Objectors were not opposed to regulation *per se*; rather, they felt as though the proposed amount to be taxed on the *legal* transfer of cannabis was exorbitant and the requisite record keeping to comply with the law would be far too cumbersome, especially considering the fact that the drug was both very rarely prescribed by physicians and, when used recreationally, almost entirely traded through illicit channels not subject to the proposed taxation. According to the law, various individuals who might work with cannabis (importers, manufacturers, producers, veterinarians, physicians, and so on) were to be charged a tax allowing them to do so. For medical professionals, this amounted to a registration fee of $1 per year (a real-dollar value in 2019 of ~$18), as well as a $1 per ounce tax on the transfer of cannabis from the medical professional to another person who had also paid a tax to allow them to possess or exchange cannabis. For those who had not registered and paid the above levy, the tax on the transfer of each ounce of cannabis was set at $100 (a real-dollar value in 2019 of ~$1800). Anyone who violated the law was to be fined not more than $2000 (a real-dollar value in 2019 of ~$36 000), imprisoned for up to 5 years, or both.[102]

The AMA Committee on Legislative Activities published a report in June of 1937, wherein they claimed, "There is positively no evidence to indicate the abuse of cannabis as a medicinal agent or to show that its medicinal use is leading to the development of cannabis addiction."[103] Rather presciently, they continued:

"Cannabis at the present time is slightly used for medicinal purposes, but it would seem worth while [*sic.*] to maintain its status as a medical agent for such purposes as it now has. There is a possibility that a restudy of the drug by modern means may show other advantages to be derived from its medicinal use."[103]

The previous month, an editorial against the act had appeared in the *Journal of the American Medical Association*. The writer argued that it would penalize the sick and injured, and that they would be forced to "contribute toward federal efforts to suppress a habit that has little or no relation to the use of cannabis for medicinal purposes and that is already within the jurisdiction of several states."[104] The author noted that the Harrison Act had not stemmed the illicit trade in opiates and cocaine, and that the Marihuana Tax Act would neither stop the smuggling of cannabis into the country nor stop its cultivation in the United States, as it "...grows wild in field and forest and along the highways in many places."[104]

Dr. William C. Woodward, the person tasked with speaking on behalf of the AMA before Congress, was the only witness to oppose the legislation before Congress.[105] He echoed the above points and openly derided many of Anslinger's claims for lacking scientific merit, but his words were largely ignored. The bill was passed and signed into law by President Roosevelt on August 2, 1937 and went into effect on October 1 of the same year.

The first person to be arrested under the new law was Samuel Caldwell, 58, who was caught selling cannabis to Moses Baca, 26, in Denver, Colorado, on October 8, 1937. Caldwell was fined $1000 (a real-dollar value in 2019 of ~$18 000) and sentenced to 4 years in Leavenworth—the same facility that, at the time, held George "Machine Gun Kelly" Barnes. Baca was also sent to Leavenworth, but only for 18 months.[106]

5.7 Regulations Until 1970

The Marihuana Tax Act effectively ended the licit cannabis trade in the United States. The vast majority of those who had participated in it, whether they were farmers, manufacturers, doctors, or veterinarians, did not want to run afoul of the new law and face the steep penalties. They reasoned that there was no point in risking major fines for possessing or transferring a drug that had ceased to be commonly prescribed by the time the law was passed. The relatively small hemp industry, which had been struggling for years, was hit particularly hard. Demand had already fallen dramatically because synthetic fibers had replaced the role of hemp, so relatively few farmers bothered growing it. Domestic production rebounded during World War II, as hemp was needed for naval purposes, but production quickly fell off after the wartime boom. By 1958, there was virtually no industrial hemp grown in the United States, and it would only see a resurgence in the 1990s when states began to take their own initiatives to explore reviving the industry.[107] These efforts were expanded by the federal 2014 farm bill.[107]

Medical research into cannabis, however, did continue to a limited extent, as the law did not forbid or make its study prohibitively expensive.[76] One of the most notable papers to take advantage of the lack of restrictions was a 1944 report commissioned by New York City Mayor Fiorello LaGuardia, *The Marihuana Problem in the City of New York*. The impetus for the study is clear in the introduction of the report, wherein Mayor LaGuardia expressed his skepticism in the panicky narrative that had been forged by individuals like Anslinger, largely because of his experience with cannabis in Panama. Recalling the 1925 report mentioned above, La Guardia wrote, "I was impressed at that time with the report of an Army Board of Inquiry which emphasized the relative harmlessness of the drug and the fact that it played a very little role, if any, in problems of delinquency and crime in the Canal Zone."[108] The LaGuardia report produced similar findings, concluding, among other things, that cannabis does not produce physical dependency in users; that the sale of cannabis was not under the control of one group; that cannabis use does not necessarily lead to cocaine or heroin use, crime, or juvenile delinquency; that cannabis smoking was not widespread among school children; and that, "The publicity concerning the catastrophic effects of marihuana smoking in New York City is unfounded."[109]

Besides infuriating many within the FBN, the report seems to have had little effect. Similarly, a 1949 study published by Davis and Ramsey on the antiepileptic qualities of THC among patients with severe symptomatic grand mal epilepsy also drew limited attention, despite concluding, "The cannabinols [*sic.*] herein reported deserve further trial in non-institutionalized epileptics."[110] There was little appetite for research into cannabis and very few studies would be conducted in the United States until the 1960s.

The Marihuana Tax Act may have severely disrupted the licit trade in cannabis, but it failed to curb the drug's illicit use. Perhaps more importantly, it turned those who smoked recreational cannabis into federal criminals and gave federal agents the authority to monitor and arrest those who did not comply with the law. One of the first group of individuals to feel the brunt of the FBN's new powers were jazz musicians, toward whom Anslinger had a well-documented personal enmity, as he believed they were partially responsible for the spread of recreational cannabis use.[111] Following the passage of the act, Anslinger began pursuing many of the genre's most prominent stars. Files were kept on jazz musicians who had reportedly smoked cannabis, such as Duke Ellington, Cab Calloway, Dizzy Gillespie, Jimmy Dorsey, Count Basie, and Thelonious Monk, and three of the biggest names in jazz were arrested for violating the Marihuana Tax Act: Louis Armstrong, Billie Holiday, and Gene Krupa.[112]

Despite numerous arrests, cannabis use continued to spread, and it had become a common fixture throughout the entire entertainment industry by the dawn of the 1950s. It would go on to become popular among the Beats, a group of writers who were the preeminent young literary voices during the era. Cannabis use is a regular feature in Jack Kerouac's 1957 *On the Road*, arguably the group's most famous novel. By the late 1950s, it was commonly used by intellectuals, pseudo-bohemians, and folk and rock musicians.[113] By the end of the 1960s, it would be ubiquitous among members of the Baby Boom generation, whether they were college students, activists, union workers, or soldiers who were introduced to the drug while stationed in Vietnam. A writer for *Life* magazine in 1967 described the use of cannabis as "the greatest mass flouting of the law since prohibition."[114]

The rapid proliferation of recreational cannabis occurred despite both the Marihuana Tax Act and two major evolutions in U.S. drug policy that occurred in the 1950s, one national and one international. Domestically, the United States began to take a more punitive approach to preventing drug use following the war, most notably by implementing mandatory minimum sentencing for drug users. The Boggs Act of 1951, later amended by the Narcotics Control Act of 1956, punished first-time cannabis possession with a mandatory minimum prison sentence of no <2 years; second-time possession with a minimum of 5 years in prison with no option for parole or probation; and third-time possession or second-offense sale in a sentence of 10-40 years without parole or probation.[114]

Internationally, greater efforts were made to crack down on the illegal drug trade. While the international community had been in favor of taking proactive steps to make it more difficult to import and export illegal drugs since at least the Shanghai International Opium Commission of 1909, the effort had typically focused on disrupting international trades in cocaine and opium—especially with the latter's regard to Asia—and several treaties had been signed to achieve this aim prior to World War II. Cannabis prohibition had never aroused the same level of urgency among many nations (with some exceptions), as it was not considered to be as significant a problem as opiate and cocaine abuse and addiction. By the early 1950s, the United States had emerged as the world's leading superpower, and their delegation was of the opinion that cannabis was a major problem that needed to be addressed. Largely at the behest of the delegation, the United Nations adopted strong language that described cannabis as having no medicinal use and recommended it be banned on an international level.[115] This position was given teeth on March 10, 1961, when the UN Single Convention on Narcotic Drugs was ratified, which consolidated several treaties prohibiting the overproduction of medicinal drugs (like opiates) and prohibiting the international trade in drugs or preparations of drugs deemed to have no medicinal value—that is, cannabis.[116] The treaty has been signed by the vast majority of UN members and remains in effect to this day, though it has been amended several times.

Anslinger, a major proponent of the international effort to combat the drug trade and the draconian sentencing, as well as an early adopter of the "gateway drug" theory, claimed that such policies were necessary to fight, among other things, organized crime and communism.[117] He also claimed that they would slash drug abuse in the United States by 60%.[117]

They did neither; they merely put more people in prison. Between 1958 and 1967, the number of individuals arrested for cannabis at the state and local level exploded from 3287 to 54 468.[117] The number of cannabis smokers, meanwhile, was estimated to be upward of 12 million by 1969.[118]

As cannabis became more prevalent and more people were incarcerated for mere possession, public opinion began to favor a less severe antidrug strategy, even if there continued to be a steady drumbeat for a war on drug abuse. Cannabis had ceased to be a drug only used by people in marginal communities and had come to the proverbial Main Streets of America. Consequently, many became wary of imposing such harsh penalties on individuals who smoked cannabis, as they had become the sons and daughters of middle- and upper-class America. A federal narcotics official described the situation succinctly: "The middle class [*sic.*] parent is waking up to the law. 'For God's sake', he says, 'throw the book at the trafficker, but don't lock up my kid'."[118]

Some policymakers began to adopt this position, as well. In 1969, Dr. Stanley F. Yolles, Director of the National Institute of Mental Health from 1964 to 1970, told a Senate subcommittee investigating juvenile delinquency that such severe penalties could ruin the life of first offenders.[119] He added, "I am convinced that the social and psychological damage caused by incarceration is in many cases far greater to the individual and to society than was the offense itself."[119] The chief health official for the Nixon administration, Dr. Roger O. Egeberg, claimed that the cannabis laws "[we]re completely out of proportion" to the drug's potency.[120]

After almost 20 years of strict antidrug policies in the United States, many states began to reverse course. By 1972, 42 states and the District of Columbia had changed their laws so that cannabis possession offenses were recognized as misdemeanors instead of felonies.[121] This by no means meant that there was popular support for legalization or that the majority of the country thought that drugs like cannabis were relatively harmless. The policies of Richard Nixon following his election in 1968 would prove this to be the case.

5.8 The Controlled Substances Act of 1970

In his first year in office, President Nixon began to create a plan that was described as a "war on drug abuse."[122] Nixon had campaigned on the notion that rampant drug use was contributing to larger cultural problems and crime, and that it had to be addressed on many fronts. While Nixon may be remembered for being a hardliner when it came to drugs, his focus extended well beyond the purview of law enforcement. His administration authorized the federal government to increase the funding for prevention research, education, training, rehabilitation, and treatment from $59 million for the fiscal year of 1970 to $462 million for the fiscal year of 1974.[123] He was the only president to dedicate more funding to preventing and treating substance abuse than on law enforcement.[124]

This is not to say that the administration was entirely earnest in its discussion of drug policies or that it deviated from previous attempts to adopt drug policies that would adversely impact specific communities. As a top Nixon aide, John Ehrlichman would later tell journalist Dan Baum in a 1994 interview: "The Nixon campaign in 1968, and the Nixon White House after that, had two enemies: the antiwar left and black people. You understand what I'm saying. We knew we couldn't make it illegal to be either against the war or black, but by getting the public to associate the hippies with marijuana and the blacks with heroin, and then criminalizing both heavily, we could disrupt those communities. We could arrest their leaders, raid their homes, break up their meetings, and vilify them night after night on the evening news. Did we know we were lying about the drugs? Of course we did."[125]

Additionally, the Nixon administration recognized that federal drug laws needed to be rewritten, in part because a Supreme Court case involving Timothy Leary, who is best known for his pioneering work with psychedelics like LSD, had ruled that some aspects of the federal laws regarding cannabis importation were unconstitutional and, consequently, unenforceable.[126] The resultant legislation was the CSA of 1970, which superseded both the Harrison Act and the Marihuana Tax Act.

The CSA created the drug scheduling system that continues to be in operation to this day and classified cannabis as being a Schedule I drug, which is defined as being a substance both with a high potential for abuse and "no currently accepted medical use in treatment in the United States."[127] It also kept minimum sentencing requirements (though the parameters were less severe than the ones in the Narcotics Control Act) and required "all persons involved in the manufacture, distribution, and dispensing of scheduled drugs to obtain a registration from the State."[128] The CSA continues to dictate federal drug policy to this day and treated all cannabis and cannabinoids, including CBD, the same until the Farm Bill of 2018 made the distinction between hemp and marijuana (see Chapter 1 [Cannabis: An Introduction]).

The CSA has made research into Schedule I drugs like cannabis extremely difficult. Even today, only one institution based at the University of Mississippi is legally allowed to grow cannabis for research purposes, and scientists are only allowed access to cannabis from this farm after obtaining approval from the DEA, the FDA, and a Public Health Service panel. Additionally, the National Institute on Drug Abuse must support the study.[129] Such encumbrances have either denied or discouraged researchers from studying cannabis in a clinical setting. Additionally, it has led to the circular logic that continues to disrupt any rational debate on the subject of cannabis' therapeutic potential. Because cannabis is a Schedule I substance, it is believed to have "no currently accepted medical use in treatment in the United States," but it only has "no currently accepted medical use in treatment in the United States" because so few clinical trials involving cannabis have been undertaken.

As very few formal studies on cannabis have been conducted, it owes its resurgence as a therapeutic agent largely to the spread of anecdotal evidence from a host of patients, including those who suffer from glaucoma, wasting diseases, and various conditions that cause neuropathic pain. Chemotherapy patients have been particularly vocal about cannabis' ability to combat nausea and to improve appetite. Word began to spread throughout the 1970s, and the groundwork for the contemporary medicinal cannabis movement began to grow. By 1982, 31 states and the District of Columbia had passed legislation that established medicinal cannabis programs in some capacity, but they ran into significant federal roadblocks and eventually expired or were repealed by the mid-1980s.[130]

There were individual patients directly addressing the federal government's policy on medical cannabis, as well, and perhaps the most notable figure to arise from the earliest stages of the movement was Robert Randall, a glaucoma patient who discovered that cannabis reduced intraocular pressure and helped with his condition in the early 1970s. After being arrested for possession of cannabis in 1975, he petitioned the government for access to cannabis grown at the aforementioned facility in Mississippi via the FDA Compassionate Investigative New Drug (IND) program. Randall eventually won his case and began receiving cannabis through this program. Others applied for the same treatment throughout the 1970s and 1980s, especially as the number of AIDS patients grew and word spread that cannabis could be used to counteract the intense nausea that is a symptom of the disease. Dronabinol, a synthetic form of THC that was released under the trade name Marinol in 1985, was meant to provide similar antiemetic effects, but many patients have said they prefer cannabis.[131]

The number of patients applying for cannabis through the Compassionate IND program continued to grow throughout the 1980s and into the 1990s. However, drug policy in the United States had become far more severe, particularly after President Ronald Reagan began his war on drugs and President George H. Bush continued it into the 1990s. Mandatory sentencing returned, police forces were increasingly militarized, and children were told to "Just say no" (for a detailed account of the effects of this drastic change in drug policy, see Michelle Alexander's *The New Jim Crow*).

Because all illegal drugs were considered unequivocally bad, the federal government did not want to look hypocritical by prescribing cannabis to patients. Consequently, the Compassionate IND program was shuttered by the Department of Health and Human Services in 1992, though existing patients were allowed to continue with the program.[132] Patients were given the option of legally treating their condition with Marinol or illegally treating their condition with cannabis. Many chose the latter and were jailed. Those who facilitated their treatment often faced a similar punishment.

5.9 The Floodgates Open

In 1991, voters in San Francisco, then a major epicenter for the AIDS epidemic, approved a local ballot initiative to name cannabis as an approved medicine for the treatment of conditions such as AIDS, glaucoma, MS, and chronic pain. The city council passed a resolution in 1992 that did not decriminalize cannabis by any means, but it placed the arresting of patients using cannabis for medicinal reasons at the lowest level of priorities for law enforcement.[133]

Four years later, California would be the first to pass a statewide initiative (Proposition 215) legalizing medical cannabis and allowing doctors to "recommend" (not prescribe) cannabis to patients.[134] Similar legislation would pass in Alaska, Washington, and Oregon 2 years later. As of this writing, 33 states and the District of Columbia have medicinal cannabis programs (see Fig. 5.3). For up-to-date information about a specific state, please see our book's Web site: cannabistextbook.com.

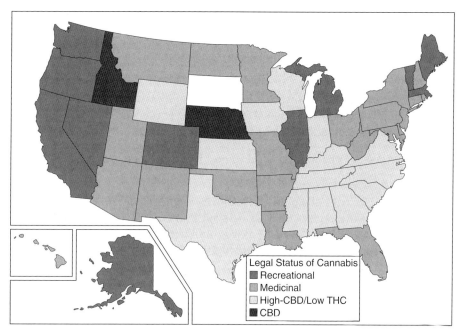

Figure 5.3 Cannabis regulations as of January 1, 2020.

In 2012, Colorado and Washington became the first states to legalize recreational cannabis. Eleven states and the District of Columbia (see Table 5.1) have passed laws legalizing the recreational use of cannabis that has been legally defined as marijuana, which the Farm Bill of 2018 defines as, "...any part of that plant, including the seeds thereof and all derivatives, extracts, cannabinoids, isomers, acids, salts, and salts of isomers, whether growing or not, with delta-9 tetrahydrocannabinol concentration" above 0.3% on a dry weight basis.[135] For up-to-date information about a specific state, please see our book's Web site: cannabistextbook.com.

To state that the floodgates have opened and that a sea change has occurred in what seems like the blink of an eye is to state the obvious. Americans have become far more accepting of cannabis, particularly as a therapeutic agent. A March 2019 poll conducted by Quinnipiac found that 93% of Americans support legalizing medical cannabis, with only 5% opposing.[136] The same poll found that support for legalizing recreational cannabis stands at 60%, while a similar poll conducted in 2006 found that 60% opposed it.[137]

This has led to a lot of confusion. The federal government has resisted calls to either *reschedule* or *deschedule* cannabis.

TABLE 5.1 State and Territory Medicinal Cannabis Timeline

1996	California passes Proposition 215, becoming the first state to legalize medical cannabis.
1996	Arizona passes Proposition 200 to legalize medicinal cannabis, but it is later overturned. Another ballot measure in 2010 allowed for medicinal cannabis to be legalized.
1998	Alaska, Oregon, and Washington legalize medical cannabis through ballot measure.
1998	The District of Columbia legalizes medical cannabis through ballot measure. Congress delayed implementation indefinitely. In 2010, the City Council passed a bill legalizing medical cannabis. Implementation of this bill was not delayed by Congress and went into effect on January 1, 2011.
1998	Nevada voters approved an initiative to amend the constitution and legalize medical cannabis. The state constitution required a second vote 2 years later, in 2000, which also passed.
1999	Maine legalizes medical cannabis through ballot measure.
2000	Hawaii legalizes medical cannabis through state legislature.
2000	Colorado legalizes medical cannabis through ballot measure.
2004	Montana legalizes medical cannabis through ballot measure.
2004	Vermont legalizes medical cannabis through state legislature.
2006	Rhode Island legalizes medical cannabis through state legislature.
2007	New Mexico legalizes medical cannabis through state legislature.
2008	Michigan legalizes medical cannabis through ballot measure.
2010	The District of Columbia legalizes medical cannabis through city council.
2010	New Jersey legalizes medical cannabis through state legislature.
2011	Delaware legalizes medical cannabis through state legislature.
2012	Connecticut legalizes medical cannabis through state legislature.
2012	Massachusetts legalizes medical cannabis through ballot measure.

TABLE 5.1 Continued

2013	New Hampshire and Illinois legalize medical cannabis through their state legislatures.
2014	Alabama, Florida, Iowa, Kentucky, Mississippi, Missouri, North Carolina, South Carolina, Tennessee, and Wisconsin pass laws allowing the use of low-THC, high-CBD oils for certain medical conditions.
2014	Guam legalizes medical cannabis through ballot measure.
2014	Maryland, Minnesota, and New York legalize medical cannabis through their state legislatures.
2014	Utah passes a law allowing the use of low-THC, high-CBD oils for certain medical conditions. They are the first state to do so.
2015	Louisiana legalizes medical cannabis through state legislature.
2015	Georgia, Oklahoma, Texas, Virginia, and Wyoming pass laws allowing the use of low-THC, high-CBD oils for certain medical conditions.
2015	Puerto Rico legalizes medical cannabis by executive order.
2016	Arkansas, Florida, and North Dakota legalize medical cannabis through ballot measures.
2016	Pennsylvania and Ohio legalize medical cannabis through their state legislatures.
2017	West Virginia legalizes medical cannabis through state legislature.
2017	Indiana passes a law allowing the use of low-THC, high-CBD oils for certain medical conditions.
2018	Indiana and Kansas legalize CBD through state legislature.
2018	Missouri, Oklahoma, and Utah legalize medical cannabis through ballot measure.
2019	Kansas passes a law allowing the use of low-THC, high-CBD oils for certain medical conditions.
2019	The U.S. Virgin Islands legalize medical cannabis through act of legislatures.

(Rescheduling cannabis would mean removing it from Schedule I status and categorizing it as either a Schedule II, Schedule III, or Schedule IV substance. Descheduling cannabis would remove it from the CSA altogether and would align more with the concept of legalization and likely result in it being treated in a fashion akin to alcohol or tobacco.) Consequently, each state that has legalized recreational cannabis has had to independently create a legal framework to facilitate the cultivation and sale of cannabis within their jurisdiction, even if federal agents can still treat cannabis as an illegal drug no matter if an individual found to be in possession of cannabis obtained it through licit channels created and sanctioned by a state. To clarify their position, the Justice Department issued what is now known as the Cole Memo in 2013, which stated, in part, that "marijuana remains an illegal drug under the CSA and that federal prosecutors will continue to aggressively enforce this statute."[138] The memo also implied federal agents would be less likely to enforce the CSA in states where regulatory systems are aligned with the priorities of the Justice Department, and that such priorities include prohibiting the use of cannabis by minors and preventing revenues from cannabis sales from going to criminal enterprises.[138] In 2014, the Justice Department issued another memo indicating that the same logic would be applicable to tribal lands and reservations across the United States.[139] The Cole Memo was rescinded by former Attorney General Jeff Sessions in 2018, but no discernible change in policy has occurred.[140]

The 2018 Farm Bill, which notably made the distinction between hemp and marijuana, allows the transfer of hemp products, but not marijuana, across state lines, and eliminates the federal prohibition of hemp and hemp-derived products, including those that contain hemp-derived CBD. Regulating hemp and hemp-derived products are now a matter to be addressed by each state individually. According to John Hudak of the Brookings Institution, the bill stipulates that "state departments of agriculture must consult with the state's governor and chief law enforcement officer to devise a plan that must be submitted to the Secretary of USDA (The United States Department of Agriculture). A state's plan to license and regulate hemp can only commence once the Secretary of USDA approves that state's plan."[141] For states that do not create a plan of their own, "the USDA will construct a regulatory program under which hemp cultivators in those states must apply for licenses and comply with a federally-run program."[141]

5.10 The Present

Since 1996, more than 33 states and the District of Columbia have created medical cannabis programs, legalized the recreational use of cannabis, or both. There are 11 states, plus the District of Columbia, where both medical and recreational cannabis is legal (see Table 5.2). There are 22 states that have legalized medical cannabis (see Table 5.1). In 14 states, medical cannabis is legal, but only for a small number of patients and in formulations that contain high levels of CBD and low levels of THC (see Table 5.1). Restrictions in these states vary significantly, both with regard to who is allowed

TABLE 5.2 State and Territory Recreational Cannabis Timeline

2012	Colorado and Washington become the first states to legalize recreational cannabis through ballot measures.
2014	Alaska, the District of Columbia, and Oregon legalize recreational cannabis through ballot measures.
2015	Tribal authorities of the Flandreau Santee Sioux tribe in South Dakota legalize recreational cannabis.
2015	The Suquamish and Squaxin Island tribes sign a tribe-state pact with Washington that allows the operation of cannabis stores on tribal land in compliance with Washington law.
2016	California, Maine, Massachusetts, and Nevada legalize recreational cannabis through ballot measures.
2016	The Puyallup Tribe signs a tribe-state pact with Washington that allows the operation of cannabis stores on tribal land in compliance with Washington law.
2018	Michigan legalizes recreational cannabis through ballot measure.
2018	Vermont becomes the first state to legalize recreational cannabis through state legislature. No provision is made to allow for legal commercial sales.
2018	The Northern Mariana Islands legalize cannabis through state legislature.
2019	Guam and Illinois legalize recreational cannabis through their state legislatures.

access to these formulations and what levels of THC are lawful. In Kansas, for example, Claire and Lola's Law went into effect on July 1, 2019 and allows patients to obtain, possess, and administer formulations that contain up to 5% THC for certain debilitating medical conditions, but it does not explicitly state that formulations containing more than 0.3% THC can be purchased legally in the state.[142] In Alabama, Leni's Law allows patients to obtain, possess, and administer formulations that contain up to 3% THC for certain debilitating medical conditions.[143] Patients must travel outside of the state to purchase these formulations. Three states, Idaho, Nebraska, and South Dakota, and one territory, American Samoa, do not explicitly allow the medicinal use of cannabis except for preparations that have been approved by the FDA.

At this time, Epidiolex is the only preparation of CBD that has been approved by the FDA, but CBD is legal in states where recreational cannabis has been legalized. In states where recreational cannabis has not been legalized, federal law applies. Federal law states that CBD is legal so long as it is hemp derived, contains <0.3% THC, and complies with state regulations. Some states have additional restrictions. Only CBD oil that contains zero THC is legal in Idaho.[144] In Iowa, CBD is only legal for individuals with state-issued registration cards until the United States Department of Agriculture (USDA) approves the plan the state submitted to comply with the 2018 Farm Bill.[145] At this time, CBD in all forms except for Epidiolex appears to be illegal in South Dakota.[146] CBD oil, which often contains trace amounts of THC, is also still considered illegal in American Samoa.[147]

As this continues to be a rapidly changing regulatory environment, it is recommended that one consult the Web site of the book cannabistextbook.com. for more up-to-date information.

REFERENCES

[1] Brownstein MJ. A brief history of opiates, opioid peptides, and opioid receptors. *Proc Natl Acad Sci U S A*. 1993;90(12):5391-5393. doi: 10.1073/pnas.90.12.5391.

[2] Agnew J. *Alcohol and Opium in the Old West*. Jefferson, NC: McFarland & Company, Inc., Publishers; 2014:35.

[3] Booth M. *Opium: A History*. New York, NY: St. Martin's Press; 1996:104.

[4] Booth M. *Opium: A History*. New York, NY: St. Martin's Press; 1996:19.

[5] Choffnes D. *Nature's Pharmacopeia: A World of Medicinal Plants*. New York, NY: Columbia University Press; 2016:84.

[6] Fay PW. *The Opium War, 1840-1842: Barbarians in the Celestial Empire in the Early Part of the Nineteenth Century and the War by Which They Forced her Gates Ajar*. Chapel Hill, NC: The University of North Carolina Press; 1997:7-8.

[7]Agnew J. *Alcohol and Opium in the Old West*. Jefferson, NC: McFarland & Company, Inc., Publishers; 2014:40.

[8]Fay PW. *The Opium War, 1840-1842: Barbarians in the Celestial Empire in the Early Part of the Nineteenth Century and the War by Which They Forced her Gates Ajar*. Chapel Hill, NC: The University of North Carolina Press; 1997:41-64.

[9]Booth M. *Opium: A History*. New York, NY: St. Martin's Press; 1996:128.

[10]Booth M. *Opium: A History*. New York, NY: St. Martin's Press; 1996:175-177.

[11]Morgan HW. *Drugs in America: A Social History, 1800-1980*. Syracuse, NY: Syracuse University Press; 1981:3.

[12]Raver A. Sowing the seeds of a felonious life. New York Times [Internet]. 1992 Mar 5:Sect. C:3(col. 1). https://timesmachine.nytimes.com/timesmachine/1992/03/05/issue.html. Accessed September 6, 2019.

[13]Morgan HW. *Drugs in America: A Social History, 1800-1980*. Syracuse, NY: Syracuse University Press; 1981:6.

[14]Booth M. *Opium: A History*. New York, NY: St. Martin's Press; 1996:69.

[15]Morgan HW. *Drugs in America: A Social History, 1800-1980*. Syracuse, NY: Syracuse University Press; 1981:7.

[16]Mikuriya TH. *Cannabis: Collected Medical Papers Volume I: Marijuana: Medical Papers 1839-1972*. Nevada City, CA: Symposium Publishing; 2007:xix.

[17]Agnew J. *Alcohol and Opium in the Old West*. Jefferson, NC: McFarland & Company, Inc., Publishers; 2014:111-112.

[18]Morgan HW. *Drugs in America: A Social History, 1800-1980*. Syracuse, NY: Syracuse University Press; 1981:27.

[19]Morgan HW. *Drugs in America: A social history, 1800-1980*. Syracuse, NY: Syracuse University Press; 1981:38-41.

[20]Golding AMB. Two hundred years of drug abuse. *J R Soc Med*. 1993;86(5):282-286.

[21]Morgan HW. *Drugs in America: A Social History, 1800-1980*. Syracuse, NY: Syracuse University Press; 1981:29.

[22]Agnew J. *Alcohol and Opium in the Old West*. Jefferson, NC: McFarland & Company, Inc., Publishers; 2014:111.

[23]Brecher EM, et al. Licit and illicit drugs. In: Belenko SR, ed. *Drugs and Drug Policy in America: A Documentary History*. Westport, CT: Greenwood Press; 2000:1.

[24]Morgan HW. *Drugs in America: A Social History, 1800-1980*. Syracuse, NY: Syracuse University Press; 1981:40.

[25]Agnew J. *Alcohol and Opium in the Old West*. Jefferson, NC: McFarland & Company, Inc., Publishers; 2014:223.

[26]Booth M. *Opium: A History*. New York, NY: St. Martin's Press; 1996:150-156.

[27]The opium habit's power. New York Times [Internet]. 1878 Jan 6:Page 5(col. 1). https://timesmachine.nytimes.com/timesmachine/1878/01/06/issue.html. Accessed September 9, 2019.

[28]Morgan HW. *Drugs in America: A Social History, 1800-1980*. Syracuse, NY: Syracuse University Press; 1981:90.

[29]Agnew J. *Alcohol and Opium in the Old West*. Jefferson, NC: McFarland & Company, Inc., Publishers; 2014:112.

[30]Courtwright DT. Dark paradise: opiate addiction in American before 1940. In: Belenko SR, ed. *Drugs and Drug Policy in America: A Documentary History*. Westport, CT: Greenwood Press; 2000:6.

[31]Brecher EM, et al. Licit and illicit drugs. In: Belenko SR, ed. *Drugs and Drug Policy in America: A Documentary History*. Westport, CT: Greenwood Press; 2000:6-7.

[32]Booth M. *Opium: A History*. New York, NY: St. Martin's Press; 1996:194-195.

[33]Agnew J. *Alcohol and Opium in the Old West*. Jefferson, NC: McFarland & Company, Inc., Publishers; 2014:92-97.

[34]Booth M. *Opium: A History*. New York, NY: St. Martin's Press; 1996:196.

[35]Morgan HW. *Drugs in America: A Social History, 1800-1980*. Syracuse, NY: Syracuse University Press; 1981:88-117.

[36]Morgan HW. *Drugs in America: A Social History, 1800-1980*. Syracuse, NY: Syracuse University Press; 1981:64-67.

[37]Agnew J. *Alcohol and Opium in the Old West*. Jefferson, NC: McFarland & Company, Inc., Publishers; 2014:176-178.

[38]Morgan HW. *Drugs in America: A Social History, 1800-1980*. Syracuse, NY: Syracuse University Press; 1981:94.

[39]Terry CE, Pellens M. The opium problem. In: Belenko SR, ed. *Drugs and Drug Policy in America: A Documentary History*. Westport, CT: Greenwood Press; 2000:6.

[40]Morgan HW. *Drugs in America: A Social History, 1800-1980*. Syracuse, NY: Syracuse University Press; 1981:95.

[41]Morgan HW. *Drugs in America: A Social History, 1800-1980*. Syracuse, NY: Syracuse University Press; 1981:62.

[42]Morgan HW. *Drugs in America: A Social History, 1800-1980*. Syracuse, NY: Syracuse University Press; 1981:43.

[43]Taylor A. American diplomacy and the narcotics traffic, 1900-1939. In: Belenko SR, ed. *Drugs and Drug Policy in America: A Documentary History*. Westport, CT: Greenwood Press; 2000:32-33.

[44]Booth M. *Opium: A History*. New York, NY: St. Martin's Press; 1996:121.

[45]Morgan HW. *Drugs in America: A Social History, 1800-1980*. Syracuse, NY: Syracuse University Press; 1981:97-98.

[46]Booth M. *Opium: A History*. New York, NY: St. Martin's Press; 1996:180.

[47]Anslinger HJ, Tompkins WF. *The Traffic in Narcotics*. New York, NY: Funk & Wagnalls Company, Inc; 1953:29.

[48]Cronon W. *Nature's Metropolis: Chicago and the Great West*. New York, NY: W. W. Norton & Company, Inc; 1991:206-259.

[49]Kantor AF. Upton Sinclair and the Pure Food and Drugs Act of 1906. "I aimed at the public's heart and by accident I hit it in the stomach". *Am J Public Health*. 1976;66(12):1202-1205. doi: 10.2105/ajph.66.12.1202.

[50]Fee E. Samuel Hopkins Adams (1871-1958): journalist and muckraker. *Am J Public Health*. 2010;100(8):1390-1391. doi: 10.2105/AJPH.2009.186452.

[51]The layman and the great American fraud. *JAMA*. 1908;L(15):1196. doi: 10.1001/jama.1908.02530410036007.

[52]Pure Food and Drug Act of 1906, Public Law 59-384, 59th Congress, Session I, June 30, 1906. In: Belenko SR, ed. *Drugs and Drug Policy in America: A Documentary History*. Westport, CT: Greenwood Press; 2000:30-31.

[53]Taylor A. American diplomacy and the narcotics traffic, 1900-1939. In: Belenko SR, ed. *Drugs and Drug Policy in America: A Documentary History*. Westport, CT: Greenwood Press; 2000:41.

[54]Morgan HW. *Drugs in America: A Social History, 1800-1980*. Syracuse, NY: Syracuse University Press; 1981:90-93.

[55]Musto DF. The American disease: origins in narcotic control. In: Belenko SR, ed. *Drugs and Drug Policy in America: A Documentary History*. Westport, CT: Greenwood Press; 2000:47-48.

[56]Musto DF. The 1937 Marijuana Tax Act. In: Mikuriya TH, ed. *Cannabis: Collected Clinical Papers Volume 1: Marijuana: Medical Papers 1839-1972*. Nevada City, CA: Symposium Publishing; 2007:419.

[57]Booth M. *Cannabis: A History*. New York, NY: Picador; 2003:162.

[58]Morgan HW. *Drugs in America: A Social History, 1800-1980*. Syracuse, NY: Syracuse University Press; 1981:110-111.

[59]Taylor A. American diplomacy and the narcotics traffic, 1900-1939. In: Belenko SR, ed. *Drugs and Drug Policy in America: A Documentary History*. Westport, CT: Greenwood Press; 2000:58-59.

[60]Kolb L, Du Mez AG. The prevalence and trend of drug addiction in the United States and factors influencing it. In: Belenko SR, ed. *Drugs and Drug Policy in America: A Documentary History*. Westport, CT: Greenwood Press; 2000:60.

[61]Morgan HW. *Drugs in America: A Social History, 1800-1980*. Syracuse, NY: Syracuse University Press; 1981:116.

[62]Poorer Drug Users in Pitiful Plight. New York Times [Internet]. 1915 April 15:Page 7(col. 2). https://timesmachine.nytimes.com/timesmachine/1915/04/15/104645259. html?pageNumber=7. Accessed September 16, 2019.

[63]Booth M. *Opium: A History*. New York, NY: St. Martin's Press; 1996:181.

[64]Anslinger HJ, Tompkins WF. *The Traffic in Narcotics*. New York, NY: Funk & Wagnalls Company, Inc; 1953:53.

[65]Anslinger HJ, Tompkins WF. *The Traffic in Narcotics*. New York, NY: Funk & Wagnalls Company, Inc; 1953:31.

[66]Musto DF. The 1937 Marijuana Tax Act. In: Mikuriya TH, ed. *Cannabis: Collected Clinical Papers Volume 1: Marijuana: Medical Papers 1839-1972*. Nevada City, CA: Symposium Publishing; 2007:422.

[67]Booth M. *Cannabis: A History*. New York, NY: Picador; 2003:143.

[68]Ludlow FH. *The Hasheesh Eater: Being Passages from the Life of a Pythagorean*. Los Angeles, CA: Enhanced Media; 2015:12.

[69]Ludlow FH. *The Hasheesh Eater: Being Passages from the Life of a Pythagorean*. Los Angeles, CA: Enhanced Media; 2015:23.

[70]Mikuriya TH. *Cannabis: Collected Medical Papers Volume I: Marijuana: Medical Papers 1839-1972*. Nevada City, CA: Symposium Publishing; 2007:31-114.

[71]McMeens RR. Report of the Ohio State Medical Committee on *Cannabis indica*. In: Mikuriya TH, ed. *Cannabis: Collected Medical Papers Volume I: Marijuana: Medical Papers 1839-1972*. Nevada City, CA: Symposium Publishing; 2007:134.

[72]Remington JP, Wood HC. The dispensatory of the United States of America. In: Mikuriya TH, ed. *Cannabis: Collected Medical Papers Volume I: Marijuana: Medical Papers 1839-1972*. Nevada City, CA: Symposium Publishing; 2007:343.

[73]Aldrich M. The history of therapeutic cannabis. In: Mathre ML, ed. *Cannabis in Medical Practice: A Legal, Historical and Pharmacological Overview of the Therapeutic Use of Marijuana*. Jefferson, NC: McFarland & Company, Inc., Publishers; 1997:35-55.

[74]Topics of the Times. New York Times [Internet]. 1914 July 30:Page 8(col. 4). https://timesmachine.nytimes.com/timesmachine/1914/07/30/119124627.html?pageNumber=8. Accessed September 18, 2019.

[75]Muzzles the Dogs All the Year Round. New York Times [Internet]. 1914 July 29: Page 6(col. 2). https://timesmachine.nytimes.com/timesmachine/1914/07/29/100099907. html?pageNumber=6. Accessed September 18, 2019.

[76]Walton RR. Marijuana: therapeutic applications. In: Mikuriya TH, ed. *Cannabis: Collected Medical Papers Volume I: Marijuana: Medical Papers 1839-1972*. Nevada City, CA: Symposium Publishing; 2007:159.

[77]Hamilton HC, Lescohier AW, Perkins RA. The physiological activity of *Cannabis sativa*. In: Mikuriya TH, ed. *Cannabis: Collected Medical Papers Volume I: Marijuana: Medical Papers 1839-1972*. Nevada City, CA: Symposium Publishing; 2007:80.

[78]Booth M. *Cannabis: A History*. New York, NY: Picador; 2003:157-158.

[79]Campos I. 'Reefer Madness' in Mexico preceded U.S. prohibition. *O'Shaughnessy's*. Winter/Spring 2013. https://www.beyondthc.com/wp-content/uploads/2013/11/CamposPaternoism.pdf. Accessed on September 18, 2019.

[80]Fehrenbach TR. *Fire & Blood: A History of Mexico*. Boston, MA: De Capo Press; 1995: 440-481.

[81]Fehrenbach TR. *Fire & Blood: A History of Mexico*. Boston, MA: De Capo Press; 1995: 521-524.

[82]Booth M. *Cannabis: A History*. New York, NY: Picador; 2003:160-161.

[83]Booth M. *Cannabis: A History*. New York, NY: Picador; 2003:161-167.

[84]Bonnie RJ, Whitebread CH. The marijuana conviction: a history of marijuana prohibition in the United States. In: Belenko SR, ed. *Drugs and Drug Policy in America: A Documentary History*. Westport, CT: Greenwood Press; 2000:138.

[85]Martin A, Rashidian N. *A New Leaf: The End of Cannabis Prohibition*. New York, NY: The New Press; 2014:40.

[86]Mexican Family Go Insane. New York Times [Internet]. 1927 July 6:Page 10(col. 6). https://timesmachine.nytimes.com/timesmachine/1927/07/06/97234614.html?pageNumber=10. Accessed September 18, 2019.

[87]Morgan HW. *Drugs in America: A Social History, 1800-1980*. Syracuse, NY: Syracuse University Press; 1981:138-140.

[88]Marijuana Smoking is Reported Safe. New York Times [Internet]. 1925 Nov 21:Sect. E:6(col. 1). https://timesmachine.nytimes.com/timesmachine/1926/11/21/issue.html. Accessed September 27, 2019.

[89]U.S. Treasury Department. Traffic in opium and other dangerous drugs for the year ended December 31, 1931. In: Belenko SR, ed. *Drugs and Drug Policy in America: A Documentary History*. Westport, CT: Greenwood Press; 2000:144.

[90]Booth M. *Cannabis: A History*. New York, NY: Picador; 2003:168.

[91]Booth M. *Cannabis: A History*. New York, NY: Picador; 2003:167-168.

[92]Mayor LaGuardia's Committee on Marihuana. *The Marihuana Problem in the City of New York*. Metuchen, NJ: Scarecrow Reprint Corporation;1973:5. https://archive.org/details/TheMarihuanaProblemInTheCityOfNewYork-19441973Edition/page/n31. Accessed on October 3, 2019.

[93]Booth M. *Cannabis: A History*. New York, NY: Picador; 2003:174-184.

[94]Martin A, Rashidian N. *A New Leaf: The End of Cannabis Prohibition*. New York, NY: The New Press; 2014:40-42.

[95]Anslinger HJ, Tompkins WF. *The Traffic in Narcotics*. New York, NY: Funk & Wagnalls Company, Inc; 1953:19.

[96]Musto DF. The 1937 Marijuana Tax Act. In: Mikuriya TH, ed. *Cannabis: Collected Clinical Papers Volume 1: Marijuana: Medical Papers 1839-1972*. Nevada City, CA: Symposium Publishing; 2007:425.

[97]Brown B. *Cannabis: The Illegalization of Weed in America*. New York, NY: First Second; 2019:107-129

[98]Booth M. *Cannabis: A History*. New York, NY: Picador; 2003:181.

[99]Booth M. *Cannabis: A History*. New York, NY: Picador; 2003:179.

[100]Booth M. *Cannabis: A History*. New York, NY: Picador; 2003:180-181.

[101]Marijuana Menace. In: Belenko SR, ed. *Drugs and Drug Policy in America: A Documentary History*. Westport, CT: Greenwood Press; 2000:156.

[102]Public Law No. 75-238 (Marihuana Tax Act). In: Belenko SR, ed. *Drugs and Drug Policy in America: A Documentary History*. Westport, CT: Greenwood Press; 2000:154.

[103]Report of the AMAM Committee on legislative activities. In: Belenko SR, ed. *Drugs and Drug Policy in America: A Documentary History*. Westport, CT: Greenwood Press; 2000:151.

[104]Federal regulation of the medicinal use of cannabis. In: Belenko SR, ed. *Drugs and Drug Policy in America: A Documentary History*. Westport, CT: Greenwood Press; 2000:150.

[105]Musto DF. The 1937 Marijuana Tax Act. In: Mikuriya TH, ed. *Cannabis: Collected Clinical Papers Volume 1: Marijuana: Medical Papers 1839-1972*. Nevada City, CA: Symposium Publishing; 2007:432.

[106]Booth M. *Cannabis: A History*. New York, NY: Picador; 2003:190-191.

[107]Johnson R. *Hemp as an Agricultural Commodity* (CRS Report No. RL32725). Congressional Research Service website. https://fas.org/sgp/crs/misc/RL32725.pdf. Accessed October 3, 2019.

[108]Mayor LaGuardia's Committee on Marihuana. *The Marihuana Problem in the City of New York*. Metuchen, NJ: Scarecrow Reprint Corporation; 1973:v. https://archive.org/details/The-MarihuanaProblemInTheCityOfNewYork-19441973Edition/page/n19. Accessed October 3, 2019.

[109]The marihuana problem in the city of New York. In: Belenko SR, ed. *Drugs and Drug Policy in America: A Documentary History*. Westport, CT: Greenwood Press; 2000: 157-158.

[110]Davis JP, Ramsey HH. Anti-epileptic action of marijuana-active substances. In: Belenko SR, ed. *Drugs and Drug Policy in America: A Documentary History*. Westport, CT: Greenwood Press; 2000:167.

[111]Brown B. *Cannabis: The Illegalization of Weed in America*. New York, NY: First Second; 2019:188-193

[112]Booth M. *Cannabis: A History*. New York, NY: Picador; 2003:207-219.

[113]Booth M. *Cannabis: A History*. New York, NY: Picador; 2003:207-274.

[114]Martin A, Rashidian N. *A New Leaf: The End of Cannabis Prohibition*. New York, NY: The New Press; 2014:43.

[115]Booth M. *Cannabis: A History*. New York, NY: Picador; 2003:249.

[116]Booth M. *Cannabis: A History*. New York, NY: Picador; 2003:250.

[117]Anslinger HJ, Oursler W. The murderers. In: Belenko SR, ed. *Drugs and Drug Policy in America: A Documentary History*. Westport, CT: Greenwood Press; 2000:184-185.

[118]Rosenthal J. A fresh look at those harsh marijuana penalties. New York Times [Internet]. 1969 October 19:Sect. E:8(col. 2). https://timesmachine.nytimes.com/timesmachine/1969/10/19/91257755.html?pageNumber=222. Accessed October 3, 2019.

[119]Schmeck HM. U.S. aide calls marijuana laws more harmful than the drug. New York Times [Internet]. 1969 September 18:Page 43(col. 4). https://timesmachine.nytimes.com/timesmachine/1969/09/18/issue.html. Accessed October 3, 2019.

[120]Laws on marijuana decried by Egeberg. New York Times [Internet]. 1969 September 3:Page 40(col. 3). https://timesmachine.nytimes.com/timesmachine/1969/09/03/88860948.html?pageNumber=40. Accessed October 3, 2019.

[121]National commission on marihuana and drug abuse. In: Belenko SR, ed. *Drugs and Drug Policy in America: A Documentary History*. Westport, CT: Greenwood Press; 2000:293.

[122]Martin A, Rashidian N. *A New Leaf: The End of Cannabis Prohibition*. New York, NY: The New Press; 2014:46.

[123]Musto DF. The American disease: origins of narcotic control. In: Belenko SR, ed. *Drugs and Drug Policy in America: A Documentary History*. Westport, CT: Greenwood Press; 2000:277.

[124]Martin A, Rashidian N. *A New Leaf: The End of Cannabis Prohibition*. New York, NY: The New Press; 2014:47.

[125]Baum D. Legalize it all: how to win the war on drugs. *Harper's Magazine*. 2016;(1991):22. https://harpers.org/archive/2016/04/?mode=microfiche. Accessed October 4, 2019.

[126]Leary v. United States. In: Belenko SR, ed. *Drugs and Drug Policy in America: A Documentary History*. Westport, CT: Greenwood Press; 2000:290-291.

[127]Comprehensive Drug Abuse Prevention and Control Act (1970). In: Belenko SR, ed. *Drugs and Drug Policy in America: A Documentary History*. Westport, CT: Greenwood Press; 2000:279.

[128]Shulgin AT. Controlled substances: chemical and legal guide to federal drug laws. In: Belenko SR, ed. *Drugs and Drug Policy in America: A Documentary History*. Westport, CT: Greenwood Press; 2000:278.

[129]Martin A, Rashidian N. *A New Leaf: The End of Cannabis Prohibition*. New York, NY: The New Press; 2014:29.

[130]Liccardo Pacula R, Chriqui JF, Reichmann DA, Terry-McElrath YM; ImpacTeen. State medical marijuana laws: Understanding the laws and their limitations. https://impacteen. uic.edu/generalarea_PDFs/medicalmarijuanapaper100301.pdf. Published October 2001. Accessed October 15, 2019.

[131]Booth M. *Cannabis: A History*. New York, NY: Picador; 2003:351-362.

[132]Booth M. *Cannabis: A History*. New York, NY: Picador; 2003:356.

[133]Aldrich M. The history of therapeutic cannabis. In: Mathre ML, ed. *Cannabis in Medical Practice: A Legal, Historical and Pharmacological Overview of the Therapeutic Use of Marijuana*. Jefferson, NC: McFarland & Company, Inc., Publishers; 1997:51.

[134]Martin A, Rashidian N. *A New Leaf: The End of Cannabis Prohibition*. New York, NY: The New Press; 2014:66.

[135]H.R.2—Agriculture Improvement Act of 2018. Congress.gov. https://www.congress.gov/ bill/115th-congress/house-bill/2/text. Updated December 20, 2018. Accessed October 4, 2019.

[136]Quinnipiac University. Quinnipiac University National Poll. Quinnipiac University. 2019. https://poll.qu.edu/national/release-detail?ReleaseID=2604. Accessed October 4, 2019.

[137]Pew Research Center. October 2017 Political Survey. Pew Research Center. 2017. http:// assets.pewresearch.org/wp-content/uploads/sites/12/2018/01/05111821/01-05-18-marijuana-topline-for-release.pdf. Accessed October 4, 2019.

[138]United States. Department of Justice. Office of the Attorney General. [Memorandum for all United States attorneys, August 29, 2013]. https://www.justice.gov/iso/opa/resour ces/3052013829132756857467.pdf. Accessed October 4, 2019.

[139]United States Department of Justice. Office of the Attorney General. [Policy statement regarding marijuana issues in Indian Country, October 28, 2014]. https://www.justice.gov/ sites/default/files/tribal/pages/attachments/2014/12/11/policystatementregardingmarijuanais-suesinindiancountry2.pdf. Accessed October 18, 2019.

[140]United States Department of Justice. Office of the Attorney General. [Memorandum for all United States attorneys, January 8, 2018]. https://www.justice.gov/opa/press-release/ file/1022196/download?utm_medium=email&utm_source=govdelivery. Accessed October 4, 2019.

[141]Hudak J (2018). The farm bill, hemp legalization and the status of CBD: An explainer. Brookings Institution website. https://www.brookings.edu/blog/fixgov/2018/12/14/the-farm-bill-hemp-and-cbd-explainer/. Accessed October 4, 2019.

[142]House Bill No. 2244. Kansas State Legislature website. http://kslegislature.com/li/ b2019_20/measures/documents/hb2244_00_0000.pdf. Accessed October 17, 2019.

[143]Cason M. Alabama Legislature approves Leni's Law to decriminalize cannabis derivative. AL.com website. https://www.al.com/news/2016/04/alabama_senate_moves_lenis_law.html. Updated January 13, 2019. Accessed October 17, 2019.

[144]Cannabidiol (CBD). Idaho Office of Drug Policy website. https://odp.idaho.gov/cannibidiol/. Accessed October 17, 2019.

[145]Ta L. CBD is still illegal in Iowa, but for how long? Des Moines Register website. https://www.desmoinesregister.com/story/news/crime-and-courts/2019/07/09/cbd-still-illegal-iowa-but-how-long-iowa-hemp-act-farm-bill-cbd-oil-candy-water-tinctures/1674292001/. Updated July 9, 2019. Accessed October 17, 2019

[146]Attorney General Ravnsborg clarifies questions regarding industrial hemp and CBD (cannabidiol) oil. Office of the South Dakota Attorney General website. https://atg.sd.gov/OurOffice/Media/pressreleasesdetail.aspx?id=2167. March 25, 2019. Accessed October 17, 2019.

[147]Court says CBD oil is illegal. Talanei website. https://www.talanei.com/2019/07/12/court-says-cbd-oil-is-illegal/. July 12, 2019. Accessed October 17, 2019.

6

The Endocannabinoid System

6.1 Overview

The endocannabinoid system (ECS) is a wide-ranging biochemical communication and regulatory system that is primarily found in the central and peripheral nervous system (PNS), as well as the immune system. Virtually every organ system in the body is affected directly or indirectly by the ECS, and its role has been characterized as being one of the body's mechanisms for maintaining physiological homeostasis. It is composed of receptors, endogenous ligands known as endocannabinoids, and enzymes that synthesize endocannabinoids and degrade both endocannabinoids and phytocannabinoids. The psychotropic and therapeutic effects of cannabis are produced when phytocannabinoids interact with the ECS.

Evidence of the ECS emerged in the 1980s as researchers attempted to explain the psychotropic effects of the primary phytocannabinoid found in cannabis, Δ^9-tetrahydrocannabinol (THC). The first cannabinoid receptor (CBR), CB_1, was discovered in the late 1980s and cloned in 1990, while a second CBR, CB_2, was cloned in 1993. CB_1 receptors are found mostly in the central nervous system (CNS) and in peripheral nerve terminals, while CB_2 receptors are particularly prevalent in the body's immune system and are responsible for the immunomodulatory effects of cannabis and endocannabinoids.[1] THC has been shown to have the highest affinity for CB_1 receptors among phytocannabinoids, which accounts for its noted psychotropic effects. Δ^8-Tetrahydrocannabinol, cannabinol (CBN), and Δ^9-tetrahydrocannabivarin (THCV) all activate both CBRs but have less affinity for CB_1 receptors than THC, thereby accounting for their slightly reduced psychotropic effects when compared to THC. Cannabidiol (CBD) does not bind to either CBR but has been shown to indirectly interact with both CB_1 and CB_2 receptors.

Evidence suggests that the ECS may be more expansive than currently believed. There may be additional CBRs, such as the orphan G protein receptor GPR55, and cannabinoids like THC have been shown to bind with peroxisome proliferator-activated receptors.[2] Additionally, research has indicated that cannabinoids indirectly interact with vanilloid signaling systems, particularly transient receptor potential vanilloid 1 (TRPV1) receptors, though the means through which these systems interact is not well understood.[3]

6.2 An Introduction to Cell Receptors and Ligands

To grasp the innerworkings of the ECS, it is imperative that one first understand how nerve cells (or *neurons*) communicate with one another. What follows is a simplified model of the nervous system that is meant more to introduce readers to some specific mechanisms of neurobiology and a few key terms than to be a comprehensive description of the entire nervous system.

To begin, the body's nervous system is divided into the CNS and the PNS. The CNS includes the brain, the brain stem, and the spinal cord. The PNS is the vast network of nerves linked to the brain and the spinal cord through spinal and cranial nerves.

There are ~100 billion neurons within the average person's CNS and an even greater number of glial cells (or *glia*), which largely support and protect neurons. Each neuron has a cell body and projections that connect it to other neurons. These projections include long, slender fibers known as *axons* and branching structures known as *dendrites*. Axons transmit electrical information between neurons. Dendrites send and receive information to and from other neurons through synaptic contacts (or *synapses*). Each neuron may be connected to as many as 10 000 other neurons via synaptic connections, and it is estimated that there are as many as 1000 trillion synaptic connections in total within the average human brain.[4]

These synaptic contacts do not touch but rather communicate with one another by sending chemical transmitters that are known as *neurotransmitters*. These neurotransmitters are sent via *synaptic vesicles* across the *synaptic cleft*, which is ~10-20 nm in width.[5] Typically, neurotransmitters are packaged into synaptic vesicles by the *presynaptic terminal* and then sent across the synaptic cleft to the receiving dendrite (the *postsynaptic element*). When these transmitters arrive at the postsynaptic element, they bind to specific proteins known as *receptors*. The flow of information can also occur in retrograde fashion, wherein transmitters are sent from the postsynaptic element back to receptors in the presynaptic terminal. Signaling in the ECS operates in this fashion, which means that endocannabinoid transmitters in the postsynaptic element are synthesized and released "on demand" by physiological and pathological stimuli and then travel back to receptors in presynaptic terminals.[6]

For the sake of visualizing this process, one can imagine that each type of receptor is like a lock and each transmitter is like a key. If the key does not fit, it cannot successfully open the lock. Similarly, if the transmitter molecule does not fit in the receptor, it cannot successfully bind with and activate it. Transmitter molecules that are capable of binding with cellular receptors are known as *ligands*. When ligands activate the receptor, they are known as *agonists*. There are both full and partial agonists. When ligands bind to receptors, but do not activate them, they are known as *neutral antagonists*. When ligands bind to receptors and deactivate them or displace agonists, thereby preventing activization, they are known as *inverse agonists* or *antagonists*.

Specific receptors are named after their ligands. There are receptors for some of the most well-known neurotransmitters in the brain, such as dopamine, serotonin, and norepinephrine. Additionally, there are other receptors that were discovered because of their affinity for molecules found in drugs, as well as endogenous neurotransmitters that also bind to these receptors. These receptors are typically named after the drugs that activate them, as is the case with nicotine receptors, opiate receptors, and CBRs. To be clear, these drugs merely mimic endogenously produced neurotransmitters that bind to their corresponding receptors.

When a transmitter activates a receptor, it sends a signal to the cell body and triggers a cellular response by an *effector*. One can think of receptors as being intermediaries between transmitters, which remain outside of cell membranes, and effectors, which remain inside of cell membranes. Free transmitters that do not immediately bind to receptors are either reabsorbed into the presynaptic terminal or degraded into inactive metabolites by enzymes in the synaptic cleft.[7]

CBRs belong to a family of receptors known as G protein-coupled receptors because they are linked to adjacent guanine nucleotide-binding proteins (G proteins).[8] They also thread through cell membranes 7 times.[9] When receptors couple with either phytocannabinoids or endocannabinoids, effectors that are subunits of the G protein (known as Gα proteins) are activated and exert effects on the cell such as altering the flow of ions into the neuron or inhibiting or promoting the release of molecules.[10] The types of Gα proteins with which cannabinoids couple are known as $G_{i/o}$ subunits and have a key role in the regulation of different types of signaling to be explored below. In addition, $G_{i/o}$ subunits are instrumental in the regulation of the enzyme adenylyl cyclase.[11]

6.3 The History of the ECS

Researchers were not clear how cannabis produced its intoxicating or therapeutic effects until relatively recently. Even in the early 1980s, it was assumed that the high lipophilicity of cannabinoids accounted for their pharmacological action and that phytocannabinoids produced their effects by modifying the membranes of neurons in a fashion akin to many anesthetics or by interfering with neural communication, as alcohol does.[12] Researchers at the time concluded that there was no need for specific CBRs or endogenous mediators and, additionally, believed that cannabinoids did not exhibit stereoselectivity, thereby precluding the possibility of receptor-type activity.[13]

As the decade progressed, it was discovered that this premise was not accurate. Cannabinoids are highly stereospecific, which led several groups to begin searching for specific receptors sites in the CNS.[13] Two findings, both by Allyn Howlett, then at St. Louis University Medical School, are monumental in this regard.

In the early 1980s, Howlett read about research that had been conducted by Pfizer on the effects of several novel cannabinoids they had been developed to study cannabis' effects on pain. When she saw that the company had abandoned the project, she reached out and asked if they would be willing to donate the compounds to her lab so she could continue the research. They complied.[14]

One of the novel cannabinoids that Howlett and her team received from Pfizer is known as CP55,940, which is significantly more potent *in vivo* than THC.[15] While conducting testing with CP55,940 and other psychotropic cannabinoids in the early 1980s, the team realized that the compounds had the ability to inhibit adenylate cyclase, a key indicator of $G_{i/o}$ protein coupling, which suggested that cannabinoids interact with these specific types of G proteins.[13] This was the first major finding by Howlett.

A few years later, in the late 1980s, Howlett's team used CP55,940 radiolabeled with tritium (then a new technology) to search for binding sites in the CNS, which would be indicative of specific CBRs. In 1988, they eventually discovered one such binding site for CP55,940 and other cannabinoids in rat brain membranes, thereby providing proof of a CBR.[16] In 1990, this receptor was cloned in Tom Bonner's laboratory at the National Institute of Health.[17] These receptors have since been named CB_1 receptors; they are the most abundant G protein-coupled receptors in the nervous system.[18]

Following the discovery of the CB_1 receptor, many researchers reasoned that it would be odd for the brain to dedicate resources to produce receptors that bind to exogenous compounds found primarily within a plant and assumed that there must be an endogenous mediator capable of binding to and activating CB_1 receptors. Researchers soon discovered the compound, N-arachidonoylethanolamide, which was isolated by Devane et al. in 1992. It parallels the effects of psychotropic phytocannabinoids like THC, though it has a lower potency at CB_1 receptors than THC and a far shorter duration of action.[19] The compound was given the nickname "anandamide" by the team, which is based on the Sanskrit word for bliss, *ananda*.[13] Later studies found that there is an entire family of anandamide-type compounds, many of which are considered putative endocannabinoids.[13]

In 1993, a second G protein-coupled CBR, CB_2, was cloned from rat spleen in Sean Munro's laboratory in Cambridge.[13] Though

CB_2 receptors are found primarily in the immune system, they have also been detected in the CNS.[3] In 1995, Mechoulam et al. identified a cannabinoid ligand in canine gut that binds to both CB_1 and CB_2 receptors and elucidated it as 2-arachidonoylglycerol (2-AG). There are other putative endocannabinoids that have been discovered that will be explored below.[20]

In addition to discovering several endocannabinoids and putative endocannabinoids, researchers have also discovered numerous synthetic cannabinoids that are capable of binding to CBRs. This includes both agonists, such as CP55,940, and antagonists that specifically target CB_1 and CB_2 receptors or both. As an example, SR 141716A (rimonabant) is a CB_1 antagonist that was developed to serve primarily as an appetite suppressant. As it is widely known that THC tends to both activate CB_1 receptors and stimulate the appetite, it was believed that blocking CB_1 receptors could produce the contrary effects (ie, satiety). While this did prove to be the case, it was also found that blocking CB_1 receptors resulted in severe mood disorders and, in some cases, suicide.[21] Though the drug was approved in Europe and is still used by cannabinoid researchers to this day, the Food and Drug Administration (FDA) rejected its use in the United States. In hindsight, interfering with anandamide (a transmitter that takes its name from the word for "joy") was bound to have negative effects on mood.

Finally, ongoing research into the extent of the ECS has indicated that many cannabinoids interact with more than just CB_1 and CB_2 receptors either directly or indirectly. Some cannabinoids have shown a relatively high affinity for the orphan G protein-coupled receptor GPR55, which suggests that it may be yet another CBR, though the exact status of GPR55 remains controversial.[22] Additionally, anandamide has been shown to bind to TRPV1 receptors (also known as vanilloid receptor 1 or the capsaicin receptor),[23] and other transient receptor potential (TRP) channels may modulate the effects of cannabinoids.[24] These subjects will be explored in greater detail below and in Chapter 8 (The Pharmacodynamics of Cannabis).

6.4 Endocannabinoids

As mentioned above, there are two primary endocannabinoids, anandamide and 2-AG, that have been the subject of the most research. At this time, at least 11 additional, putative endocannabinoids have been found in humans. They include 2-arachidonoyl glycerol ether (2-AGE or noladin ether), oleamide, N-arachidonoyl dopamine (NADA), N-docosahexaenoyl ethanolamide (DHEA), eicosapentaenoyl ethanolamide (EPEA), O-arachidonoyl ethanolamine (virodhamine), N-oleoyl dopamine, dihomo-γ-linolenoyl ethanolamide, docosatetraenoyl ethanolamide, sphingosine, and haemopressin.[25]

6.4.1 Anandamide

Apart from being discovered as the first endocannabinoid, anandamide (Fig. 6.1) is the most researched cannabinoid. It binds to both CB_1 and CB_2 receptors, though its affinity for CB_1 receptors is fourfold that of CB_2 receptors.[9] (K_i CB_1 – 89 nM; K_i CB_2 = 371 nM).[20] Anandamide has also been shown to activate GPR55 receptors with a half maximal effective concentration (EC50) of 18 nM.[26] It also activates TRPV1 receptors but has a low binding affinity for the latter despite being a full agonist.[9]

Anandamide is found throughout the nervous system, and its highest levels of concentration occur in the parts of the CNS and PNS that have the largest number of CBRs.[9] Exogenous anandamide produces antinociception (reduced sensitivity to pain), hypothermia, hypomobility, and catalepsy in mice following either intravenous, intraperitoneal, or intrathecal administration. Of note, the manipulation of the ECS by modulating enzymes associated with the synthesis or breakdown (catabolism) of endocannabinoids did not affect body temperature.[27] Despite significant molecular differences, many of the effects of anandamide are akin to THC, though THC has a notably longer-lasting effect,[10] especially when it comes to pain suppression.[20]

Evidence suggests that some anandamide is stored inside neurons, but most of it is synthesized on demand in the postsynaptic neuron in a Ca^{2+}-dependent manner and then transmitted to presynaptic terminals.[28] As mentioned above, it has a relatively short duration of action and is quickly hydrolyzed by fatty acid amide hydrolase (FAAH) into ethanolamine and arachidonic acid.[9]

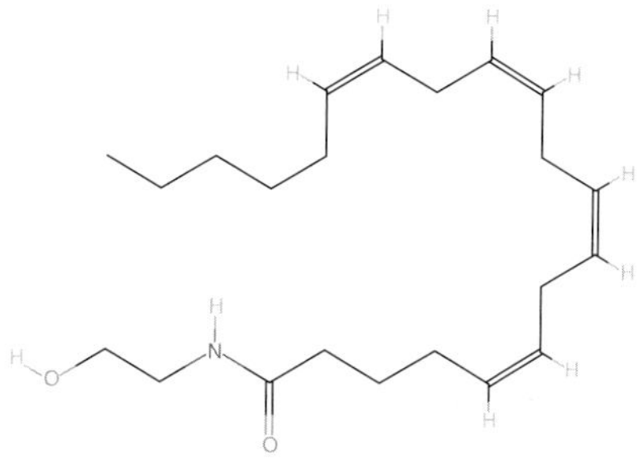

Figure 6.1 Anandamide.

6.4.2 2-Arachidonoylglycerol

2-AG (Fig. 6.2) has been proposed as the true natural ligand for the CBRs, as concentrations of 2-AG in the brain are 170-fold higher than those of anandamide.[20] However, it has a lower affinity for CB_1 receptors than anandamide, even though it is a full agonist.[9] Compared to anandamide, it is a more potent agonist at CB_2 receptors, though research indicates that the agonistic activity of 2-AG is attenuated by the presence of anandamide.[29] 2-AG has also been shown to bind to GPR55 receptors with an EC50 value of 3 nM[26] and is also a TRPV1 receptor agonist.[30]

The biological activities with which 2-AG is believed to be involved include immune and cardiovascular functions, inflammatory responses, neuroprotection, neuromodulation, as well as cell proliferation, embryo development, and hippocampal function.[9] It may also be associated with pain modulation[20] and, like anandamide, is believed to be synthesized on demand in postsynaptic neurons and undergo retrograde transmission to presynaptic terminals.[31]

As 2-AG is an ester, it is easily hydrolyzed by the body, but this process is inhibited by the presence of fatty acid esters of glycerol (palmitoyl glycerol and linoleoyl glycerol), which occur in greater concentrations compared to 2-AG.[13] These two compounds are not considered to be endocannabinoids, despite their interaction with 2-AG, and the enzyme monoacylglycerol lipase is responsible for the presynaptic degradation of 2-AG.[32]

6.4.3 Putative Endocannabinoids

Research into the putative endocannabinoids is ongoing, with more studies needed to support and expand upon the limited data that is available at this time. What follows is a general overview of the 11 aforementioned compounds.

- 2-AGE (noladin ether) has a significantly higher affinity for CB_1 receptors than CB_2 receptors and is found in highest concentrations in the thalamus and hippocampus.[9] Noladin ether has also been shown to activate GPR55 receptors.[32]
- Oleamide is a sleep-inducing fatty acid amide

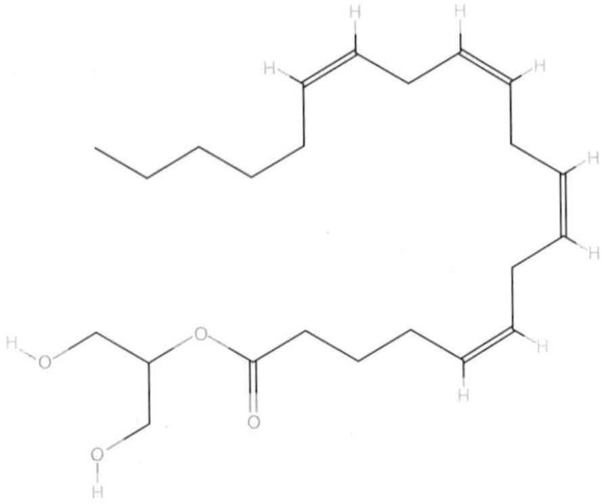

Figure 6.2 2-Arachidonoylglycerol.

within the same family as anandamide. Both are synthesized in the brain and hydrolyzed by FAAH. Conflicting reports about the independent binding affinity of oleamide at CBRs have led some to believe that it may not be an endocannabinoid in its own right, but rather a potentiator for other cannabinoids.[33]

- NADA activates CB_1 receptors and TRPV1 receptors, with the highest concentrations in the striatum and hippocampus.[9]
- DHEA is a structural analog to anandamide that binds weakly to CBRs and has a higher affinity for CB_1 than CB_2 receptors.[34] DHEA has been detected in human plasma and may play a role in suppressing the production of proinflammatory cytokine MCP-1.[35]
- EPEA binds weakly to CBRs and has a higher affinity for CB_1 than CB_2 receptors.[34]
- O-Arachidonoyl ethanolamine (virodhamine) is a partial agonist of CBRs, as well as a partial agonist of GPR55.[9,36]
- N-Oleoyl dopamine is a TRPV1 ligand and CB1 agonist.[37]
- Dihomo-γ-linolenoyl ethanolamide and docosatetraenoyl ethanolamide have been found in mammalian tissues and have been shown to bind to CB_1 receptors.[38]
- Sphingosine may act as a CB_1 receptor antagonist.
- Haemopressin may also be a CB_1 receptor antagonist/inverse agonist.[25]

More research into these putative endocannabinoids needs to be conducted to establish how they interact with the ECS.

6.5 Cannabinoid Receptors

Though research into the ECS is ongoing, and evidence suggests that it may be far more complex than currently acknowledged, it is currently accepted that there are only two CBRs found within the ECS—CB_1 and CB_2. Human CB_1 receptors contain 472 amino acids and CB_2 receptors contain 360 amino acids.[18] The two receptors share 44% amino acid sequence identity and the gene loci for CB_1 and CB_2 receptors have been localized to position 6q14-q15 in chromosome 6 and position 1p36 in chromosome 1, respectively.[9]

Both receptors are found in broad range of animals, including mammals, birds, reptiles, and fish.[39] As mentioned above, CBRs couple with G_i or G_o proteins and are most frequently found in presynaptic terminals where they are activated by the retrograde transmission of endocannabinoids from postsynaptic neurons or, as explained below, immune cells.[9] The expression of more or fewer CBRs appears to be influenced by stressors.[40]

More will be said about the mechanisms of action of both CB$_1$ and CB$_2$ receptors in Chapter 8 (The Pharmacodynamics of Cannabis).

6.5.1 CB$_1$ Receptors

CB$_1$ receptors are found primarily in the CNS and tend to be located on presynaptic terminals but can also be found on postsynaptic neurons and glia.[9] The highest concentrations of CB$_1$ receptors in the CNS are found in areas associated with thinking, memory, pleasure, time perception, and coordination, which is consistent with the psychological effects of THC.[2] The areas of distribution of CB$_1$ receptors in the CNS can be found in Table 6.1. CB$_1$ receptors are also found, though in smaller concentrations, in the male and female reproductive systems, the cardiovascular system, the gastrointestinal tract, and bones.[2,9]

Other than being instrumental in generating the psychological and cognitive effects of cannabis, CB$_1$ receptors also play a role in psychomotor activity, gastrointestinal functions, itching, and the regulation of body temperature and muscle tone.[2] Additionally, the distribution of CB$_1$ receptors in pain pathways within the brain, spinal cord, and PNS reflects the role the ECS plays in pain modulation and is consistent with the reported antinociceptive (decreased attentiveness to pain) effects of cannabis.[20]

CB$_1$ receptors in the CNS play a significant role in the regulation of other neurotransmitters such as dopamine, serotonin, and glutamate.[2] One could envision the interaction between CB$_1$ receptors and endocannabinoids as being akin to a dimmer switch. When the signal flow of certain transmitters from presynaptic neurons is too high, endocannabinoids are released from postsynaptic neurons to stem the flow of presynaptic transmitters. Considered from a therapeutic perspective, this could be a very useful means of treating certain forms of nerve-based pain caused by the excessive release of neurotransmitters, particularly glutamate. Considered from a biological perspective, the ECS is an extremely important neuroprotective system, as excessive amounts of certain transmitters, such as glutamate, can cause neuronal necrosis.[41]

6.5.2 CB$_2$ Receptors

The highest concentrations of CB$_2$ receptors are found in the immune system, particularly in the spleen, tonsils, monocytes, and B and T cells. They are also located in various parts of the CNS

TABLE 6.1 Distribution of CB$_1$ in the Nervous System

Brain Part	Dense	Moderate	Low
Cerebrum:	• Primary somatosensory cortex (layers II, III, and VI) • Cingulate cortex (layer II) • Entorhinal cortex (layers II and IV) • Piriform cortex (layer III) • Frontal lobe (associational cortical regions) • Hippocampus (fields CA1, CA2, and CA3; subicular complex) • Outer molecular layer of dentate gyrus • Olfactory bulb (ependymal and subependymal layers) • Anterior olfactory nucleus • Olfactory tract • Anterior commissure (olfactory fibers) • Amygdala nucleus • Basal ganglia (internal portion of the globus pallidus, putamen, caudate nucleus, striatonigral pathway, and entopeduncular nucleus)	• Somatosensory cortex (layer V) • Temporal association cortex • Secondary somatosensory cortex • Supplementary motor cortex • Visual cortex • Auditory cortex • Inner polymorphic layer of dentate gyrus • Basal forebrain • Basal ganglia (external portion of the globus pallidus, ventral pallidum, and claustrum)	• Somatosensory cortex (layer IV) • Primary motor cortex • Granule cell layer of dentate gyrus • Olfactory tubercle • Basal ganglia (nucleus accumbens)

(Continued)

TABLE 6.1 Continued

Brain Part	Dense	Moderate	Low
Cerebellum:	All regions		
Diencephalon:		• Thalamus (anterior, dorsomedial, and intralaminar nuclei) • Stria terminalis • Epithalamus (habenular nucleus) • Hypothalamus (lateral and paraventricular nuclei) • Infundibular stem	• Thalamus (medial geniculate, lateral geniculate, ventral posterior, and ventral lateral nuclei) • Subthalamic nucleus
Brain stem:	• Substantia nigra (pars reticulata) • Periaqueductal gray (PAG) • Gray matter around the fourth ventricle • Spinal trigeminal nucleus and spinal tract of the trigeminal nucleus	• Solitary nucleus • Nucleus ambiguus • Inferior olivary nucleus	• Ventral tegmental area • Substantia nigra (pars compacta)
Spinal cord:	• Dorsal horn • Lamina X • Dorsal root ganglions	• Deep dorsal horn • Thoracic intermediolateral nucleus	

From Svíženská I, Dubový P, Šulcová A. Cannabinoid receptors 1 and 2 (CB1 and CB2), their distribution, ligands and functional involvement in nervous system structures—a short review. *Pharmacol Biochem Behav.* 2008;90(4):501-511. doi: 10.1016/j.pbb.2008.05.010.

and PNS, as illustrated in Table 6.2.[20] Changes in CB_2 receptor expression and endocannabinoid levels have been associated with a wide range of conditions affecting parts of the body beyond the immune system, including the CNS, kidney, liver, bone, skin, lung, gastrointestinal tract, and cardiovascular system.[40]

CB_2 receptors operate in a fashion similar to CB_1 receptors, as they suppress signaling from immune cells to neurons.[42] A key difference to note, however, is that CB_2 receptors in the immune system do not suppress the signaling of neurotransmitters, but of *cytokines*, which are proteins that are the means of communication for immune cells.[43] Cytokines can be proinflammatory or anti-inflammatory.[43]

Proinflammatory cytokines fight against infections, neutralize irritants, and remove dead or dying cells, thereby resulting in inflammation. Seen in this light, inflammation is a natural and ordinarily healthy response to threats detected by the immune system. Unfortunately, this phenomenon can at times become exacerbated by a variety of other factors, which results in damage to healthy cells. This, in turn, generates discomfort, pain, and other serious symptoms that are often dependent upon where the inflammation is taking place.

The ECS acts to attenuate inflammation through the retrograde transmission of endocannabinoids from neurons to CB_2 receptors in immune cells, which instruct these cells to slow or stop the release of cytokines. By virtue of this mechanism, the ECS, and CB_2 receptors in particular, appears to play a major role in mitigating the symptoms of disorders that arise due to unhealthy levels of inflammation (specifically autoimmune disorders).[9] Evidence suggests that CB_2 receptors in the CNS may play a similar role in combatting neuroinflammatory and neurodegenerative disorders like Alzheimer disease and amyotrophic lateral sclerosis (ALS).[3]

6.5.3 Putative Endocannabinoid Receptors

While the CB_1 and CB_2 receptors have been definitively shown to be core components of the ECS, they are not the only receptors that respond to cannabinoids. In fact, several receptors appear to bind to cannabinoids, while some crosstalk between the ECS and other systems (particularly the vanilloid signaling system), has also been observed.[3] Despite these observations, there is still some debate about whether it is accurate to include them as part of the ECS.

The one receptor that has garnered the most attention is the orphan G protein-coupled receptor GPR55. GPR55 receptors

TABLE 6.2 Distribution of CB$_2$ in the Nervous System

Brain Part	Dense	Moderate	Low
Cerebrum:	• Orbital cortex (layers III and V) • Visual cortex (layers III and V) • Auditory cortex (layers III and V) • Motor cortex (layers III and V) • Piriform cortex (layers III and V) • Islands of Calleja • Hippocampus (pyramidal neurons in fields CA2 and CA3) • Anterior olfactory nucleus • Amygdala nucleus • Basal ganglia (striatum nucleus)		
Cerebellum:	• Purkinje cells • Granule cells	• Purkinje dendrites in the molecular layer	
Diencephalon:	• Thalamus (ventral posterior, lateral posterior, posterior, and paracentral nuclei)	• Thalamus (lateral geniculate nucleus)	• Thalamus (paraventricular and mediodorsal nuclei) • Hypothalamus (ventromedial and arcuate nuclei)

Brain stem:
- Dorsal cochlear nucleus
- Facial motor nucleus

- Substantia nigra (pars reticulata)
- Periaqueductal gray (PAG)
- Inferior colliculus
- Interpeduncular, paratrochlear, and red nuclei
- Lateral lemniscus (paralemniscal and dorsal nuclei)
- Pontine nucleus
- Medial and lateral vestibular nuclei
- Parvocellular reticular nucleus
- Spinal tract of the trigeminal nucleus

From Svíženská I, Dubový P, Šulcová A. Cannabinoid receptors 1 and 2 (CB1 and CB2), their distribution, ligands and functional involvement in nervous system structures—a short review. *Pharmacol Biochem Behav*. 2008;90(4):501-511. doi: 10.1016/j.pbb.2008.05.010.

are found primarily in the adrenals, the gastrointestinal tract (particularly the ileum and jejunum), and parts of the CNS. Ryberg et al. found that concentrations of GPR55 receptors in mouse CNS tissues were highest in the frontal cortex, striatum, hypothalamus, brain stem, hippocampus, and cerebellum but were notably lower than CB_1 receptors. They also discovered that GPR55 appears to be G_{13} coupled rather than $G_{i/o}$ coupled, as is the case with CB_1 and CB_2 receptors.[26]

GPR55 receptors bind with various endocannabinoids including anandamide and 2-AG; putative endocannabinoids noladin ether and virodhamine; naturally occurring phytocannabinoids such as THC and CBD (as an antagonist); and synthetic cannabinoids such as CP55,940 and HU210. Virodhamine and 2-AG are extremely potent GPR55 ligands when compared to their activity at CB_1 and CB_2 receptors, while nonendocannabinoids, particularly palmitoylethanolamide (PEA), have also been shown to be potent and selective agonists of GPR55.[26]

It appears that GPR55 plays a regulatory role in vascular tone control, immune cell function, and cell migration.[26] Shi et al. have suggested that GPR55 receptors may also modulate feelings of anxiety,[44] while these findings are promising, more research into the function of GPR55 receptors is needed before one can definitively make the claim that GPR55 receptors are part of the ECS.

6.6 Tolerance to Cannabinoids

Finally, frequent users of cannabis have been known to develop a tolerance to the psychotropic effects of THC. The mechanism behind this phenomenon is most likely related to CB_1 receptor down-regulation. Receptor down-regulation is a process by which a cell limits the number of receptors on its surface that can be coupled with ligands. Because there are fewer available receptors to which ligands can bind, this translates into a reduced sensitivity to the drug.

The down-regulation of CB_1 receptors has been observed in the human CNS after chronic exposure to THC. Observations have also shown that different parts of the brain may down-regulate less quickly than others.[9] Conversely, D'Souza et al. observed that CB_1 up-regulation began within merely 2 days of abstinence and continued for over 4 weeks, which was the length of the study.[45] Of note, within this timeframe, CB_1 receptor availability did not reach parity with the study's healthy controls, and it is unclear if a more prolonged period of abstinence would allow chronic users to reestablish CB_1 receptor sensitivity comparable to individuals who do not frequently use cannabis.

6.7 Conclusion

In just 30 years, our understanding of the scope and the mechanisms underlying the ECS has grown tremendously. It is now clear that the ECS plays a vital role in the regulation of signal flow between neurons in the CNS and between neurons and immune cells in the PNS. More research is still needed to determine if the putative endocannabinoids are indeed cannabinoids, if putative CBRs are CBRs, and how much crosstalk, if any, there is between the ECS and other systems, such as the vanilloid signaling system. An elucidation of how these systems interact could provide far more insight into if or how the terpenic compounds and minor phytocannabinoids described in Chapter 4 (Constituents of Cannabis) produce their reputed synergistic effects, as studies have shown most are not CBR ligands. No matter the answer, the next decade of research into the ECS will likely produce some illuminating and potentially groundbreaking data.

REFERENCES

[1]Turcotte C, Blanchet MR, Laviolette M, Flamand N. The CB2 receptor and its role as a regulator of inflammation. *Cell Mol Life Sci*. 2016;73(23):4449-4470. doi: 10.1007/s00018-016-2300-4.

[2]Small E. *Cannabis: A Complete Guide*. Boca Raton, FL: CRC Press; 2017:305.

[3]Onaivi ES, Ishiguro H, Qing-Rong L. Cannabinoid CB2 receptor mechanism of *Cannabis sativa L.* In: Chandra S, et al., eds. *Cannabis sativa L.—Botany and Biotechnology*. Cham, Switzerland: Springer International Publishing AG; 2017:227-247.

[4]Brain neurons & synapses. The Human Memory website. https://human-memory.net/brain-neurons-synapses/. Updated September 27, 2019. Accessed November 11, 2019.

[5]Nolte J. *The Human Brain: An Introduction to Its Functional Anatomy*. Philadelphia, PA: Mosby Elsevier; 2009:1-19.

[6]Small E. *Cannabis: A Complete Guide*. Boca Raton, FL: CRC Press; 2017:304.

[7]Nolte J. *The Human Brain: An Introduction to Its Functional Anatomy*. Philadelphia, PA: Mosby Elsevier; 2009:178-182.

[8]Nolte J. *The Human Brain: An Introduction to Its Functional Anatomy*. Philadelphia, PA: Mosby Elsevier; 2009:185.

[9]Svíženská I, Dubový P, Šulcová A. Cannabinoid receptors 1 and 2 (CB1 and CB2), their distribution, ligands and functional involvement in nervous system structures—a short review. *Pharmacol Biochem Behav*. 2008;90(4):501-511. doi: 10.1016/j.pbb.2008.05.010.

[10]Small E. *Cannabis: A Complete Guide*. Boca Raton, FL: CRC Press; 2017:303.

[11]Gilman AG. G proteins: transducers of receptor-generated signals. *Annu Rev Biochem.* 1987;56:615-649. doi: 10.1146/annurev.bi.56.070187.003151.

[12]Martin A, Rashidian N. *A New Leaf: The End of Cannabis Prohibition.* New York, NY: The New Press; 2014:18-19.

[13]Mechoulam R, Hanuš L. A historical overview of chemical research on cannabinoids. *Chem Phys Lipids.* 2000;108(1-2):1-13. doi: 10.1016/s0009-3084(00)00184-5.

[14]Martin A, Rashidian N. *A New Leaf: The End of Cannabis Prohibition.* New York, NY: The New Press; 2014:18.

[15]Herkenham M, Lynn AB, Little MD, et al. Cannabinoid receptor localization in brain. *Proc Natl Acad Sci U S A.* 1990;87(5):1932-1936. doi: 10.1073/pnas.87.5.1932.

[16]Devane WA, Dysarz FA III, Johnson MR, Melvin LS, Howlett AC. Determination and characterization of a cannabinoid receptor in rat brain. *Mol Pharmacol.* 1988;34(5):605-613.

[17]Pertwee RG. Cannabinoid pharmacology: the first 66 years. *Br J Pharmacol.* 2006;147:S163-S171. doi: 10.1038/sj.bjp.0706406.

[18]Nolte J. *The Human Brain: An Introduction to Its Functional Anatomy.* Philadelphia, PA: Mosby Elsevier; 2009:190.

[19]Justinova Z, Solinas M, Tanda G, Redhi GH, Goldberg SR. The endogenous cannabinoid anandamide and its synthetic analog R(+)-methanandamide are intravenously self-administered by squirrel monkeys. *J Neurosci.* 2005;25(23):5645-5650. doi: 10.1523/JNEUROSCI.0951-05.2005.

[20]Hohmann AG, Suplita RL II. Endocannabinoid mechanisms of pain modulation. *AAPS J.* 2006;8(4):E693-E708. doi: 10.1208/aapsj080479.

[21]Sam AH, Salem V, Ghatei MA. Rimonabant: from RIO to ban. *J Obes.* 2011;2011:432607. doi: 10.1155/2011/432607.

[22]Lauckner JE, Jensen JB, Chen HY, et al. GPR55 is a cannabinoid receptor that increases intercellular calcium and inhibits M current. *Proc Natl Acad Sci U S A.* 2008;105(7): 2699-2704. doi: 10.1073/pnas.0711278105.

[23]Ross RA. Anandamide and vanilloid TRPV1 receptors. *Br J Pharmacol.* 2003;140(5): 790-801. doi: 10.1038/sj.bjp.0705467.

[24]Mueller C, Morales P, Reggio PH. Cannabinoid ligands targeting TRP channels. *Front Mol Neurosci.* 2019;11:487. doi: 10.3389/fnmol.2018.00487.

[25]Pertwee RG. Endocannabinoids and their pharmacological actions. *Handb Exp Pharmacol.* 2015;231:1-37. doi: 10.1007/978-3-319-20825-1_1.

[26]Ryberg E, Larsson N, Sjögren S, et al. The orphan receptor GPR55 is a novel cannabinoid receptor. *Br J Pharmacol.* 2007;152(7):1092-1101. doi: 10.1038/sj.bjp.0707460.

[27]Nass SR, Long JZ, Schlosburg JE, et al. Endocannabinoid catabolic enzymes play differential roles in thermal homeostasis in response to environmental or immune challenge. *J Neuroimmune Pharmacol.* 2015;10(2):364-370. doi: 10.1007/s11481-015-9593-1.

[28]Cascio MG, Marini P. Biosynthesis and fate of endocannabinoids. In: Pertwee RG, ed. *Endocannabinoids.* Cham, Switzerland: Springer International Publishing AG; 2015:39-58

[29]Gonsiorek W, Lunn C, Fan X, et al. Endocannabinoid 2-arachidonyl glycerol is a full agonist through human type 2 cannabinoid receptor: antagonism by anandamide. *Mol Pharmacol.* 2000;57(5):1045-1050.

[30]Muller C, Morales P, Reggio PH. Cannabinoid ligands targeting TRP channels. *Front Mol Neurosci.* 2019;11:487. doi: 10.3389/fnmol.2018.00487. eCollection 2018.

[31]Small E. *Cannabis: A Complete Guide.* Boca Raton, FL: CRC Press; 2017:307.

[32]Reggio PH. Endocannabinoid binding to the cannabinoid receptors: what is known and what remains unknown. *Curr Med Chem.* 2010;17(14):1468-1486.

[33]Leggett JD, Aspley S, Beckett SRG, et al. Oleamide is a selective endogenous agonist of rat and human CB_1 cannabinoid receptors. *Br J Pharmacol.* 2004;141(2):253-262. doi: 10.1038/sj.bjp.0705607.

[34]Brown I, Gascio MG, Wahle KWJ. Cannabinoid receptor-dependent and -independent anti-proliferative effects of omega-3 ethanolamides in androgen receptor-positive and -negative prostate cancer cell lines. *Carcinogenesis*. 2010;31(9):1584-1591. doi: 10.1093/carcin/bgp151.

[35]Brown I, Gascio MG, Rotondo D, et al. Cannabinoids and omega-3/6 endocannabinoids as cell death and anticancer modulators. *Prog Lipid Res*. 2013;52(1):80-109. doi: 10.1016/j.plipres.2012.10.001.

[36]Sharir H, Console-Bram L, Mundy C, et al. The endocannabinoids anandamide and virodhamine modulate the activity of the candidate cannabinoid receptor GPR55. *J Neuroimmune Pharmacol*. 2012;7(4):856-865. doi: 10.1007/s11481-012-9351-6.

[37]Grabiec U, Dehghani F. *N*-arachidonoyl dopamine: a novel endocannabinoid and endovanilloid with widespread physiological and pharmacological activities. *Cannabis Cannabinoid Res*. 2017;2(1):183-196. doi: 10.1089/can.2017.0015.

[38]Bradshaw HB, Walker JM. The expanding field of cannabimimetic and related lipid mediators. *Br J Pharmacol*. 2005;144(4):459-465. doi: 10.1038/sj.bjp.0706093.

[39]McPartland JM, Agraval J, Gleeson D, Heasman K, Glass M. Cannabinoid receptors in invertebrates. *J Evol Biol*. 2006;19(2):366-373. doi: 10.1111/j.1420-9101.2005.01028.x.

[40]Small E. *Cannabis: A Complete Guide*. Boca Raton, FL: CRC Press; 2017:306.

[41]Small E. *Cannabis: A Complete Guide*. Boca Raton, FL: CRC Press; 2017:306-308.

[42]Small E. *Cannabis: A Complete Guide*. Boca Raton, FL: CRC Press; 2017:308.

[43]Zhang JM, An J. Cytokines, inflammation and pain. *Int Anesthesiol Clin*. 2007;45(2):27-37. doi: 10.1097/AIA.0b013e318034194e.

[44]Shi QX, Yang LK, Shi WL, et al. The novel cannabinoid receptor GPR55 mediates anxiolytic-like effects in the medial orbital cortex of mice with acute stress. *Mol Brain*. 2017;10(1):38. doi: 10.1186/s13041-017-0318-7.

[45]D'Souza DC, Cortes-Briones JA, Ranganathan M, et al. Rapid changes in CB1 receptor availability in cannabis dependent males after abstinence from cannabis. *Biol Psychiatry Cogn Neurosci Neuroimaging*. 2016;1(1):60-67. doi: 10.1016/j.bpsc.2015.09.008.

7

The Pharmacology of Cannabis

7.1 Overview

The pharmacology of cannabis is shrouded in mystery, largely due to its various constituents and numerous cultivars. This adds to the complexity of studying cannabis because there are a seemingly infinite variety of chemovars with varying concentrations of phytocannabinoids, terpenic compounds, flavonoids, and other potentially therapeutic compounds. Most of these compounds have not been adequately studied either on their own or in conjunction with the other constituents of cannabis, and there are only limited data about the pharmacokinetics, pharmacodynamics, and potential therapeutic uses of these compounds. Consequently, this chapter will focus on and provide a pharmacological overview of the pharmacokinetics of the two phyto-cannabinoids that have been studied the most: Δ^9-tetrahydrocananbinol (THC) and cannabidiol (CBD).

Historically, pharmacology encompasses pharmacodynamics, but considering the complexity of the endocannabinoid system, the pharmacodynamics and mechanisms of action of THC and CBD will be explored in Chapter 8 (The Pharmacodynamics of Cannabis).

7.2 History of Pharmaceutical Cannabis

As discussed in Chapters 2 (The History of Cannabis) and 5 (U.S. Cannabis Regulations From Past to Present), cannabis has been used as both a medicine and a recreational intoxicant for millennia, though an understanding of its mechanism of action and pharmacokinetics remained elusive until the latter half of the 20th century. As more information about cannabis has become available, it has become clear that herbal cannabis should not be considered a single drug, but many drugs due to the presence of myriad phytocannabinoids that can be subdivided into eleven classes: cannabigerol (CBG), cannabichromene (CBC), cannabidiol (CBD), Δ^9-tetrahydrocananbinol (THC), Δ^8-tetrahydrocananbinol (Δ^8-THC), cannabicyclol (CBL), cannabielsoin (CBE), cannabinol (CBN), cannabinodiol (CBND), cannabitriol (CBT), and a class for miscellaneous cannabinoids. Many of the most common cannabinoids were not isolated until the 1960s and 1970s, and while the discovery of the endocannabinoid system (ECS) did not take place until the 1980s and 1990s (as described in Chapter 6 [The Endocannabinoid System]), research into the extent of this system is ongoing.

The first phytocannabinoid believed to be isolated was CBN (Fig. 7.1) by Wood, Spivey, and Easterfield in the 1890s, and it was believed to be the primary psychoactive agent in cannabis for several decades.[1] CBN was

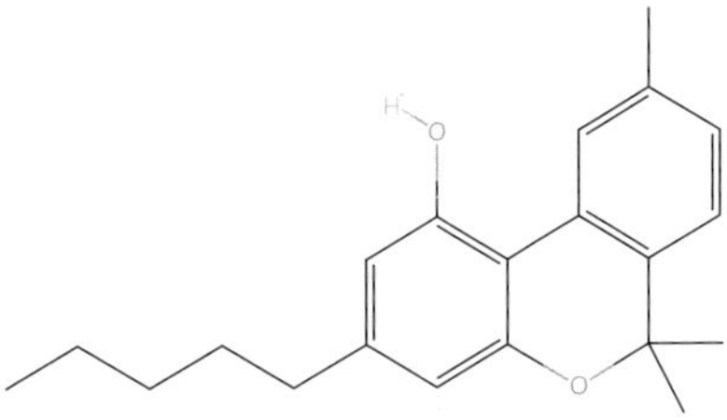

Figure 7.1 Cannabinol (CBN).

synthesized for the first time by Adams et al. in 1940,[2] and he was also credited with isolating CBD (Fig. 7.2) in the same year.[3] Raphael Mechoulam and Yechiel Gaoni isolated THC (Fig. 7.3) in 1964,[4] and together they then synthesized CBD and THC for the first time in 1965.[2] Additional cannabinoids have been isolated since then, and a full listing of known phytocannabinoids and their structures can be found in Table 4.1 of Chapter 4 (Constituents of Cannabis).

Between 1964 and 1978, ~2000 research articles were published exploring the effects of these cannabinoids with specific focus on THC, which was confirmed to be the primary psychoactive agent in cannabis.[5] This was highlighted in 1965 in an article by Mechoulam and Gaoni.[6] Researchers also believed that THC, apart from being the primary psychoactive agent, was the sole analgesic component in cannabis. Later studies would reveal that CBD also possesses analgesic qualities, particularly when administered in conjunction with THC and other cannabinoids.[2] Beyond examining the analgesic qualities of THC, many studies during the 1970s focused on THC's potential as a treatment for conditions such as glaucoma (Helper and Frank, 1971), wasting diseases (Salan et al., 1975), and hypertension (Benowitz and James, 1975).[5] Cannabis was also found to have antiasthmatic, anti-inflammatory, and soporific effects, but the intoxicating effects of THC, as well as the risk of tachycardia, were considered to be unacceptable side effects considering what was then believed to be its limited efficacy in treating these conditions.[5]

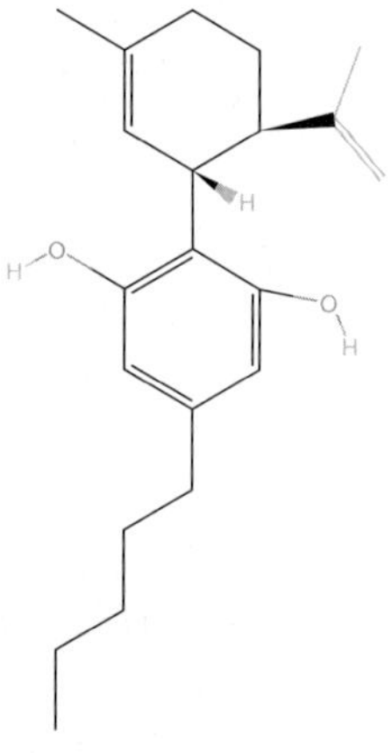

Despite these concerns, studies confirmed that it was a potent antiemetic and that it could be used to stimulate the appetite of patients who were often unable to eat due to extreme nausea, particularly after undergoing chemotherapy. In the 1980s, THC (dronabinol) marketed under the name Marinol, and its synthetic analog, nabilone (marketed

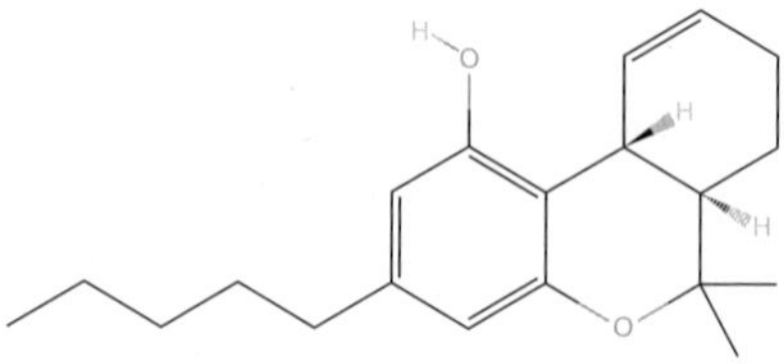

Figure 7.2
Cannabidiol (CBD).

Figure 7.3 Δ^9-Tetrahydrocannabinol (THC).

under the name Cesamet), received Food and Drug Administration (FDA) approval, and were used as medicines to suppress nausea and vomiting among patients undergoing chemotherapy and to improve the appetites of patients with HIV and acquired immune deficiency syndrome (AIDS).[2]

Soon after, CBD was shown to be effective as an anticonvulsant,[5] which corroborated claims from the 1940s that cannabis was an effective antiepileptic.[7] More recently, this has been corroborated by additional studies and anecdotal data.[8] Since then, a number of products have been developed and are available, perhaps most notably nabiximols (Sativex). This formulation was manufactured in the 2000s by GW Pharmaceuticals and consists of a 1:1 ratio of THC and CBD, as well as additional cannabinoid and noncannabinoid components. It has been shown to be effective at treating spasticity associated with multiple sclerosis.[9] Nabiximols has been approved for use in 25 countries and is currently undergoing phase III trials in the United States.[10] In 2018, a formulation that contains CBD as its sole active ingredients marketed under the name Epidiolex received approval from the FDA for the treatment of seizures associated with Lennox-Gastaut syndrome (LGS) and Dravet syndrome (DS).[11]

Besides FDA-approved medications like those mentioned above, there has been significant growth in the use of myriad preparations of cannabis that have not received FDA approval, though any product that contains more than 0.3% THC is still illegal at the federal level. Under federal law, hemp-derived preparations that contain <0.3% THC and high concentrations of CBD can be legally purchased, though states may place additional restrictions on the sale of these products. Many states have legalized the sale and distribution of medicinal cannabis for eligible patients as long as they obtain a *recommendation** from a medical professional and comply with any additional state laws. Some states have legalized the recreational and medicinal use of cannabis, thereby allowing individuals over the age of 21 to either grow their own cannabis or purchase cannabis

---

*Only FDA approved formulations containing cannabis extracts from marijuana-derived sources or synthetic cannabinoids can be prescribed by medical professionals. In states where medical cannabis programs have been implemented, medical professionals are allowed to recommended cannabis to patients. As most hemp-derived CBD formulations that contain no THC can now be purchased over the counter (formulations specially created to treat seizures excepted), it is not necessary for patients to obtain a prescription before purchasing these preparations.

products from a licensed distributor. For an overview of existing regulations, please see 5.10 in Chapter 5 (U.S. Cannabis Regulations From Past to Present). For a state-by-state list of qualifying conditions, please see Table 7.1 or consult this book's Web site: www.cannabistextbook.com.

In recent years, there has been growing interest in other cannabinoids, particularly CBN, CBG (Fig. 7.4), and CBC (Fig. 7.5). There has also been a spike in interest in how the numerous cannabinoids found within cannabis plants interact with the terpenic compounds and flavonoids that are also found in cannabis (for a partial listing of the most common terpenic compounds and flavonoids, see Chapter 4 [Constituents of Cannabis]). Apart from giving cannabis its unique smell, the terpenic compounds found in herbal cannabis may also contribute to what is known as the "entourage effect," wherein some of the therapeutic aspects of individual cannabinoids are augmented by their interaction with other cannabinoids and terpenoids.[65] There continues to be some controversy surrounding the subject, as the mechanisms that give rise to the entourage effect are not well understood, and a 2019 study that tested six of the most common terpenic compounds found in cannabis (α-pinene, β-pinene, α-caryophyllene, linalool, limonene, and β-myrcene) showed that none of them directly activated CB_1 or CB_2 receptors or modulated the effects of THC at receptors.[66] Apart from disputing the existence of the entourage effect, the paper contradicts other studies that show β-caryophyllene to be a CB_2 agonist.[67] Dr. Ethan B. Russo, an authority on the subject of the entourage effect, has characterized the study as being misleading, as he says that the mechanism of action behind the entourage effect is not restricted to the two cannabinoid receptors, and that the synergistic effects produced by terpenic compounds could arise due to their interaction with other receptors in the body.[68] More will be said about the entourage effect in Chapter 8 (The Pharmacodynamics of Cannabis).

Research into the potential therapeutic uses of lesser known cannabinoids and additional constituents like terpenes and terpenoids is ongoing, and, at this time, there are only limited data on their absorption, distribution, and metabolism in the body. Consequently, this chapter will focus on the two most common cannabinoids, THC and CBD.

(text continues on page 201)

TABLE 7.1 Qualifying Conditions by State and Territory

State/Territory	THC Limit	Flower or Extract	Conditions
Alabama	3%	Extract only	Cachexia, severe or chronic pain, severe nausea, seizures, severe and persistent muscle spasms, and any other condition that is severe and resistant to conventional medicine.[12]
Alaska	No	Both	Cancer, glaucoma, HIV/AIDS cachexia, severe pain, severe nausea, seizures, muscle spasms, and multiple sclerosis.[13]
American Samoa	0%	Neither	CBD and THC are both illegal in American Samoa.[14]
Arizona	No	Both	HIV/AIDs, Alzheimer disease, amyotrophic lateral sclerosis (ALS), cancer, Crohn disease, glaucoma, hepatitis C, posttraumatic stress disorder, or to alleviate symptoms such as cachexia, nausea, seizures, severe and chronic pain, and severe or persistent muscle spasms.[15]
Arkansas	No	Both	ALS, Alzheimer disease, cachexia, cancer, chronic or debilitating disease, Crohn disease, fibromyalgia, glaucoma, hepatitis C, HIV/AIDS, intractable pain, MS, peripheral neuropathy, PTSD, seizures, severe arthritis, severe nausea, severe and persistent muscle spasms, Tourette syndrome, and ulcerative colitis. Additional conditions may qualify, subject to approval by the Department of Health.[16]
California	No	Both	Any debilitating illness where cannabis has been deemed appropriate and recommended by a physician. Specific examples include anorexia, arthritis, cachexia, cancer, chronic pain, HIV/AIDS, glaucoma, migraines, nausea, persistent muscle spasms, and seizures.[17]

(Continued)

TABLE 7.1 Continued

State/Territory	THC Limit	Flower or Extract	Conditions
Colorado	No	Both	Debilitating medical conditions: cachexia, cancer, chronic pain, chronic nervous system disorders, glaucoma, HIV/AIDS, nausea, persistent muscle spasms, and seizures. Disabling medical conditions: autism spectrum disorder, PTSD, and any condition for which a physician could provide an opioid.[18]
Connecticut	No	Both	ALS, cachexia, cancer, cerebral palsy, chronic neuropathic pain, complex regional pain syndrome, Crohn disease, cystic fibrosis, epilepsy, glaucoma, hydrocephalus, HIV/AIDS, interstitial cystitis, intractable headache syndromes, irreversible spinal cord injury, medial arcuate ligament syndrome (MALS), MS, muscular dystrophy, neuropathic pain, osteogenesis imperfecta, Parkinson disease, neuralgia, persistent muscle spasms, postlaminectomy syndrome, PTSD, severe psoriasis and psoriatic arthritis, rheumatoid arthritis, sickle cell disease, Tourette syndrome, ulcerative colitis, vulvodynia, and other medical conditions pending approval by the Department of Consumer Protection.[19]
Delaware	18+: No Minors: 7%	Both	Alzheimer disease, ALS, cachexia, cancer, chronic pain, cirrhosis, epilepsy, glaucoma, HIV/AIDS, migraine, MS, nausea, PTSD, seizures, persistent muscle spasms, or any debilitating condition as determined by a physician.[20]
District of Columbia	No	Both	Attending physician's discretion.[21]

Florida	No	Both	ALS, cancer, Crohn disease, chronic pain due to a qualifying medical condition, epilepsy, glaucoma, HIV/AIDS, MS, Parkinson disease, PTSD, seizures, terminal illnesses (<12 mo to live), and other debilitating diseases.[22]
Georgia	5%	Extract only	AIDS, autism spectrum disorder, Alzheimer disease, ALS, autism, cancer, Crohn disease, epidermolysis bullosa, intractable pain, mitochondrial disease, MS, Parkinson disease, PTSD, severe or end-stage peripheral neuropathy, seizures, sickle cell disease, and Tourette syndrome. Patients in hospice care may also qualify.[23]
Guam	No	Both	Cancer, epilepsy, glaucoma, HIV/AIDS, MS, PTSD, rheumatoid arthritis, spinal cord injury, and any condition for which the patient's physician may feel medical cannabis may relief.[24]
Hawaii	No	Both	ALS, cachexia, cancer, chronic pain, Crohn disease, epilepsy, glaucoma, HIV/AIDS, lupus, MS, nausea, persistent muscle spasms, PTSD, rheumatoid arthritis, and seizures.[25]
Idaho	0%	Neither	There is no medical cannabis program of any kind in Idaho.[26]

(Continued)

TABLE 7.1 Continued

State/Territory	THC Limit	Flower or Extract	Conditions
Illinois	No	Both	Autism, Alzheimer disease, HIV/AIDS, ALS, anorexia nervosa, Arnold-Chiari malformation, cancer; cachexia/wasting syndrome, causalgia, chronic inflammatory demyelinating polyneuropathy, chronic pain, Crohn disease, CRPS (complex regional pain syndrome type II), dystonia, Ehlers-Danlos syndrome, epilepsy, fibrous dysplasia, glaucoma, hepatitis C, hydrocephalus, hydromyelia, interstitial cystitis, inflammatory bowel disease (IBD), lupus, migraines, MS, muscular dystrophy, myasthenia gravis, myoclonus, nail-patella syndrome, neuro-Behcet autoimmune disease, neurofibromatosis, neuropathy, osteoarthritis, Parkinson disease, polycystic kidney disease (PKD), postconcussion syndrome, PTSD, reflex sympathetic dystrophy, residual limb pain, rheumatoid arthritis, seizures, severe fibromyalgia, Sjögren syndrome, spinal cord diseases, spinal cord injuries, spinocerebellar ataxia, superior canal dehiscence syndrome, syringomyelia, Tarlov cysts, Tourette syndrome, traumatic brain injury, and ulcerative colitis.[27]
Indiana	0.3%	N/A	At this time, only patients with treatment-resistant epileptic conditions, such as Dravet syndrome and Lennox-Gastaut syndrome, qualify for low-THC, high-CBD preparations.[28]
Iowa	3%	Extract only	ALS, autism spectrum disorder; cachexia, cancer; chronic pain, Crohn disease, epilepsy, MS, cancer-related nausea, Parkinson disease, terminal illnesses, and ulcerative colitis.[29]
Kansas	5%	Extract only	A debilitating medical condition causing serious impairment, including one that produces seizures, for which the patient is under current and active treatment by an MD or DO licensed to practice in the state of Kansas.[30]

Kentucky	Not defined	N/A	Individuals participating in a clinical trial or expanded access program through a hospital or associated clinic affiliated with a public university in Kentucky that has a college or school of medicine.[31]
Louisiana	No	Extract only	Cachexia, cancer, Crohn disease, epilepsy, glaucoma, HIV/AIDS, intractable pain, MS, muscular dystrophy, Parkinson disease, PTSD, seizure disorders, and spasticity. Additionally, some symptoms associated with autism spectrum disorder may qualify.[32]
Maine	No	Both	Attending physician's discretion.[33]
Maryland	No	Both	Anorexia, cachexia or wasting syndrome, chronic pain, glaucoma, PTSD, seizures, severe nausea, severe or persistent muscle spasms, or other conditions that have been severe and for which other treatments have proven ineffective.[34]
Massachusetts	No	Both	ALS, cancer, Crohn disease, glaucoma, HIV/AIDS, hepatitis C, MS, Parkinson disease, or for other conditions to be determined in writing by a qualifying physician.[35]
Michigan	No	Both	Alzheimer disease, ALS, arthritis, autism spectrum disorder, cachexia, cancer, cerebral palsy, colitis, chronic pain, Crohn disease, glaucoma, HIV/AIDS, IBD, hepatitis C, nail-patella, nausea, obsessive-compulsive disorder (OCD), Parkinson disease, PTSD, seizures, severe and persistent muscle spasms, spinal cord injury, Tourette syndrome, and ulcerative colitis.[36]

(Continued)

TABLE 7.1 Continued

State/Territory	THC Limit	Flower or Extract	Conditions
Minnesota	No	Extract only	ALS, cancer, cachexia, Crohn disease, glaucoma, HIV/AIDS, MS, nausea or severe vomiting, seizures, severe and persistent muscle spasms, severe or chronic pain, Tourette syndrome, and terminal illnesses with a probable life expectancy of <1 y, provided the treatment produces cachexia, chronic pain, and nausea.[37]
Mississippi	0.5%	Extract only	Epilepsy and seizures.[38]
Missouri	No	Both	ALS, Alzheimer disease, autism spectrum disorder; cachexia, cancer; Crohn disease, chronic pain or neuropathy, epilepsy, glaucoma, hepatitis C, HIV/AIDS, Huntington disease, IBD, intractable migraines, MS, opioid substitution, Parkinson disease, PTSD or other debilitating psychiatric disorders, Tourette syndrome, sickle cell anemia, seizures, symptoms or conditions associated with any terminal illness, and any chronic, debilitating medical condition that may be ameliorated in the professional judgment of the physician.[39]
Montana	No	Both	Cachexia, cancer, Crohn disease, epilepsy, glaucoma, HIV/AIDS, intractable nausea or vomiting, peripheral neuropathy, PTSD, severe and chronic pain, severe and persistent muscle spasms, and admittance into hospice care in accordance with hospice rules.[40]
Nebraska	0%	Neither	There is no medical cannabis program of any kind in Nebraska, but no regulations explicitly contradicting federal law, which would suggest that CBD is legal so long as it complies with federal law. It is not clear if this is the case at this time, as state officials have made claims to the contrary.

State			
Nevada	No	Both	Anorexia, anxiety, autism spectrum disorder, autoimmune disorders, AIDS/HIV, cachexia, cancer, chronic pain, glaucoma, opioid dependency, muscle spasms, neuropathic conditions, PTSD, seizures, severe nausea or pain, or other conditions subject to approval.[41]
New Hampshire	No	Both	ALS, Alzheimer disease, cachexia, cancer, chemotherapy-induced anorexia, chronic pain, chronic pancreatitis, Crohn disease, Ehlers-Danlos syndrome, elevated intraocular pressure, epilepsy, glaucoma, hepatitis C, HIV/AIDS, lupus, MS, muscular dystrophy, nausea or vomiting, Parkinson disease, persistent muscle spasms, PTSD, seizures, severe pain, spinal cord injury or disease, and traumatic brain injury or disease.[42]
New Jersey	No	Both	ALS, anxiety, cancer, chronic pain, Crohn disease, dysmenorrhea, epilepsy, glaucoma, HIV/AIDS, IBD, migraines, MS, muscular dystrophy, opioid dependency, PTSD, seizure disorders, spasticity disorders, Tourette disorder, and any terminal illness if a physician has determined that the patient has less than a year to live.[43]
New Mexico	No	Both	ALS, Alzheimer disease, anorexia, arthritis, autism spectrum disorder, cancer, cachexia, Crohn disease, epilepsy, Friedrich ataxia, glaucoma, hepatitis C, HIV/AIDs, hospice care, Huntington disease, inclusion body myositis, intractable nausea/vomiting, Lewy body disease (LBD), MS, obstructive sleep apnea, opioid use disorder; peripheral neuropathy, Parkinson disease, PTSD, severe chronic pain, spasmodic torticollis, spinal cord injury, spinal muscular atrophy, and ulcerative colitis.[44]
New York	No	Extract and nonsmokable forms of flower cannabis	ALS, cancer, chronic pain, epilepsy, HIV/AIDS, Huntington disease, IBD, Parkinson disease, PTSD, MS, neuropathies, opioid substitution, and spinal cord damage.[45]

(Continued)

TABLE 7.1 Continued

State/Territory	THC Limit	Flower or Extract	Conditions
North Carolina	0.9%	Extract	Intractable epilepsy.[46]
North Dakota	No	Both	Alzheimer disease, ALS, anorexia, arthritis, autism spectrum disorder, brain injury, bulimia, cachexia, cancer, chronic or debilitating disease, Crohn disease, Ehlers-Danlos syndrome, endometriosis, epilepsy, fibromyalgia, glaucoma, hepatitis C, HIV/AIDS, interstitial cystitis, intractable nausea, neuropathy, migraine, MS, PTSD, seizures, severe and persistent muscle spasms, severe debilitating pain, spinal injury, spinal stenosis, and Tourette syndrome.[47]
Northern Mariana Islands	No	Both	There is no medical cannabis program in the Northern Mariana Islands.
Ohio	No	Both	ALS, Alzheimer disease, cancer, chronic traumatic encephalopathy, Crohn disease, fibromyalgia, glaucoma, hepatitis C, HIV/AIDS, IBD, MS, chronic or intractable pain, Parkinson disease, PTSD, sickle cell anemia, spinal cord injury or disease, Tourette disease, traumatic brain injury, and ulcerative colitis.[48]
Oklahoma	No	Both	Attending physician's discretion.[49]
Oregon	No	Both	Alzheimer disease, cancer, glaucoma, HIV/AIDS, or treatment for a medical condition that produces cachexia, persistent muscle spasms, seizures, severe nausea, and severe pain.[50]

Pennsylvania	No	Extract and nonsmokable forms of flower cannabis	ALS, anxiety disorders, autism spectrum disorder; cancer; Crohn disease, dyskinetic/spastic movement disorder; epilepsy, glaucoma, HIV/AIDS, Huntington disease, IBD, MS, intractable pain, intractable seizures, intractable spasticity, MS, opioid dependency, neurodegenerative disorders, neuropathies, Parkinson disease, PTSD, sickle cell anemia, Tourette disease, and terminal illnesses.[51]
Puerto Rico	No	Extract and nonsmokable forms of flower cannabis	ALS, Alzheimer disease, anorexia, anxiety, arthritis, cancer; Crohn disease, epilepsy, fibromyalgia, hepatitis C, HIV/AIDS, or other diseases that cause cachexia, migraines, MS, Parkinson disease, PTSD, severe pain, or spinal cord injury.[52]
Rhode Island	No	Both	Alzheimer disease, autism spectrum disorder; cachexia, cancer; chronic pain, Crohn disease, glaucoma, hepatitis C, HIV/AIDs, nausea, persistent muscle spasms, PTSD, and seizures.[53]
South Carolina	0.9%	Extract	Forms of epilepsy including Dravet syndrome, Lennox-Gastaut syndrome, and refractory epilepsy.[54]
South Dakota	0%	Neither	There is no medical cannabis program of any kind in South Dakota, but no regulations explicitly contradicting federal law, which would suggest that CBD is legal so long as it complies with federal law. It is not clear if this is the case at this time, as state officials have made claims to the contrary.
Tennessee	0.9%	Extract	Intractable seizures.[55]
Texas	0.5%	Extract	ALS, autism spectrum disorder; incurable neurodegenerative disorders, intractable epilepsy, MS, seizure disorders, and terminal cancer.[56]

(Continued)

TABLE 7.1 Continued

State/Territory	THC Limit	Flower or Extract	Conditions
U.S. Virgin Islands	No	Both	Alzheimer disease, ALS, arthritis, cancer, Crohn disease, diabetes, epilepsy, hepatitis C, HIV/AIDS, Huntington disease, MS, neuropathy, Parkinson disease, PTSD, spinal cord injury, traumatic brain injury, or any condition that either requires hospice care or causes cachexia, nausea, seizures, or severe muscle spasms.[57]
Utah	0.3%	Extracts	Intractable epilepsy and individuals with terminal illnesses who have <6 mo to live.[58]
Vermont	No	Both	Cachexia, cancer, Crohn disease, glaucoma, HIV/AIDS, MS, Parkinson disease, PTSD, seizures, severe or chronic pain, severe nausea, and any patient receiving hospice care.[59]
Virginia	10%	Extract	Attending physician's discretion.[60]
Washington	No	Both	Cachexia, cancer, Crohn disease, glaucoma, hepatitis C, HIV/AIDS, intractable pain, muscle spasms, nausea, PTSD, seizures, traumatic brain injury, or "any terminal or debilitating condition."[61]
West Virginia	No	Extract	ALS, cancer, Crohn disease, HIV/AIDS, epilepsy, Huntington disease, intractable seizures, MS, neuropathies, Parkinson disease, PTSD, severe chronic or intractable pain, sickle cell anemia, spinal cord damage, and terminal illnesses.[62]
Wisconsin	0.3%	Extract	Attending physician's discretion.[63]
Wyoming	0.3%	Extract	Intractable epilepsy.[64]

7.3 Pharmacology of FDA-Approved Cannabis-Based Preparations

7.3.1 Dronabinol[69] (Marinol)

Description

The active ingredient in Marinol is dronabinol, a synthetic version of Δ^9-tetrahydrocannabinol, that has been chemically designated (6aR,10aR)-6a,7,8,10a-Tetrahydro-6,6,9-trimethyl-3-pentyl-6H-dibenzo[b,d]-pyran-1-ol. Dronabinol has an empirical formula of $C_{21}H_{30}O_2$ and a molecular weight of 314.46. Its chemical structure is shown in Figure 7.6.

Dronabinol is a resinous oil that is sticky at room temperature and is not soluble in water. Marinol is formulated in sesame oil and is dispensed in the form of a capsule.

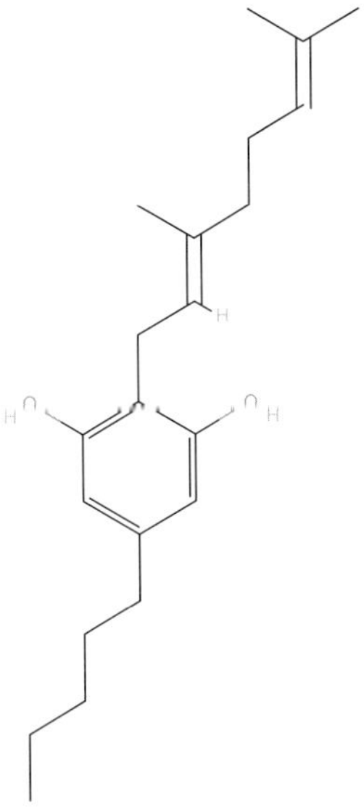

Pharmacological Action

Mechanism of Action

Figure 7.4 Cannabigerol (CBG).

Dronabinol has a complex set of effects on the central nervous system (CNS) via the ECS, particularly the CB$_1$ receptor. This subject will be explored in greater detail in Chapter 8 (The Pharmacodynamics of Cannabis).

Pharmacokinetics

Absorption

Between 90% and 95% of dronabinol is absorbed after a single oral dose, but only 10%-20% reaches systemic circulation due to a combination of first-pass hepatic metabolism and high lipid

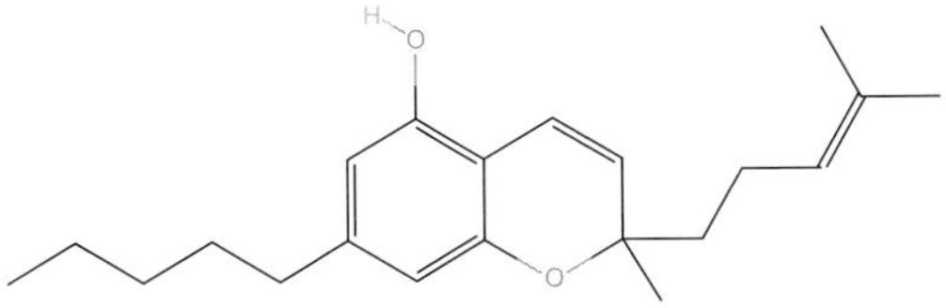

Figure 7.5 Cannabichromene (CBC).

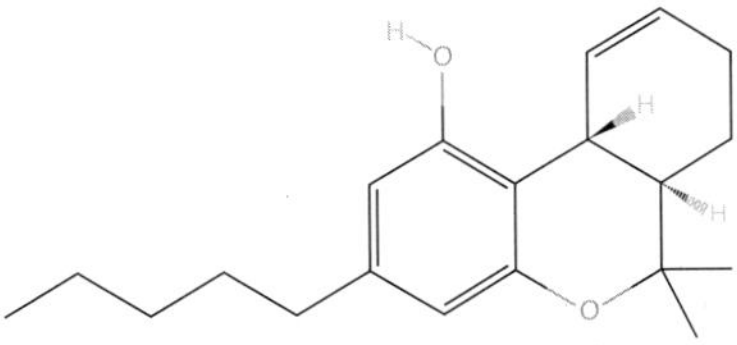

Figure 7.6 Dronabinol.

TABLE 7.2 Mean PK Parameter Values for Dronabinol in Healthy Subjects (*n* = 34; 20-45 years; fasted)

Twice Daily Dose	C_{max} ng/mL	Median T_{max} h (range)	$AUC_{(0-12)}$ ng•h/mL
2.5 mg	1.32 (0.62)	1.00 (0.50-4.00)	2.88 (1.57)
5 mg	2.96 (1.81)	2.50 (0.50-4.00)	6.16 (1.85)
10 mg	7.88 (4.54)	1.50 (0.50-3.50)	15.2 (5.52)

solubility. Concentrations of dronabinol and its major active metabolite, 11-hydroxy-Δ9-tetrahydrocannabinol (11-OH-THC), peak between 0.5 and 4 hours and decline over the course of several days. Plasma concentrations are dose dependent; for details, please refer to Table 7.2. For a comparison of pharmacokinetic data between dronabinol and nabilone, see Table 7.3.

TABLE 7.3 Pharmacokinetic Data for Dronabinol and Nabilone

Preparation (dosage)	Dronabinol (5 mg)	Nabilone (2 mg)
Absorption	90%-95%	100%
Bioavailability	N/A	N/A
Volume of distribution	10 L/kg	12.5 L/kg
Peak plasma concentration (C_{max})	0.62 ng/mL	2 ng/mL
Median time to peak plasma (T_{max})	1.00 h (range: 0.5-4.0 h)	2 h
Initial half-life	4 h	2 h
Terminal half-life	25-36 h	35 h
Plasma clearance	0.2 L/kg-h	N/A
Onset of action	0.5-1 h	1-1.5 h[a]
Duration of action	4-6 h[a]	8-12 h[a]

[a]Additional data obtained from Davis M, Malda V, Daeninck P, Pergolizzi J. The emerging role of cannabinoid neuromodulators in symptom management. *Support Care Cancer*. 2007;15(1):63-71. doi: 10.1007/s00520-006-0180-0.

Food intake, particularly a high-fat/high-calorie meal, delays absorption by about 4 hours and causes a 3-fold increase in total exposure (AUC_{inf}).

Distribution and Bioavailability

Dronabinol has a high protein binding of 97% with apparent volume of distribution of ~10 L/kg. The bioavailability of dronabinol is not available at this time, and a discussion on the bioavailability of orally administrated THC will be discussed below.

Elimination

The initial half-life of dronabinol is ~4 hours, and the terminal half-life ranges from 25 to 36 hours. Additionally, the plasma clearance is highly variable due to complexity of cannabinoid distribution and metabolism.

Metabolism

Dronabinol undergoes extensive first-pass hepatic metabolism, with CYP2C9 and CYP3A4 being the primary enzymes. A more detailed discussion of the metabolism of THC will follow below.

Excretion

Dronabinol and its metabolites are excreted in both feces and urine, though biliary excretion is the primary route of elimination.

Low levels of dronabinol metabolites may continue to be excreted in urine and feces for long periods of time, with reported metabolites still detectable for upward of 5 weeks.

Pharmacodynamics

The onset of action of dronabinol is ~0.5-1 hours, with peak subjective effects occurring within 2-4 hours, though psychoactive effects typically abate after 4-6 hours. Dronabinol may stimulate appetite for up to 24 hours after administration.

Dronabinol may produce many of the effects associated with THC and may impact mood, cognition, memory, and perception. Such effects are dose dependent with a great deal of interpatient variability. Dronabinol may affect the cardiovascular system, resulting in tachycardia or orthostatic hypotension, and syncope has been reported.

Tachyphylaxis and tolerance to some of the pharmacological effects develop with chronic use. Patients may develop a tolerance to the cardiovascular and CNS effects of dronabinol, and the initial tachycardia may be replaced by normal sinus rhythm followed by bradycardia.

Of note, tachyphylaxis and tolerance do not develop with regard to the appetite stimulant effect.

Therapeutic Indications

There are two indications for dronabinol:

1. Anorexia associated with weight loss in patients with AIDS.
2. Nausea and vomiting associated with cancer chemotherapy in patients who have failed to respond to other antiemetic treatments.

Off-Label Uses

Based on data from a phase II trial, dronabinol has been found to have therapeutic value in moderate to severe obstructive sleep apnea though more studies are required to validate this finding.[70]

Dosage and Administration

Dronabinol marketed under the name Marinol is administered orally and is available as a soft, round gelatin capsule in 2.5, 5, and 10 mg doses. It is also available as oral solution in 5 mg/mL dose. The dosing strategy for the two main indications is described below.

Anorexia Associated With Weight Loss in Patients With AIDS

The recommended starting dosage of dronabinol is 2.5 mg twice daily, preferably 1 hour before lunch and dinner. For patients who are unable to tolerate 2.5 mg twice daily, an initiating dose of 2.5 mg once daily an hour before dinner or bedtime is recommended.

If a dose higher than 5 mg/d is warranted, a gradual increase by 2.5 mg in a stepwise manner once a day to a maximum dose of 10 mg twice a day is recommended.

Nausea and Vomiting Associated With Chemotherapy

For patients who are experiencing nausea and vomiting associated with chemotherapy and are also unresponsive to other antiemetic treatments, the recommended starting dose of dronabinol is 5 mg/m^2 1-3 hours before chemotherapy, and repeating every 2-4 hours following chemotherapy, for a total of 4-6 doses per day. For patients unable to tolerate a high dosage due to adverse CNS effects, consider an initiating dose of 2.5 mg/m^2 mg once daily 1-3 hours prior to chemotherapy. In both instances, the first (or only) dose should be administered at least 30 m prior to eating or on an empty stomach. Doses later in the day can be taken without regard to meals.

Dosage can be titrated as tolerated to achieve therapeutic effects in increments of 2.5 mg/m². Note that adverse reactions are dose related and that the subjective effects of dronabinol increase significantly as one approaches the maximum dose. The maximum dose is 15 mg/m² and can be administered 4-6 times per day.

Obstructive Sleep Apnea, Moderate to Severe (Off-Label Use)

The recommended starting does is 2.5 mg before bedtime and gradual titration to a maximum of 10 mg may be necessary, but dose escalation in increments of 2.5-5 mg every week is required.

Adverse Reactions

Dronabinol has significant effects on CNS, especially in elderly patients who may show increased susceptibility to the psychoactive effects of the drug. The most commonly reported adverse in patients who received dronabinol for AIDS-related weight loss and for nausea and vomiting related to cancer chemotherapy can be found in Table 7.4. The most frequently reported adverse experiences involved the CNS, especially during the first 2 weeks of use.

The most commonly reported adverse reactions were euphoria, confusion, fast heartbeat (tachycardia), severe dizziness, nausea, and vomiting. Additional adverse reactions include

- General: Fatigue.
- Hypersensitivity reactions: Burning sensation on the skin, flushing, hives, oral lesions, rash, swollen lips, and throat tightness. (See Contraindications below.)
- Injury: Fall. (See Specific Populations below.)

TABLE 7.4 Adverse Reactions to Dronabinol

Rate of Incidence 3%-10%	Rate of Incidence 1%-3%	Rate of Incidence >1%
• Abnormal thinking	• Asthenia	• Conjunctivitis
• Abdominal pain	• Amnesia	• Depression
• Dizziness	• Anxiety	• Diarrhea
• Euphoria	• Ataxia	• Fecal incontinence
• Nausea	• Confusion	• Flushing
• Paranoia	• Depersonalization	• Hypotension
• Somnolence	• Hallucination	• Myalgia
• Vomiting		• Nightmares
		• Speech difficulties
		• Tinnitus
		• Vision difficulties

- Nervous system: Disorientation, loss of consciousness, movement disorder, and seizures. (See Warnings and Precautions below.)
- Psychiatric disorders: Delirium, insomnia, panic attack.
- Vascular disorders: Syncope. (See Warnings and Precautions below.)

Drug Interactions

Dronabinol is metabolized by CYP2C9 and CYP3A4 isoenzymes, and inhibition of either CYP will result in higher plasma concentrations of dronabinol and increase the probability of adverse reactions. Conversely, inducers of CYP2C9 and CYP3A4 may lower dronabinol plasma concentration. Clinicians may need to adjust dosages when coadministered with an inhibitor or inducer of either isoenzyme.

Additive CNS Effects

When administered concomitantly with drugs that have a similar effect on the CNS, such as CNS depressants (eg, antihistamines, barbiturates, benzodiazepines, buspirone, ethanol, lithium, muscle relaxants, opioids, scopolamine, tricyclic antidepressants, other anticholinergic agents), additive CNS effects such as confusion, sedation, or dizziness may occur.

Additive Cardiovascular Effects

When administered concomitantly with drugs that have a similar effect on the cardiovascular system (eg, amphetamines, anticholinergic agents, antihistamines, tricyclic antidepressants, atropine, scopolamine, sympathomimetic agents), additive effects such as hypotension, hypertension, syncope, and tachycardia may occur.

Highly Protein-Bound Drugs

Dronabinol is highly protein bound and may displace and increase the free portion of other highly protein-bound drugs (eg, warfarin, cyclosporine, amphotericin B) that have been administered concomitantly. Clinicians should monitor patients for potential adverse effects when initiating treatment or increasing dosages of dronabinol.

Contraindications

Dronabinol is contraindicated in patients who have a history of hypersensitivity to dronabinol or sesame oil. Reported hypersensitivity reactions include a burning sensation in the skin, flushing, hives, oral lesions, rash, swollen lips, and throat tightness.

Warnings and Precautions

Psychiatric Adverse Reactions

Dronabinol may exacerbate existing psychiatric conditions such as schizophrenia, bipolar disorder, and depression. Clinicians should screen patients for existing psychiatric conditions before initiating treatment with dronabinol and use of the drug should be avoided in patients with a history of mental illness. If use of the drug cannot be avoided, clinicians should monitor patients for new or worsening symptoms. Additionally, clinicians should avoid concomitant use of dronabinol with other drugs associated with similar psychiatric effects.

Cognitive Adverse Reactions

Dronabinol has been associated with cognitive impairment and may produce an altered mental state. If symptoms or signs of cognitive impairment develop, reduce the dosage or discontinue the use of dronabinol.

Hazardous Activities

Dronabinol can drastically reduce one's ability to operate heavy machinery or to drive a motor vehicle, and it is highly recommended that patients avoid these activities while taking dronabinol.

Hemodynamic Instability

As noted above, patients on dronabinol may experience hypotension, hypertension, syncope, or tachycardia, and patients with existing cardiac disorders may be at a higher risk for these adverse effects. Additionally, drugs with similar effect on the cardiovascular system (eg, amphetamines, anticholinergic agents, antihistamines, tricyclic antidepressants, atropine, scopolamine, sympathomimetic agents) may result in additive effects and should consequently be avoided if possible. When first administering or adjusting dosages of dronabinol, clinicians should monitor patients for changes in blood pressure, heart rate, and incidence of syncope.

Seizures

Some patients have reported incidents of seizure and seizure-like activity following administration of dronabinol. Clinicians should consider patients' previous histories of seizures, including those who have received antiepileptic medications, before prescribing dronabinol, and should monitor these patients for increased frequency or severity of seizure after treatment with dronabinol has begun. If patients with no history of seizures experience a seizure following the administration of dronabinol, clinicians should discontinue use.

Multiple Substance Abuse

Patients may potentially abuse dronabinol, especially if they have a history of abusing substances like cannabis or alcohol. Clinicians should assess the potential for abuse prior to prescribing dronabinol and monitor those who have a history of abuse.

Paradoxical Nausea, Vomiting, or Abdominal Pain

Dronabinol may cause some patients to experience nausea, vomiting, or abdominal pain, and in rare cases, this may lead to severe adverse reactions such as dehydration and electrolyte abnormalities. These symptoms are akin to cannabinoid hyperemesis syndrome, which is typically observed in chronic cannabis users.

Patients who are being treated for nausea may not immediately recognize these adverse effects as abnormal, so it is important to explicitly tell patients or their caregivers to report any worsening nausea, vomiting, or abdominal pain after treatment with dronabinol has begun. If patients do experience these adverse reactions while taking dronabinol, clinicians should consider a reduction in dosage or the discontinuation of the drug.

Specific Populations

Pregnant Women

There is limited information on the effects of synthetic cannabinoids like dronabinol during pregnancy, though the use of nonsynthetic cannabis has been associated with adverse fetal/neonatal outcomes. Consequently, pregnant women should not be prescribed or take dronabinol.

Nursing Women

There are not adequate data on the risks associated with the use of synthetic cannabinoids like dronabinol while breast-feeding, but there is a potential for adverse effects. Consequently, women should not breast-feed during treatment with dronabinol or for 9 days after last dose.

Pediatric Use

The safety and efficacy of dronabinol has not been established for pediatric patients.

Geriatric Use

The antiemetic effects of dronabinol are no different in younger patients than patients over the age of 55, but elderly patients may be more sensitive to the psychotropic and cardiovascular effects of dronabinol. Additionally, elderly patients with dementia may experience exacerbated CNS effects of somnolence or dizziness, thereby increasing the risk of injury from a fall.

Clinicians should be advised to exercise caution with dose selection and to opt for a lower dosing range when initiating treatment.

Effect of CYP2C9 Polymorphism

CYP2C9 genetic polymorphism may diminish the systemic clearance of dronabinol and increase plasma concentrations. It is recommended that clinicians monitor patients known to carry genetic variants associated with reduced CYP2C9 function for increased adverse reactions.

Abuse and Dependence

Dronabinol is a Schedule III drug and may pose a potential risk of abuse, though this risk may be quite low. In an open-label study lasting 5 months, no instances of abuse, diversion, or systematic change in personality or social functioning were observed in patients with AIDS who received dronabinol. Still, patients should be aware that there is a risk of abuse and should also be advised to keep dronabinol in a secure location to avoid use by individuals for whom the drug has not been prescribed.

Continued administration of dronabinol may lead to dependency or addiction. Withdrawal syndromes were reported upon discontinuation in patients who had received 210 mg/d for 12-16 consecutive days. Symptoms appeared within 12 hours of discontinuation and included irritability, insomnia, and restlessness. Twenty-four hours after discontinuation, withdrawal symptoms worsened, with patients describing periods of "hot flashes," hiccoughs, loose stools, loss of appetite, rhinorrhea, and sweating. Most symptoms dissipated after 48 hours of discontinuation, though some patients reported sleep disturbances for several weeks following treatment.

7.3.2 Nabilone[71] (Cesamet)

Description

The active ingredient in Cesamet is nabilone, a synthetic cannabinoid that is similar to Δ^9-tetrahydrocannabinol, which has been chemically designated (±)-*trans*-3-(1,1-dimethylheptyl)-6,6a,7,8,10,10a-hexahydro-1-hydroxy-6-6-dimethyl-9*H*-dibenzo[b,d]pyran-9-one. Nabilone has an empirical formula of $C_{24}H_{36}O_3$ and a molecular weight of 372.55. Its chemical structure is shown in Figure 7.7.

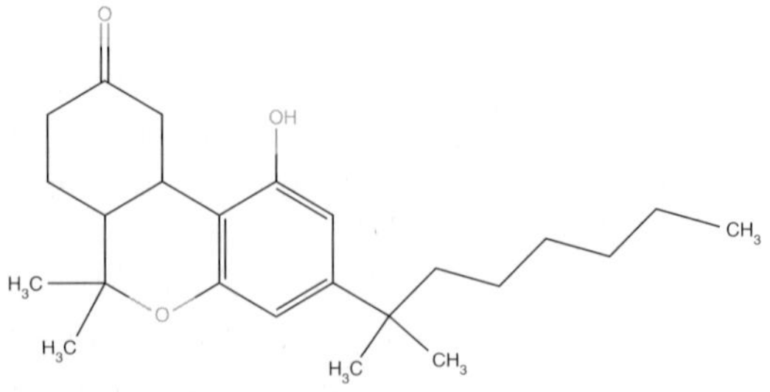

Figure 7.7 Nabilone.

Nabilone is a white or whitish polymorphic crystalline powder with low water solubility (>0.5 mg/L) and a pH value ranging from 1.2 to 7.

Cesamet capsules contain 1 mg of nabilone.

Pharmacological Action

Mechanism of Action

Nabilone has a complex set of effects on the CNS via the ECS, particularly the CB_1 receptor.

Pharmacokinetics—Distribution, Bioavailability, Elimination, and Excretion

Nabilone is completely absorbed in the gastrointestinal tract with peak plasma concentrations of 2 ng/mL reached within 2.0 hours, and the bioavailability is not available at this time. It has an apparent volume of distribution of ~12.5 L/kg with a plasma half-life between 2 and 35 hours and food intake did not significantly alter the rate of absorption. Within 7 days of oral or intravenous administration of nabilone, ~60%-70% is excreted in feces while 20%-25% is eliminated through the urine.

Metabolism

The precise information regarding the metabolism of nabilone and the accumulation of its metabolites is not currently available, though available evidence suggests that at least one nabilone metabolite has a terminal elimination half-life that exceeds that of the parent compound.

At least two metabolic pathways associated with the biotransformation of nabilone have been confirmed, and two metabolites have been identified. Like other cannabinoids, cytochrome P450 enzyme isoforms play a major in its metabolism.

Nabilone has not been shown to significantly inhibit CYP1A2, CYP2A6, CYP2C19, CYP2D6, or CYP3A4; had a weak inhibitory effect on CYP2E1 and CYP3A4; and had a moderate inhibitory effect on CYP2C8 and CYP2C9. Of note, when coadministered with other drugs, nabilone is unlikely to interfere with P450-mediated degradation.

Pharmacodynamics

Nabilone may produce many of the subjective effects associated with THC, thereby impacting patients' mood, perception, memory, and ability to control impulses. Like THC, higher doses tend to result in more pronounced effects, but even doses within the lower therapeutic range may produce substantial subjective effects, particularly among patients who have limited experience with cannabis. Tolerance to these effects develops quickly and can be reversed with cessation.

In addition to CNS effects, nabilone has effects on the cardiovascular system including increased supine and standing heart rate, as well as orthostatic hypotension. It may also cause an extremely mild decrease in airway resistance, but no effects have been observed in patients with asthma.

Therapeutic Indications

Nabilone is indicated for nausea and vomiting associated with cancer chemotherapy in patients who have failed to respond to other antiemetic treatments.

Dosage and Administration

Nabilone marketed under the name Cesamet is administered orally and is available in capsule formulation containing 1 mg of nabilone.

Treatment with 1 or 2 mg of nabilone may be administered 2 or 3 times daily during each cycle of chemotherapy. Clinicians should begin low when initiating treatment and only increase as necessary. Nabilone can be administered either 1-3 hours prior to chemotherapy or taken the night before with the maximum daily dose of 6 mg/d administered in three divided doses (tid).

If necessary, nabilone may be administered up to 48 hours following the last dose of each cycle of chemotherapy.

Adverse Reactions

The most common adverse effects include drowsiness, vertigo, dry mouth, euphoria, ataxia, headache, and difficulty concentrating. Less common adverse reactions are listed in Table 7.5.

TABLE 7.5 Adverse Reactions to Nabilone

Rate of Incidence >10%	Rate of Incidence <10%
• Vertigo/dizziness	• Dysphoria
• Drowsiness	• Hypotension
• Dry mouth	• Asthenia
• Ataxia	• Anorexia
• Depression	• Headache
• Visual disturbance	• Nausea
• Difficulty concentrating	• Sedation
• Euphoria	• Disorientation
• Sleep disturbance	• Depersonalization
	• Increased appetite

Following the approval of nabilone, additional adverse reactions were reported. These reactions were reported voluntarily, and frequency of occurrence cannot be determined.

- Blood and hematopoietic: Leukopenia.
- Nervous system: CNS depression, CNS stimulation, stupor, and circumoral paresthesia.
- Psychiatric: Somnolence, psychosis, and emotional lability.
- Miscellaneous: Abnormal thinking, lack of feeling, and facial edema.

Drug Interactions

Nabilone is highly bound to plasma proteins and may displace other protein-bound drugs, so clinicians may need to adjust dosages of nabilone or coadministered medications and exercise caution when administering combinations of nabilone and any CNS depressant.

Published reports on the drug/drug interactions involving cannabinoids are summarized in Table 7.6.

Contraindications

Nabilone is contraindicated in patients who have a history of hypersensitivity to cannabinoids.

Warnings and Precautions

Nabilone has a high degree of interpatient variability, and patients should be supervised during initial use and following dose adjustments. Additionally, the effects of nabilone may persist for upward of 48-72 hours.

TABLE 7.6 Published Reports on Drug/Drug Interactions With Cannabinoids[72]

Coadministered Drug(s)	Clinical Effect(s)
Amphetamines, cocaine, other sympathomimetic agents	Additive hypotension, tachycardia, possibly cardiotoxicity
Atropine, scopolamine, antihistamines, other anticholinergic agents	Additive or super-additive tachycardia, drowsiness
Amitriptyline, amoxapine, desipramine, other tricyclic antidepressants	Additive tachycardia, hypertension, drowsiness
Barbiturates, benzodiazepines, ethanol, lithium, opioids, buspirone, antihistamines, muscle relaxants, other CNS depressants	Additive drowsiness and CNS depression
Antipyrine, barbiturates	Decreased clearance presumably due to competitive inhibition of metabolism
Theophylline	Increased theophylline metabolism
Opioids	Cross-tolerance and mutual potentiation
Naltrexone	THC effects were enhanced by opioid receptor blockade
Alcohol	Heightened subjective mood effects

As is the case with THC, nabilone can drastically reduce one's ability to operate heavy machinery or to drive a motor vehicle, and it is highly recommended that patients avoid these activities while taking nabilone.

Psychiatric Adverse Reactions

Nabilone may exacerbate existing psychiatric conditions such as schizophrenia, bipolar disorder, and depression. Clinicians should screen patients for existing psychiatric conditions before initiating treatment with nabilone, and use of the drug should be avoided in patients with a history of mental illness. If use of the drug cannot be avoided, clinicians should monitor patients for new or worsening symptoms. Additionally, clinicians should avoid concomitant use of nabilone with other drugs associated with similar psychiatric effects.

Additive Reactions With Sedatives, Hypnotics, and Other Psychoactive Drugs

Nabilone may affect the CNS, which may cause feelings of dizziness, drowsiness, euphoria, anxiety, ataxia, disorientation, depression, hallucinations, and even psychosis. It may also cause tachycardia and hypotension. Alcohol, hypnotics, sedatives, or other psychoactive substances may exacerbate some of these effects, and nabilone should be used with caution if patients are receiving these therapies.

Hepatic and Renal Impairment

The safety of prescribing nabilone to patients with hepatic or renal impairment has not been adequately studied.

Patients With Hypertension

Nabilone may elevate supine and standing heart rates and may also cause postural hypotension. Elderly patients or patients with existing cardiac disorders, particularly hypotension, may be at a higher risk for these adverse effects. When first administering or adjusting dosages of nabilone, clinicians should monitor patients for changes in blood pressure, heart rate, and incidence of syncope.

Multiple Substance Abuse

Patients may potentially abuse nabilone, which is a Schedule II drug, especially if they have a history of abusing substances like cannabis or alcohol. Clinicians should assess the potential for abuse prior to prescribing nabilone and monitor those who have a history of abuse.

Specific Populations

Pregnant Women

There is limited information on the effects of nabilone during pregnancy. Pregnant women should not be prescribed or take nabilone unless the benefit justifies the risk of potential harm to the fetus.

Nursing Women

There are no adequate data on the risks of breast-feeding, and consequently, it is not recommended that women breast-feed during treatment with nabilone.

Pediatric Use

The safety and efficacy of nabilone has not been established in patients under 18 years of age. Clinicians should exercise extreme caution in prescribing this medication to children due to its psychoactive effects.

Geriatric Use

Clinicians should exercise caution before prescribing nabilone to elderly patients, as they may be more sensitive to its psychotropic and cardiovascular effects.

Abuse and Dependence

Nabilone is a Schedule II drug, which means it has a high potential for abuse and dependence. Prescriptions should be limited to an amount corresponding to a single cycle of chemotherapy.

7.3.3 Cannabidiol[73] (Epidiolex)

Description

The active ingredient in Epidiolex is CBD, a phytocannabinoid that occurs naturally in *Cannabis sativa*. It has been chemically designed 2-[(1R,6R)-3-Methyl-6-(1-methylethenyl)-2-cyclohexen-1-yl]-5-pentyl-1,3-benzenediol (IUPAC/CAS). CBD has an empirical formula of $C_{21}H_{30}O_2$ and a molecular weight of 314.46. Its chemical structure is shown in Figure 7.2.

CBD is a white or pale yellow crystalline solid that is insoluble in water and soluble in organic solvents.

The Epidiolex (cannabidiol) solution is a clear, colorless to slightly yellow liquid that contains CBD at a concentration of 100 mg/mL.

Pharmacological Action

Mechanism of Action

The precise mechanism of action of CBD is unknown, and its anticonvulsant effects are not due to its interaction with cannabinoid receptors. It is likely that the anticonvulsant effects are due to the cumulative effects arising from the modulation of synaptic and extrasynaptic GABA channels and intracellular calcium in receptors such as GPR55, VDAC, and TPRV, as well as possible anti-inflammatory effects.

This subject will be explored in greater detail in Chapter 8 (The Pharmacodynamics of Cannabis).

Pharmacokinetics

In patients, CBD exhibits an increase in exposure that is less than dose proportional over the range of 5-20 mg/kg/d.

Absorption

Maximum plasma concentration (T_{max}) occurs between 2.5 and 5 hours, and food, particularly a high-fat/high-calorie meal, increases the C_{max} 5-fold and AUC_{inf} by 4-fold.

Distribution

In healthy volunteers, CBD and its metabolites exhibit *in vitro* protein binding >94%.

Bioavailability

The bioavailability of this preparation of CBD is not available at this time.

Elimination

The half-life of CBD in plasma is between 56 and 61 hours after twice a day dosing for 7 days, with a plasma clearance of 1111 L/h following a single dose 1.1 times the maximum recommended daily dosage of 1500 mg.

Metabolism

CBD is metabolized primarily by cytochrome P450 enzyme (CYP) system, specifically CYP2C19 and CYP3A4 enzymes, as well as UGT1A7, UGT1A9, and UGT2B7 isoforms.

Excretion

The majority of CBD is excreted through feces, with only minor renal clearance.

Pharmacodynamics

The precise pharmacodynamics of CBD is not known, though the anticonvulsant effects of the drug do not appear to be through direct interaction with endocannabinoid receptors. This subject will be explored in greater detail in Chapter 8 (The Pharmacodynamics of Cannabis).

Therapeutic Indications

CBD is indicated for the treatment of seizures associated with LGS and DS. This indication is based on two randomized, double-blind, placebo-controlled studies in 396 patients with LGS and a single randomized, double-blind, placebo-controlled trial in 120 patients with DS.

Dosage and Administration

CBD is marketed under the brand name Epidiolex. For this preparation, it is administered orally with a starting dosage of 2.5 mg/kg twice daily (total: 5 mg/kg/d). Following the initial period of 1 week, this can be increased to a maintenance dosage of 5 mg/kg twice daily (total: 10 mg/kg/d). For further seizure reduction, patients who tolerate the 5 mg/kg twice daily dosage may benefit from a dosage increase to the maximum recommended maintenance dosage of 10 mg/kg twice daily (total: 20 mg/kg/d), with weekly increments of 2.5 mg/kg twice daily (5 mg/kg/d). If deemed necessary, a more rapid titration from 10 to 20 mg/kg/d may be warranted, though dosage increases should occur no more frequently than every other day. It should be noted that 20 mg/kg/d dosages did reduce seizure rates at a level above the recommended daily dosage of 10 mg/kg/d, but there was a concomitant rise in adverse reactions.

Each bottle of Epidiolex contains 100 mL of solution. The solution should be administered with a calibrated measuring device such as a 5- or 1-mL oral syringe, and not a household teaspoon or tablespoon. Any solution remaining 12 weeks after opening should be disposed.

As is the case when discontinuing any antiepileptic drugs, dosages should be gradually reduced when discontinuing the use of CBD, as an abrupt cessation may risk an increase in seizure frequency.

Adverse Reactions

The discontinuation rate secondary to adverse reactions are dose proportional with 2.7% of patients taking 10 mg/kg/d of Epidiolex, 11.8% for those taking 20 mg/kg/d, and 1.3% for placebo. Transaminase elevation was the most common reason for discontinuation and occurred at a rate of 1.3% for patients receiving 10 mg/kg/d, 5.9% for patients receiving 20 mg/kg/d doses, and 0.4% of patients on placebo. The next most common reason for discontinuance was somnolence or lethargy, which was the reason for discontinuation among 3% of patients taking doses of 20 mg/kg/d, but 0% for patients taking either 10 mg/kg/d doses or the placebo. A listing of the most frequently observed adverse reactions are listed in Table 7.7.

TABLE 7.7 Adverse Reactions to Cannabidiol

Rate of Incidence ≥10% and Greater Than Placebo	Rate of Incidence ≥3% and Greater Than Placebo
• Decreased appetite • Diarrhea • Fatigue, malaise, asthenia • Infection • Insomnia, sleep disorder, poor sleep quality • Rash • Somnolence • Transaminase elevation	• Abdominal pain, discomfort • Aggression, anger • Decrease in weight • Drooling, salivary hypersecretion • Gait disturbance • Gastroenteritis • Hypoxia, respiratory failure • Irritability, agitation • Lethargy • Sedation

Decreased Weight

Weight loss was observed, particularly in patients who were given doses of 20 mg/kg/d. A total of 18% of patients given this dosage experienced weight loss of ≥5% from their baseline weight, while only 9% of patients on 10 mg/kg/d experienced similar weight loss. In total, 16% of patients saw a decrease in weight of ≥5% from their baseline weight, while only 8% patients who were given placebo experienced similar weight loss

Hematologic Abnormalities

Decreases in hemoglobin and hematocrit were observed in controlled studies of CBD, with the mean decrease in hemoglobin being −0.42 g/dL and in hematocrit of −1.5% from baseline to end of treatment, and 30% developed laboratory-defined anemia.

Increases in Creatine

CBD was observed to cause elevations in serum creatine, though the mechanisms behind the phenomenon are unclear. In controlled studies with LGS and DS patients, as well as healthy adults, serum creatine increased ~10% within 2 weeks of beginning the medication. The increase was reversible in healthy adults, but not assessed in patients with LGS and DS.

Drug Interactions

In the liver, CBD is metabolized by CYP3A4 and CYP2C19 isoenzymes, and consequently, inhibition of either CYP will result in higher plasma concentrations of CBD and increase the probability of adverse reactions. Conversely, inducers of CYP3A4 and CYP2C19 may lower the CBD plasma concentration. Clinicians may need to decrease or increase dosages of CBD when coadministered with an inhibitor or inducer of either isoenzyme.

Numerous other drug-drug interactions exist secondary to inhibition of other cytochrome P450 isoenzymes including CYP2C8 and CYP2C9 as well UGT1A9 and UGT2B7. Coadministration of substrates and potential inhibitions of enzyme activity by CBD may necessitate reducing dosages of these substrates.

Clobazam

Administration of CBD with clobazam, a benzodiazepine, results in a threefold increase in plasma concentrations of the active metabolite in clobazam (N-desmethylclobazam), which is a substrate of CYP2C19, and increases the risk of clobazam-related adverse reactions requiring a reduction in dosage of clobazam.

Valproate

Concomitant use of CBD with valproate increases the incidence of liver enzyme elevations, and a reduction or discontinuation of either CBD or valproate may be warranted. Insufficient data exist to fully assess the risks of coadministration of CBD and other hepatotoxic drugs.

Alcohol and Other CNS Depressants

The use of either alcohol or another CNS depressant concomitantly with CBD may increase the risk of sedation and somnolence.

Contraindications

CBD is contraindicated in patients who have a history of hypersensitivity to CBD, sesame oil, or any other ingredient in the medication.

Warnings and Precautions

Hepatocellular Injury

Dose-related elevations in liver transaminases (alanine aminotransferase [ALT] or aspartate aminotransferase [AST]) may occur with CBD and elevations of 3 times the upper limit of normal (ULN) without elevated bilirubin without an alternative explanation are potential indications of severe liver injury. Of note, these elevations occurred primarily early and within the first 2 months of treatment though there have been cases up to 18 months after initiation. Concomitant administration with valproate and clobazam may increase the risk of transaminase elevation and dose adjustment or discontinuation of valproate or clobazam may be necessary. A total of 17% of patients had transaminase elevations compared to 1% on placebo.

Baseline Measurement and Monitoring

Baseline transaminase levels are strong indicators of subsequent elevations. Higher dosage of 20 mg/kg/d in patients with baseline measurements above 3 times the ULN had more frequent (30%) treatment-emergent ALT elevations compared to 12% who had normal baseline transaminase levels. Of note, none of the patients taking lower dosage of 10 mg/kg/d had >3 times ALT elevations. These data suggest that clinicians should obtain baseline serum transaminases (ALT and AST) prior to initiation of CBD and subsequently be tested at 1, 3, and 6 months and as clinically indicated after the initiation of CBD.

Levels should also be obtained 1 month following any adjustment to dosage or introduction of medications known to impact liver function. Consider more frequent monitoring if the patient is taking valproate or clobazam, or if they have elevated liver enzymes at baseline.

In two-thirds of cases, liver transaminase levels returned to normal following either the discontinuance of CBD or a reduction in dosage. In one-third of cases, liver transaminase levels returned to normal without altering dosage.

Clinicians should be vigilant and monitor patients for signs and symptoms of liver dysfunction (nausea, jaundice, vomiting, fatigue, anorexia, etc.) and accordingly suspend or discontinue CBD treatment and measure serum transaminase and total bilirubin. CBD treatment should be discontinued in patients with elevations of liver transaminases 3 times the ULN or bilirubin levels >2 times the ULN, as well as in patients with elevations of liver transaminases 5 times the ULN.

Somnolence

As noted above, somnolence or sedation (with lethargy) is a common adverse effect of CBD and appears to be dose dependent, with 34% of patients who received 20 mg/kg/d reporting somnolence or sedation, compared to 27% of patients who received 10 mg/kg/d. Additionally, the rate of incidence was higher among patients who were also taking clobazam compared to those who were not.

Alcohol and other CNS depressants appear to increase incidence of somnolence or sedation and patients should not drive or operate heavy machinery until they know whether or not CBD affects their ability to do so.

Suicidal Behavior and Ideation

Antiepileptic drugs have been shown to increase the risk of suicidal thoughts or behaviors in patients taking these drugs. Before prescribing CBD or any other antiepileptic drug, clinicians must balance the risk of suicidal ideation or behaviors and the risks associated with the untreated illness.

Hypersensitivity Reactions

Patients with cannabis allergies may experience unpleasant symptoms like pruritus, erythema, and angioedema. If a patient develops hypersensitivity reactions to CBD, treatment should be discontinued.

Withdrawal of Antiepileptic Drugs

Like discontinuing any other antiepileptic drug, CBD should be gradually lowered and discontinued to minimize the risk of seizures. In case of a serious adverse event, rapid discontinuation can be considered.

Specific Populations

Pregnant Women

At this time, there are no adequate data on the development risks associated with the use of CBD in pregnant women.

Nursing Women

There are no adequate data on the risks associated with the use of CBD while breast-feeding.

Pediatric Use

CBD safety and efficacy for treatment of seizures in patients 2 years of age and older with LGS and DS has been established, though this has not been the case in patients younger than 2 years of age.

Geriatric Use

Dose selection for elderly patients should begin at the lower end of the dosing range due to the higher probability that the patient may have reduced hepatic, renal, or cardiac function.

Abuse and Dependence

Patients who were given two daily doses of 750 mg of CBD for 4 weeks did not show signs or symptoms of withdrawal over the 6-week period following drug discontinuation. Meanwhile, in a human abuse potential study, administration of CBD at doses of 750, 1500, and 4500 mg in the fasted state produced positive subjective measures within the accepted placebo range and significantly lower than small doses (10 or 30 mg) of dronabinol or 2 mg of alprazolam (a Schedule IV benzodiazepine marketed under the name Xanax). The results of these studies suggest that CBD does not produce physical dependence and that the risk of abuse is low.

7.4 Pharmacokinetics of Non–FDA-Approved Cannabis Preparations

In the majority of cultivars found in the United States, the most prevalent phytocannabinoids at harvest are Δ^9-tetrahydrocannabinolic acid-A (THCA-A) for drug-type cultivars or cannabidiolic acid (CBDA) for fiber-type cultivars. Raw cannabis that has been classified as marijuana (above 0.3% THC, per the 2018 Farm Bill) contains significantly more THCA-A than either the isomer Δ^9-tetrahydrocannabinolic acid-B (THCA-B) or CBDA.[74] Raw cannabis that has been classified as hemp (below 0.3% THC) contains significantly more CBDA (Fig. 7.8) than either

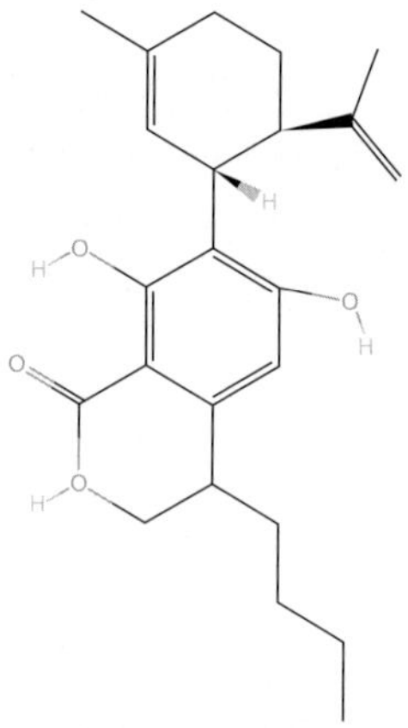

Figure 7.8 Cannabidiolic acid (CBDA).

THCA-A (Fig. 7.9) or THCA-B (Fig. 7.10). The cannabinoid acids CBDA, THCA-A, and THCA-B do not produce intoxicating effects.[75]

7.4.1 Decarboxylation

Cannabinoid acids are converted to THC or CBD following decarboxylation, which is a chemical reaction wherein carboxylic acid groups are removed from their parent compounds and carbon dioxide (CO_2) is released. Decarboxylation occurs when cannabis is introduced to heat or light, and THCA-A is particularly notorious for its instability.[74] When it is introduced to moderate heat or light,

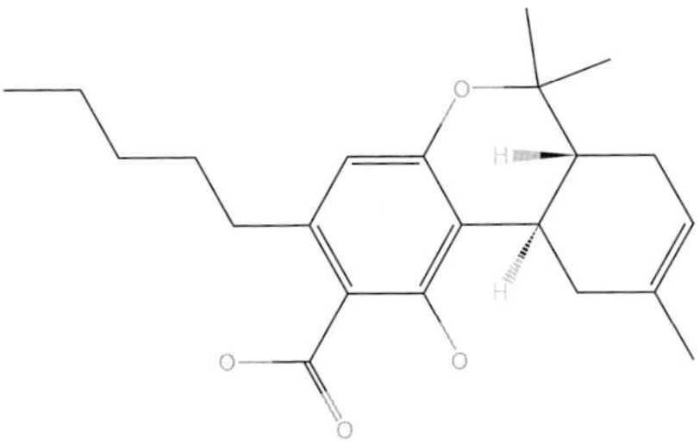

Figure 7.9 Δ^9-
Tetrahydrocannabinolic acid A
(THCA-A).

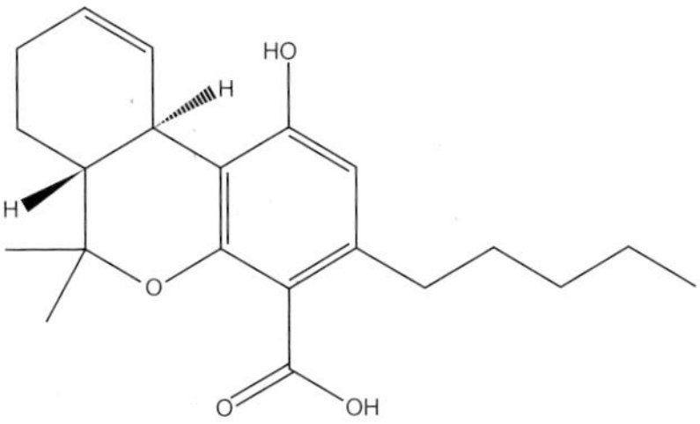

Figure 7.10 Δ^9-
Tetrahydrocannabinolic acid B
(THCA-B).

THCA-A undergoes decarboxylation, even when stored at room
temperature in solvents, as well as when stored in darkness and
at temperatures as low as $-18°C$.[76] Decarboxylation appears to be
less rapid in hashish or when cannabis is stored in its herbal or
raw state. Studies indicate that undisturbed terpenoid compounds
and glandular trichomes inhibit the oxidative decarboxylation of
THCA-A and remain mostly intact even when cannabis is processed
into hashish.[74] The range of Δ^9-THC acids to THC in leaves and
flowers of drug-type cannabis can range anywhere from 2:1 to 17:1,
while the same ratio in hashish has been reported to range from
6.1:1 to 0.5:1, and that hotter climates tend to produce cannabis
samples that have higher concentrations of THC in relation to
Δ^9-THC acids.[77] Less prevalent cannabinoids like CBG and CBC
also exist in acid form prior to decarboxylation, and CBN is formed
via the oxidation of THC and occurs in higher concentrations in
older cannabis.[78]

Almost all common routes of administration utilize some
means of decarboxylation to maximize THC or CBD levels.
Additionally, due to cannabinoids' limited solubility in water,
preparations are commonly made using vehicles such as alcohol or
various oils.

7.4.2 Routes of Administration and Absorption Overview

There are many routes of administration for cannabis with the
two most popular being inhalation and oral administration.
Less popular routes include sublingual, dermal, and rectal
administration. Juicing herbal cannabis has also become popular
with some groups.

Not all routes of administration produce the same therapeutic
or intoxicating effects in patients, and bioavailability and

absorption rates can vary widely depending on how cannabis is administered. The juice of raw, drug-type cannabis contains very low levels of THC and high levels of Δ^9-THC acids since the cannabis has not been decarboxylated. Conversely, oral administration may produce a more potent form of intoxication because THC undergoes first-pass liver metabolism into 11-hydroxy-THC (11-OH-THC), which has been shown to generate a more intense level of intoxication than its parent compound, THC.[79] Routes of administration that bypass the gastrointestinal tract result in significantly lower first-pass metabolism and, consequently, far lower levels of 11-OH-THC. Additionally, CBD, when taken in conjunction with THC, may mitigate the intoxicating effects of THC and 11-OH-THC while also potentiating some of the therapeutic effects of these compounds.[80] Consequently, the data from the sections above on dronabinol (which is chemically no different than THC) and CBD may not always match the data below, as the studies described below were conducted with cannabis (and not medications containing solely dronabinol or CBD).

Inhalation

In the United States since the 1930s, inhalation has been the most common route of administration for drug-type cannabis. The dried leaves and flowers of the female cannabis plant are either rolled into a cigarette or inserted into a pipe and then smoked. Vaporizing cannabis became popular much later and is often preferred by some cannabis users, especially medical patients. Vaporizers do not rely on combustion and instead vaporize the numerous compounds found within cannabis (see Table 7.8). Vaporization occurs at heats well below the point at which cannabis combusts, ~445°F (230°C)[81] and prevents the inhalation of myriad polynuclear aromatic hydrocarbons (PAHs), which are by-products of combustion and often carcinogenic.

Vaporizers have existed for decades but were often prohibitively expensive or difficult to transport on one's person in a convenient fashion until the 2010s, though more affordable and less cumbersome options have been developed within the last decade and have largely allayed these grievances. Even some handheld vaporizers allow users to manipulate the temperature of devices, thereby offering more control over the vaporization process, and, due to these technological advances, vaporizers have become extremely common among both medicinal and recreational users.

TABLE 7.8 Boiling Points of Common Constituents

Compound Type	Compound Name	Boiling Point (°C)
Cannabinoid	Δ^9-Tetrahydracannibinol (THC)	157[a]
	Cannabidiol (CBD)	160-180[a]
	Cannabinol (CBN)	185[a]
	Cannabichromene (CBC)	220[a]
	Cannabigerol (CBG)	N/A
	Δ^8-Tetrahydracannibinol (Δ^8-THC)	175-178[a]
	Tetrahydrocannabivarin (THCV)	<220[a]
Terpenoid	β-Myrcene	166-168[a]
	β-Caryophyllene	119[a]
	Limonene	177[a]
	Linalool	198[a]
	α-Pinene	156[a]
	Borneol	210[a]
	Δ-3-Carene	168[a]
	Terpinolene	186[b]
	β-Pinene	163-166[b]
	Humulene	123[b]
	Nerolidol	236-266[b]
Flavonoid	Cannflavin-A	182[a]

[a]Russo EB, McPartland JM. Cannabis and cannabis extracts: greater than the sum of their parts? In: Russo EM, Grotenhermen F, eds. *Handbook of Cannabis Therapeutics: From Bench to Bedside*. Binghamton, NY: Hawthorn Press, Inc; 2010:171-204. https://saltonverde.com/wp-content/uploads/2017/09/17-Handbook_cannabis_therapeutics_from_bench_to_bedside.pdf#page=190. Accessed October 8, 2019.
[b]Obtained from Praxis Laboratories. https://praxis-laboratory.com/terpene-analysis/. Accessed October 8, 2019.

Not all portable vaporizers are designed to vaporize flower cannabis, and many are manufactured solely for the purposes of vaporizing concentrated cannabis oil or distillate. However, to create these substances, solvents such as butane or carbon dioxide are used to extract the cannabinoids from the plant matter, which is then discarded.[82] Some concentrates contain a carrier oil, such as vegetable glycerin, as well as the concentrated cannabinoids that have been extracted from the plant. These concentrates are oil based because cannabinoids are lipophilic.[83]

Oils often come in premade cartridges that are then inserted into a device—most commonly a "vape pen," so-called because these devices resemble pens (Box 7.1). The contents are heated to the point of vaporization, and the vapors are then inhaled. Some concentrates contain only carrier oils and specific cannabinoids. Others contain carrier oils and cannabinoids, as well as the terpenoids and flavonoids commonly found in certain cultivars of cannabis. In many cases, this is done by manufacturers to recreate the flavors and aromas of preferred cultivars (often referred to as "strains").

More concentrated forms of cannabis are known as dabs and may look like wax, butter, honey, or even glass. They do not come in cartridges and do not utilize carrier oils. Users heat the concentrate on a hot surface, and then use what is known as a "dab rig" to inhale the resultant fumes. As the name suggests, only a dab will suffice to produce a high level of intoxication, as these concentrates tend to be extremely potent. Some concentrates,

---

BOX 7.1 A Note on E-cigarette, or Vaping, Product Use Associated Lung Injury (EVALI)

Recently, the use of vape pens has become a public health concern, largely due to a string of illnesses and fatalities linked to the use of cartridges purchased on the illicit market. The Centers for Disease Control and Prevention (CDC) found that these cartridges used vitamin E acetate as a carrier oil, and that this additive, while safe for topical use, appears to be strongly linked to e-cigarette, or vaping, product use associated lung injury (EVALI), which can be fatal, and has been linked to 47 fatalities at the time of this writing. The CDC conducted tests on bronchoalveolar lavage (BAL) fluid samples collected from the lungs of 29 EVALI patients and found that they all tested positive for vitamin E acetate. Consequently, it is highly recommended that patients avoid all vaping products obtained through illicit or even informal sources, as they may contain vitamin E acetate or another adulterant.[84]

such as shatter (which gets its name because the cannabis oil has been concentrated to the point that it resembles amber glass), may contain upward of 90% THC.[82] Flower cannabis, by comparison, is significantly lower in THC, with literature claiming that the most potent cultivars top out closer to 30% THC. The average level of THC in confiscated flower cannabis in 2014 was 12%.[85]

Cannabis users who opt to smoke or use a vaporizer (vape) find this route of administration affords multiple benefits. Most notably, it is far easier to self-titrate, as both methods of inhalation produce a rapid onset and deliver cannabinoids directly into the bloodstream via the lungs. Concentrations of THC in plasma are detectable within seconds and peak between 3 and 10 minutes after smoking, and the intoxicating effects of THC can be felt within 1 minute of administration and typically peak within about half an hour of inhalation.[77] A moderate dosage of 5-10 mg tends to result in intoxication lasting upward of an hour or 2, while stronger doses of 20-25 mg may last for upward of 3 hours or more.[86] Patients may experience drowsiness or grogginess after this time, thereby making it potentially dangerous to drive or operate heavy machinery even after the acute effects of intoxication have subsided. A review on the effects of cannabis and driving published by Neavyn et al. in 2014 recommends patients abstain from driving for a minimum of 8 hours after the onset of cannabis intoxication.[87]

Bioavailability

Though inhalation offers rapid onset, a significant portion of the THC may be lost during the smoking process, with ~30% of the THC contained within a cannabis cigarette being destroyed by combustion (pyrolysis), and much of the remaining smoke is cast off as side-stream smoke or lost due to incomplete absorption.[88] Some studies have found that the amount of THC transferred to the user can be increased by means of a pipe instead of a cigarette or joint.[89]

The bioavailability of THC is highly variable when cannabis is smoked or vaped, with some studies placing the range between 18% and 50%.[88] Other studies have placed the range of smoking even lower, at between 16% and 19%.[89] Still others have found that bioavailability depends on how familiar one is with cannabis, with occasional users receiving either 10% ± 7% or 14% ± 1%, and heavy users receiving either 23% ± 16% or 27% ± 10%.[89] Intra- and intersubject variability in smoking dynamics—that is, frequency of intake, intake volume, intake duration—is the likely reason for the wide range in reported bioavailability.[88] THC plasma concentrations, AUC values, and half-lives were observed to be higher among habitual cannabis users than infrequent users.[90]

Vaping tends to produce more pronounced effects than smoking. Spindle et al. found that vaporizing cannabis with a device known as a Volcano[†] resulted in higher concentrations of THC in blood when compared to equal doses of cannabis inhaled by means of smoking a pipe, with a 25 mg dose resulting in a peak THC concentration of 14.4 ng/mL compared with a peak THC concentration of 10.2 ng/mL when the cannabis was smoked in a pipe.[91] It is likely that vaporizer and concentrate/distillate quality may also impact the amounts of cannabinoids absorbed, which is yet another reason to avoid concentrates obtained through the illicit market beyond those noted above.

Using a vaporizer to inhale concentrates that are high in CBD and low in THC presents similar pros and cons, though there are some significant differences. Systematic bioavailability of inhaled CBD appears to be higher than THC and is ~31% (range: 11%-45%).[92] The average peak blood plasma level after five individuals smoked cigarettes containing ~19 mg of CBD was 110 ng/mL (range: 42-191 ng/mL), occurring 3 minutes after administration.[92]

While bioavailability may be higher, it is often difficult to recognize when one has ingested an appropriate dosage of CBD because it does not produce an intoxicating effect like THC. While the danger of overdosing on or consuming a toxic amount of CBD is not a significant worry, the possibility that patients may be consuming products that contain no CBD or far less CBD than indicated on product labeling is a concern.

Researchers have found that CBD products purchased online often contain significantly less CBD than advertised, especially among vaporization liquids. Bonn-Miller et al. discovered that, of the 24 vaporization liquids tested, 18 contained less CBD than stated on product packaging, 3 contained more CBD, and only 3 products contained a concentration correctly corresponding with the product's label.[93] Products manufactured by some less reputable companies have been found to contain no CBD whatsoever, and many of them have received formal warning letters from the FDA.[94] Consequently, it is highly recommended that patients only purchase CBD products from licensed distributors.

[†]Literature suggests that the Volcano® is often regarded as one of the best nonportable (desktop) vaporizers on the market.

Oral Administration

Oral doses of cannabis are another common route of administration. Oral administrations may come in the form of capsules, as is the case with pharmaceuticals like dronabinol (a synthetic form of THC and the active ingredient in Marinol) discussed above. More commonly, oral administrations come in the form of food products infused with cannabis extracts, which are often referred to as "edibles." Edibles come in a wide range of forms, such as gummies, chocolates, or other sweets, and have varying concentrations and formulations of cannabinoids. Evidence suggests that edibles have become very popular in markets where recreational cannabis has been legalized, with anecdotal evidence indicating that many consumers favor edibles because they can be consumed discreetly.[79]

Consuming cannabis via oral administration results in far slower onset than inhalation, with maximal plasma cannabinoid concentrations of THC typically occurring between 60 and 120 minutes after ingestion, though maximal plasma levels have been observed as long as 6 hours following initial administration, with some subjects showing multiple plasma peaks.[77,89] THC levels taper off at a far slower pace than when cannabis is smoked, and the protracted effect may be preferable for some patients who experience issues like chronic pain, nausea, or anxiety.[89] Conversely, the long onset may lead inexperienced users to administer multiple doses before realizing that they have taken far too much. Reports of "cannabis-induced psychosis" following the consumption of edibles have been well documented, and the experience, while not life threatening, can be extremely unpleasant.[79] For more information about the effects of overdosing, see the Dosage section below, as well as Chapter 22 (Adverse Side Effects and Health Risks of Cannabis).

Absorption rates of oral consumption of THC are ostensibly high, and Wall et al. found that 95% of radiolabeled THC was absorbed by the gastrointestinal tract when THC was delivered through a carrier oil, while Lemberger et al. found that between 90% and 95% of the THC was absorbed through a cherry syrup vehicle.[95]

Bioavailability

Despite seemingly high absorption rates, much of the THC is converted into breakdown products, such that the amount of THC that reaches the bloodstream is actually quite low. Oral administrations of dronabinol showed an overall systemic bioavailability of between 4% and 12% THC, while oral administration of a chocolate cookie containing 20-mg THC showed higher individual variation of between 2% and 14%.[95] A variety of factors, including weight, metabolism, gender, and eating habits, may contribute to bioavailability and the intensity and duration of the edible's intoxicating effects.[79] Additionally, the amount of THC contained within one product may vary from batch to batch and even among samples taken from the same batch.[79]

A great deal of THC is degraded by acids in the stomach and converted to Δ^8-tetrahydrocannabinol.[95] Much of the THC that passes through the stomach then undergoes first-pass metabolization in the liver, where it is converted to 11-OH-THC by the cytochrome P450 enzyme system.[79] Plasma concentrations of 11-OH-THC may range from 50% to 100% of THC concentrations after oral administration compared to 10% following inhalation.[88] As stated above, the effects of 11-OH-THC are distinct from the effects of THC and may produce a more significant level of intoxication. An independent report commissioned by the Colorado Department of Revenue found that 1 mg of THC contained in an edible produced behavioral effects similar to smokable cannabis with a THC content of 5.71 mg.[79]

Edible products that contain either THC and CBD or just CBD have become very popular and are available in the form of oils, gummies, or chocolates. When CBD is administered orally, bioavailability tends to range between 13% and 19%.[96] Maximum plasma concentrations are dose dependent, though there appears to be a saturation effect when extremely high doses are administered. Manini et al. administered 400 and 800 mg doses of CBD and found that mean peak plasma levels occurred at 3 hours postdose, reaching 181.2 ± 39.8 ng/mL and 221.1 ± 35.6 ng/mL, respectively.[97]

Products that do not explicitly contain THC should not produce any intoxicating effects, though some may contain trace amounts of THC, and, in most cases, this will not be sufficient to cause intoxication.[93] Furthermore, CBD will not become THC when introduced to stomach acids and claims to the contrary are not valid. One research paper suggests that lab-simulated gastric fluid converted CBD to THC, but no *in vivo* study has ever shown that this conversion takes place in humans.[98]

Consumers should practice some degree of due diligence before deciding on CBD products. As noted above, CBD does not produce an intoxicating effect like THC, and many consumers may not be able to determine if they have taken an appropriate dosage. Studies have indicated that edible CBD products purchased online often contain significantly less CBD than advertised, though the problem of mislabeling is more pronounced in products designed to be inhaled via vaporization. Bonn-Miller et al. tested 40 products containing CBD in oil form and found 10 contained less CBD than stated on product packaging, 12 contained more CBD, and 18 products could be said to contain a concentration correctly corresponding with the product's label.[93] Products manufactured by some less reputable companies have been found to contain no CBD whatsoever, and many of them have received formal warning letters from the FDA.[94]

Sublingual Administration

Should a patient want another alternative, sublingual tinctures (oil- and alcohol-based), lozenges, or oromucosal sprays are yet another option for administration. Onset is more rapid than with oral administration, but slower than inhalation. Additionally, sublingual administration avoids most first-pass metabolism by the liver, particularly when oromucosal sprays are utilized, thereby preventing reflex swallowing. Some reflex swallowing of other mediums may result in higher levels of 11-OH-THC due to liver metabolism.

Bioavailability

Information concerning the bioavailability of THC and CBD administered sublingually is scant, but research conducted by GW Pharmaceuticals found similar absorption levels and bioavailability when comparing nabiximols with oral THC. Additionally, this study illustrates that when sublingual THC and CBD are administered simultaneously in the same amounts, THC levels in plasma are always higher than CBD levels, and 45 minutes after dosing, concentrations of 11-OH-THC surpassed THC levels.[99]

As is the case with all cannabis products, consumers should be vigilant when purchasing sublingual CBD products, as the market is not well regulated, and many products do not contain the amount of CBD as advertised. Of the 20 CBD tinctures tested by Bonn-Miller et al., 8 contained less CBD than advertised, 7 contained more, and only 5 products contained the amount of CBD on the product's packaging. Additionally, some products were found to contain trace amounts of other cannabinoids, including THC.[93] Many products contained no CBD whatsoever. To avoid bad actors, patients should only purchase formulations from companies that provide data on their products.

Transdermal/Topical Administration

Topical administration of cannabis is yet another option for patients who wish to avoid inhalation or oral administration. Research into dermal patches that used the more stable Δ^8-THC instead of Δ^9-THC showed that transdermal delivery is possible, despite cannabinoids being highly hydrophobic. Touitou et al. (1988) found that skin permeability is enhanced by water and oleic acid in propylene glycol and ethanol.[89] A later study by Valiveti et al. found that transdermal delivery of Δ^8-THC produced steady-state plasma levels of 4.4-ng/mL THC in hairless guinea pigs. This level was maintained for more than 48 hours after application and only began to decline 24 hours after the removal of the patch.[100] (Hairless guinea pigs were chosen because *in vitro* studies showed similar permeability of hairless guinea pig skin and human skin, whereas Δ^8-THC permeability was 13-fold higher in rats compared to humans.)[100] Furthermore, CBD and CBN permeabilities have been found to sssbe 10-fold higher than Δ^8-THC.[101]

The transdermal administration of cannabinoids is still in the early stages of evaluation, and data for the bioavailability of this route in humans have not been validated at this time.[102]

Apart from transdermal application via patch, there are several formulations of lotions, balms, and ointments containing various cannabinoids (especially CBD) available on the market. Murine models show that CBD may be effective at treating some forms of inflammation, chronic pain, and dermatological conditions, and anecdotal evidence about the efficacy of topical CBD is widespread.[102] At this time, clinical data are still unclear, and more evidence is required to determine the bioavailability and efficacy of topical administrations of CBD.

Rectal Administration

Though uncommon today, there is historical precedent of administering cannabis smoke via the rectum in Ayurveda traditions.[103] More modern techniques have employed suppositories, which, like some other routes of administration, do not undergo first-pass metabolism, though cultural barriers remain firmly in place to restrict this route of administration.

Though research is limited, preliminary data suggest that cannabinoid bioavailability is high for suppositories, and that those containing THC hemisuccinate have a high bioavailability (roughly double that of an oral administration), and have been used to treat spasticity and pain, but data are limited to only two patients.[104] Far more research is needed to confirm these results, and studies on the rectal administration of other cannabinoids, such as CBD, appear to be lacking.[105]

Raw Cannabis

The consumption of raw, undecarboxylated cannabis is uncommon and is consumed solely for its reputed health benefits, typically after it has been juiced. Those who consume raw cannabis do not experience significant psychoactive effects. There are numerous anecdotal claims about the benefits of juicing raw cannabis, but they are not currently corroborated by scientific analysis.[106] More research in a controlled environment or clinical setting needs to be conducted. Additionally, due to the instability of THCA-A, which makes THC contamination common even in the best conditions, these studies need to be especially rigorous. At this time, there is only one study that suggests that THCA-A reduced lithium chloride–induced vomiting in murine subjects.[107]

It is possible that the benefits of juicing raw cannabis may come from the consumption of terpenic compounds, which are found in greater concentrations in raw cannabis because many of these compounds degrade during the drying and curing process, as well as during storage. This hypothesis has not been sufficiently tested; it is merely food for thought.[65]

7.4.3 Distribution of THC

THC reaches the bloodstream through the routes of administration described above and, from there, is distributed to tissues throughout the body without specific transport processes or barriers that affect its concentration in tissues.[89] Upward of 90% of THC in the blood is distributed into plasma, of which 95%-99% is bound to plasma proteins—mainly lipoproteins and to a lesser extent albumin—and the remaining 10% is distributed into red blood cells.[89] THC is particularly adept at penetrating highly perfused tissues throughout the body, including organs such as the brain, liver, heart, lung, jejunum, kidney, and spleen; thyroid, pituitary, and mammary glands; and in adipose (fat) and muscle tissues. This rapid uptake into tissues is one of the reasons for the early decline of THC in plasma.[108] Hunt and Jones calculated that 30% of THC is converted to metabolites when administered intravenously, while 70% of THC is absorbed into tissues. Its gradual redistribution, from the more perfuse tissues to the less perfuse, prolongs the process of elimination.[108] The same authors hypothesized that over 99% of THC would be metabolized within 30 minutes if it remained in the blood.[108]

The initial volume of THC distribution is equivalent to the plasma volumes between 2.5 and 3 L, with significant variance between drug-free users and chronic users—2.55 ± 1.93 L and 6.38 ± 4.1 L, respectively.[89] Kelly and Jones reported steady-state volumes of distribution at levels as low as 1 L/kg, while other data[108] (Lemberger et al., 1971; Wall et al., 1983) suggest steady-state distribution levels of 10 L/kg.[75]

Due to the high lipophilicity of THC and its metabolites, as well as its retention rates in various types of tissues, the distribution patterns of THC and THC metabolites change over time, and both have a relatively long terminal elimination half-life in plasma. Certain organs are more prone to retaining THC and its metabolites, with equilibrium of THC (and THC metabolite levels) between blood and tissue taking place 6 hours after an intravenous dose.[99] As a consequence of its quick penetration into tissues, only 5% or less of the THC in the blood is available for pharmacological activity.[109] Only 1% is found in the brain, even at peak concentrations when THC is administered intravenously, though the penetration of its metabolite, 11-OH-THC, has been found to be faster and higher than its parent compound at a ratio as high as 6:1.[75]

Brunet et al. found that, 0.5 hours following the intrajugular administration of 200 µg/kg THC in pigs, concentrations were as follows:

- Lung: 1888 ng/g
- Kidney: 272 ng/g
- Heart: 178 ng/g
- Liver: 155 ng/g
- Fat cells: 91 ng/g
- Muscle: 55 ng/g
- Brain: 49 ng/g
- Spleen: 34 ng/g
- Blood: 24 ng/g
- Vitreous humor: 1.2 ng/g
- Bile: 0.4 ng/g

The authors found that, within 6 hours of administration, THC concentrations had dropped to below 5% of the levels observed at 0.5 hours in all organs, with elimination fastest in the liver, but 6.8% of the THC found in the blood at 0.5 hours could still be detected, while the levels in fat cells had only fallen to 37.2% of where they were 0.5 hours after administration. Inversely, THC content spiked in bile to 675% of its initial concentration 0.5 hours after administration.

Twenty-four hours after administration, trace amounts of THC were still observable in the lungs (2.5% of levels 0.5 hours after administration) and blood (0.8% of levels 0.5 hours after administration). Adipose tissues still retained 34.7% of their 0.5 hours levels, and bile levels were still 275% higher than they had been 0.5 hours after administration. Ultimately, terminal half-life of elimination was judged to be 10.6 hours, and the authors calculated a distribution of 32 L/kg. Plasma kinetics were determined to be comparable to those observed in human models.[110]

As mentioned above, a significant portion of THC is distributed into adipose tissues and slowly redistributes THC back into the body. Adipose tissue is not only a short-term storage site for THC but also accumulates THC over the long term. Kreuz and Axelrod's murine study found that THC and THC metabolite levels continued to accrue after 4 weeks of daily subcutaneous administration, and that THC concentrations in fat increased fourfold from the concentration following initial administration.[111] The majority of the THC metabolites that are stored in fat deposits appear to be long-chain fatty acid conjugates of 11-OH-TIIC.[75]

Distribution of THC in Fetus and Breast Milk

It is established that, in animal and human models, THC crosses the placenta, while THC metabolites 11-OH-THC and 11-nor-9-carboxy-Δ^9-tetrahydrocannbinol (THC-COOH) do so with much less efficiency. It is possible that the placental transfer of THC-COOH does not occur at all.[99]

Plasma level concentrations have been found to be lower in fetuses than in maternal blood in various animal models, and the route of administration has been shown to strongly affect fetus plasma concentrations. Hutchings et al. (1989) found that for orally administered THC, the ratio of fetus plasma concentrations to maternal plasma concentrations to be 1:10, while Martin et al. (1977) and Abrams et al. (1985-1986) found the same ratio to be 1:3 when THC was administered intravenously or through inhalation.[75] In human models, a greater transfer appears to take place in early pregnancy than in later pregnancy, and the ratio of THC concentrations in cord blood compared to maternal blood was found to be between

1:3 and 1:6.[75] Additionally, there is significant variation in fetal exposure, with observational studies finding notable discrepancies in THC levels among dizygotic twins (fraternal twins) based on meconium and hair samples, suggesting that the placenta may play a role in modulating the amount of THC that reaches fetuses.[112]

THC passes into breast milk, and due to its high lipophilicity, chronic use leads to accumulation. THC concentrations have been found to be upward of 8 times higher in human milk than in plasma, and Bertrand et al. found that THC was detectable in 63% of the 54 breast milk samples taken during a study of breast milk levels in cannabis users even 6 days after last reported use.[113] 11-OH-THC, which is less lipophilic than its parent compound, was found in only five samples. The Bertrand et al. study suggests that, on average, THC half-life is 27 hours in human milk with an estimated reduction in THC concentration of 3% per hour.[113]

The Bertrand et al. study did not measure the plasma concentrations of the infants, but the authors estimated that infant plasma concentrations of THC are ~1000 times lower than the plasma concentration of an adult following one 10 mg dose of THC.[113] Despite a low rate of transfer, the feces of nursing infants who were exposed to cannabis via breast milk did contain THC and its metabolites.[114] This indicates not only that infants absorb and metabolize THC but that they may accumulate it in fat stores, thereby exposing nursing infants to a constant stream of THC.

Effects of THC on Fetal Brain Development

There have not been enough studies showing how THC affects developing human fetuses or infants in a manner that removes potential environmental biases, but preclinical animal models have indicated that THC does have a pernicious effect on the developing brain. In rodent models, prenatal exposure to THC has been associated with cognitive impairment, reductions in working memory, and an increase in vulnerability to seizures, while postnatal exposure has been associated with anxiety-like symptoms.[112]

Until more studies are conducted to show how THC exposure affects fetuses and infants, *it is not recommended that pregnant or nursing women consume THC*.

7.4.4 Metabolism of THC

THC is primarily metabolized in the liver via the cytochrome P450 (CYP) enzyme system, with other organs such as the brain, intestine, and lung contributing to metabolism to a lesser extent.[88]

At least 100 metabolites have been identified for THC, with biotransformation producing di- and tri-hydroxy compounds, as well as ketones, aldehydes, and carbolic acids.[99]

The psychoactive 11-OH-THC is the principal first-pass metabolite of THC, while smaller but still significant amounts of 8β-OH-THC and, to a lesser extent, 8α-OH-THC are formed.[115] 11-OH-THC is produced by hydroxylation at C9 by CYP2C9, CYP2C19, and CYP3A4 enzymes.[99] Plasma levels of 11-OH-THC depend on the route of administration, with concentrations following inhalation being 10% of concentrations observed following oral administration, which produces nearly equivalent plasma concentrations of 11-OH-THC and THC.[99] *In vitro* studies conducted by Yamaori et al. have found that CBD may hinder the conversion of THC to 11-OH-THC by inhibiting CYP enzymes CYP1A2, CYP2B6, CYP2C9, CYP2D6, and CYP3A4, and that this may result in higher levels of THC concentrations in plasma.[116]

Further oxidation of 11-OH-THC results in THC-COOH and its glucuronide conjugate 11-nor-9-carboxy-THC beta-glucuronide (THC-COOH-glucuronide), which are both inactive and the major end products of biotransformation in humans.[99] Plasma THC-COOH levels typically reach parity with and surpass THC levels within 30-45 minutes following inhalation and ~1 hour after oral administration.[99]

Significant variance in plasma clearance levels have been reported. Ohlsson et al. observed a rate of 760-1190 mL/min when THC was administered via inhalation, while Hunt and Jones described a notable disparity between infrequent and chronic users, 605 ± 149 mL/min and 977 ± 304 mL/min, respectively. Hunt and Jones hypothesized that, since only 2% of the absorbed oral dose of THC they administered reached the blood unchanged, THC should have a hepatic clearance comparable to liver blood flow (1500 mL/min).[108]

Additionally, THC or one of its metabolites (most notably THC-COOH) is retained in fat for long periods of time and is gradually released into the bloodstream; they may be detectible in the blood of chronic users for long periods of time following cessation.[99] (This phenomenon may be exaggerated in individuals who rapidly lose weight, though evidence to support this claim appears to be more theoretical and anecdotal than backed up by observational data.) THC half-life for infrequent users vs chronic users is ~1.3 days and 5-13 days, respectively, while the metabolite THC-COOH has been detected in plasma for 2-7 days in infrequent users and upward of 25 days in those who use it frequently.[83] Meanwhile, THC and the metabolite THC-COOH were detectable in saliva for an average of 34 hours (range: 1-72 hours) and 13 hours (range: 1-24 hours), respectively, with the study defining "detectable" as above 0.5 mg/mL.[75]

Other studies have found that the terminal half-life of THC is significantly longer, and confounding data can vary widely. Hunt and Jones described a range from 13.8 to 26.0 hours, while Wall et al. observed a range among men and women of 25-36 hours, and Lemberger et al. found that mean half-life for regular users was 28 hours, but that the mean half-life for naïve users was 57 hours.[117] Suffice to say, there are numerous variables that can impact the terminal half-life of THC, and frequency of cannabis use is not the only factor.

7.4.5 Elimination of THC

Routes of administration affect the rates of excretion of THC and its primary metabolites, 11-OH-THC and THC-COOH. Within 3 days of consumption, overall rates have been found to be 65% following oral administration and 45% following intravenous administration.[75] Regardless of administration method, between 80% and 90% of THC and its metabolites are excreted within 5 days.[115] More than 65% is excreted in feces and ~20% is eliminated in urine—11-OH-THC being the predominate metabolite in the former, while THC-COOH glucuronide conjugates being the primary metabolites eliminated through the latter.[115] Less than 5% of unadulterated THC is found in feces.[75]

As mentioned above, the high lipophilicity of THC and its metabolites means that small but measurable amounts may remain in adipose tissues for extended periods of time and may fluctuate. Ellis et al. found that THC metabolites were detectable (>20 ng/mL) for a range of 3-18 days (mean: 8.5 days) for infrequent users vs 3-46 days (mean: 19.1 days) for regular users. In at least one case, Ellis et al. found that it took 77 days for an individual to go 10 consecutive days without a positive result.[118]

7.4.6 Distribution of CBD

The plasma concentration, terminal half-life, and other aspects of distribution of CBD are similar to THC, though distribution volume for CBD was calculated at 30 L/kg.[75] At this time, no published data exist on the tissue distribution of CBD in humans. Although studies that have examined persistent dosing do not show accumulation in plasma, it is possible that there may be tissue accumulation.[96]

The effects of CBD on fetuses have not been adequately studied at this time, though Feinshtein et al. have found that CBD could affect placenta permeability.[119] Currently, there are no published data on how CBD affects nursing infants, though it is generally accepted that CBD is transmitted via breast milk in a manner similar to THC due to its high lipophilicity. Some tissue accumulation in infants would seem reasonable for similar reasons, but the level at which such accumulation takes place (if it takes place at all) has not been studied.

Ultimately, more research is needed to determine how CBD exposure affects fetuses and infants before it can be deemed safe to use. Until relevant data are produced on the subject, *it is not recommended that pregnant or nursing women consume CBD*.

7.4.7 Metabolism and Elimination of CBD

Like THC, CBD is primarily metabolized by the liver. Unlike THC, CBD undergoes extensive hepatic metabolism at multiple sites, with more than 100 metabolites identified from myriad organisms.[105] *In vitro* studies conducted by Jiang et al. found that CBD is metabolized by cytochrome P450 enzyme system, including CYP1A1, CYP1A2, CYP2C9, CYP2C19, CYP2D6, CYP3A4, and CYP3A5 enzymes.[120]

The most prevalent CBD metabolite in humans is 7-hydroxy-CBD (7-OH-CBD), with ~90% of dioxygenated material being found to be 7-hydroxylated metabolites, with CBD-7-olic acid (7-COOH-CBD), 6α-hydroxy-CBD (6α-OH-CBD), and 6β-hydroxy-CBD (6β-OH-CBD) being found to be some of the more prevalent minor metabolites.[117] Though there are no publications that describe the biological activity of CBD metabolites in humans at this time, *in vitro* animal studies have indicated that 7-OH-CBD and 7-COOH-CBD may have anti-inflammatory properties.[105]

Terminal half-life for CBD appears to be affected by route of administration. A study by Ohlsson et al. showed that when 20 mg of CBD was administered intravenously, the mean half-life was found to be 31 ± 4 hours.[92] The half-life of CBD appears to be significantly lower when administered orally. Guy and Flint found the half-life of a single 10 mg oral administration of CBD to be 1.09 hours, while Guy and Robson found the half-life of a single 20 mg oral administration of CBD to be 1.97 hours. Atsmon et al.

found that the half-life of 10-mg oral lipid capsules to range between 2.95 and 3.21 hours. Consroe et al. found that when large doses (700 mg) are consumed chronically, CBD half-life stretches to 2 and 5 days.[96]

Unlike THC, a large amount of free CBD is excreted through feces,[105] with 30%-35% of CBD or its metabolites being eliminated within 72 hours,[121] while the excretion rate of CBD or its glucuronide through urine is similar to that of THC—16% in 72 hours.[117]

7.5 Indications

As documented in Chapter 2 (The History of Cannabis) and Chapter 5 (U.S. Cannabis Regulations From Past to Present), both fiber-type cannabis, which is high in CBD, and drug-type cannabis, which is high in THC, have historically been used to treat a variety of conditions. Despite enjoying wide usage in the past, federal regulations have limited the number of conditions for which medications containing cannabinoids (whether natural or synthetic) can be legally prescribed by medical professionals to the three FDA-approved medications described above: dronabinol, nabilone, and the CBD formulation marketed under the name Epidiolex. To reiterate, indications for these medications are as follows.

Dronabinol (Marinol)[122]

- Anorexia or weight loss associated with AIDS;
- Nausea and vomiting associated with cancer chemotherapy, provided patients have failed to adequately respond to conventional antiemetic treatments.

Nabilone (Cesamet)[72]

- Nausea and vomiting associated with cancer chemotherapy, provided patients have failed to adequately respond to conventional antiemetic treatments.

Cannabidiol (Epidiolex)[123]

- Seizures associated with LGS or DS in patients 2 years of age or older.

While these are the only three FDA-approved medications available in the United States, medical cannabis programs that operate at the state level do allow practitioners to recommend cannabis to patients with qualifying conditions, and these change from state to state. For a full listing of the qualifying conditions by state, please see Table 7.1. Hemp-derived CBD has become legal at the federal level, though some states have placed additional regulations on the sale of CBD at the state level. Please consult Figure 5.1 or this book's Web site to ensure compliance with all local regulations (www.cannabistextbook.com).

7.5.1 A Note on CBD Products

Many CBD products are characterized as supplements, and according to the Dietary Supplement Health and Education Act of 1994, supplements are not subject to the same level of scrutiny as FDA-approved medications. As a result, consumers are not guaranteed the same level of protections for medicines that were put into place by the 1906 Pure Food and Drug Act and supplemental amendments (see Chapter 5 [U.S. Cannabis Regulations From Past to Present]). As noted above, many of these products either contain less CBD than advertised or may contain foreign substances that are harmful to consumers. Products containing THC are typically better regulated, as they do face some scrutiny from state agencies.

There is some evidence that CBD may be useful as a treatment for conditions beyond epilepsy associated with LGS or DS. For most indications, however, there are only preclinical or limited clinical data to support what has become an enormous amount of anecdotal evidence. While many of these anecdotal claims may turn out to be based in fact, they have not been properly scrutinized at this time. A review by Pisanti et al. studied the available literature on CBD, and the conditions for which it may have therapeutic benefits can be found in Table 7.9.[124]

It is recommended that patients seeking to use CBD not purchase products manufactured by companies that do not provide data documenting quality assurance. It is beyond the purview of this book to make recommendations or to endorse brands, but a partial listing of companies that manufacture THC or CBD products and provide data can be found in Appendix B and on this book's Web site: www.cannabistextbook.com.

7.6 Dosage

One of the reasons that cannabis has been used as a recreational drug for millennia is that, similar to alcohol, some individuals find the experience to be relaxing when they consume an amount of

Table 7.9 Potential Therapeutic Applications of CBD

Alzheimer's disease	Cheng et al. (2014),[125] Esposito et al. (2006),[126] Esposito et al. (2006),[127] Martin-Moreno et al. (2011),[128] Scuderi et al. (2014)[129]
Anxiety	Almeida et al. (2013),[130] Bergamaschi et al. (2011),[131] de Mello Schier et al. (2014),[132] Lemos et al. (2010),[133] Marinho et al. (2015),[134] Moreira et al. (2006)[135]
Cancer	Ligresti et al. (2006),[136] McAllister et al. (2011),[137] Pisanti et al. (2013),[138] Ramer et al. (2014),[139] Rocha et al. (2014),[140] Scott et al. (2014),[141] Shrivastava et al. (2011)[142]
Cardiovascular disease	Booz (2011),[143] Durst et al. (2007),[144] Stanley et al. (2013)[145]
Depression	El-alfy et al. (2010),[146] Hsiao et al. (2012),[147] Shoval et al. (2016)[148]
Diabetic complications	Kozela et al. (2010),[149] Rajesh et al. (2010),[150] Weiss et al (2006)[151]
Huntington's disease	Consroe et al. (1991),[152] Iuvone et al. (2009),[153] Sagredo et al. (2011)[154]
Hypoxia-ischemia injury	Hayakawa et al. (2007),[155] Hayakawa et al. (2009),[156] Pazos et al. (2012),[157] Pazos et al. (2013),[158] Ruiz-Valdepeñas et al. (2011)[159]
Infection	Appendino et al. (2008)[160]
Inflammatory diseases	Kozela et al. (2010)[149], Kozela et al. (2011),[161] Mecha et al. (2012),[162] Mecha et al. (2013),[163] Ribeiro et al. (2012),[164] Ribeiro et al. (2015)[165]
Inflammatory bowel and Crohn's disease	De Filippis et al. (2011),[166] Naftali et al. (2011),[167] Sacerdote et al. (2005)[168]
Multiple sclerosis	Buccellato et al. (2011),[169] Giacoppo et al. (2015),[170] Kozela et al. (2011)[161], Kozela et al. (2015),[171] Mecha et al. (2013)[163]
Nausea	Parker et al. (2002),[172] Rock et al. (2008)[173]
Pain	Boychuck et al. (2015)[174]

TABLE 7.9 Continued

Parkinson's disease	Chagas, et al. (2014)[175] Lastres-Becker et al. (2015)[176]; Zuardi et al. (2009)[177]
Psychosis	Crippa et al. (2015),[178] Gomes et al. (2015),[179] Zuardi et al. (2006),[180] Zuardi et al. (2012)[181]
Rheumatoid arthritis	Malfait et al. (2000)[182]

THC with which they are comfortable. Inversely, an amount of THC in excess of one's comfort zone can produce effects that range from unsettling to extremely unpleasant.

Additionally, the effects of identical dosages of cannabis can vary widely from person to person, as one's temperament, mood, and surroundings can impact how one responds to cannabis. Timothy Leary famously described this as "set and setting." The "set" is the mindset of the individual consuming the drug, while the "setting" is the social environment in which they are consuming the drug.[183] Furthermore, those who regularly use cannabis develop a tolerance for it, and the same amount that may produce a very intense experience in someone new to cannabis may barely effect a more frequent user.

It is recommended that those who have limited experience with drug-type cannabis start low and go slow. In other words, patients should consume cannabis that is low in THC before experimenting with cannabis that is high in THC, and that they should exercise caution when titrating. When taken in low doses, the psychotropic effects of THC may be minimal, with common experiences being a heightened attentiveness of sensory stimuli, mild giddiness, or a pleasant sense of light-headedness. Some of the more commonly reported descriptions of the effects of higher doses of THC include

- The subjective sense that time is moving slowly;
- Increased interest in food and music;
- Hyperactivity, restlessness, and loquacity;
- Dizziness;
- Rapid, tangential thoughts that are often associated in a loose or esoteric manner;
- Mild hallucinations;

- A feeling of extreme heaviness and lethargy often characterized as "couch lock";
- Inability to concentrate and disruption of short-term memory;
- Impaired executive decision-making abilities.[184]

These effects are typically described as being "high." As they subside, some may feel drowsy or groggy, but these residual effects typically disappear following a night of sleep.

As mentioned in Section 5 (Vernacular Taxonomy—Sativa, Indica, and Ruderalis) of Chapter 3 (The Classification of Cannabis), some cultivars are said to accentuate certain sensations more so than others, though evidence of this phenomena seems to be largely anecdotal. Additionally, cultivars that are Sativa dominant are often said to produce a "head high," meaning that they accentuate the psychological effects of THC, while cultivars that are Indica dominant are said to produce a "body high," meaning that they accentuate the physical effects of THC.[185]

All products purchased within a dispensary should contain packaging that clearly states the amount of THC or CBD per serving in milligrams. Individuals who are not accustomed to consuming THC should start with a low dose of either 2.5 or 5 mg. CBD does not have an intoxicating effect, and even large doses have shown no interference with psychomotor and psychological functions. Bergamaschi et al. reported that doses as high as 600 mg did not affect blood pressure, heart rate, or performance in a learning test measured by recall score.[186] While this may be the case, some individuals do experience hypersensitivity or somnolence following the administration of CBD, and, as with THC, it is advisable to start with a relatively modest dose, preferably 10 or 20 mg.

Determining the CBD and THC content is relatively easy for edibles purchased in a dispensary, as product packaging should indicate dosage and serving size, but discerning the cannabinoid content of flower cannabis is more difficult. In a dispensary, the packaging of flower cannabis will specify the THC content, as well as the name of the cultivar (though the packaging may refer to it as a "strain") and whether it is Indica or Sativa. Older patients who may have experimented with cannabis in their youth should be aware that THC content has risen significantly in the past 50 years, with the trend accelerating over time. As of 1968, herbal or raw cannabis containing ~0.9% THC was considered average quality.[187] By 1997, average THC levels in confiscated cannabis had risen to 4.47%,[188] increased in 2008 to 8.8%,[189] and by 2014, it was ~12%.[85] To put this in some perspective, nonalcoholic beers are allowed to contain up to 0.5% alcohol by volume (ABV), even if they are marketed as nonalcoholic; the average American beer contains 5% ABV; and the average wine contains between 11% and 13% ABV.[190]

To better understand the dosage contained in smokable or vaporized cannabis, it is recommended that one consult the "Smoke Calculator" created by the University of California Annenberg and the *Los Angeles Times* (a link to the calculator can be found in the links section of the textbook Web site: www.cannabistextbook.com). The calculator can account for variations in serving size and cultivar potency to estimate the amount of THC that will be inhaled in milligram via either smoking or vaporizing. For example, an individual who smokes a 0.3-g cannabis cigarette containing 11% THC will inhale 12 mg of THC, according to the calculator. Using a vaporizer to consume the same amount of flower cannabis of the same cultivar will produce an estimated amount of 17 mg of inhaled THC.[191]

7.7 Adverse Effects and Contraindications

Typically, cannabis does not cause severe adverse physical reactions and side effects when dosed correctly, though there are significant exceptions. The most commonly reported side effects of cannabis are dry mouth, increased heart rate (tachycardia), increased supine blood pressure, orthostatic hypotension, and conjunctival reddening.[192] Some patients have also experienced diarrhea, nausea, and hypotonia.[193] Weight gain is not a common side effect, even though cannabis is used to treat anorexia.[193] The adverse reactions to dronabinol described above or in Table 7.4 apply to THC, while the adverse reactions to Epidiolex described above or in Table 7.7 apply to CBD.

Of particular note, allergic reactions to cannabis pollen, cannabis seeds, flower cannabis, and extracted cannabinoids have all been documented. Individuals who are allergic to cannabis may experience rashes, hives, or angioedema after handling it, while those who inhale either cannabis pollen or cannabis smoke may feel an itching sensation (pruritus), develop a runny nose, experience swollen and watery eyes, or feel a shortness of breath. Cases of anaphylactic shock have also been reported, most frequently following hempseed consumption.[194] Cross-reactivity between cannabis and tomatoes, peaches, and hazelnuts has also been found.[194] As mentioned above, hypersensitivity to CBD has been reported and causes unpleasant symptoms like pruritus, erythema, and angioedema.[123]

The more serious side effects of cannabis tend to develop with chronic THC usage. These include addiction, cognitive decline, amnesia, and amotivation syndrome.[193] Cannabinoid hyperemesis syndrome, which appears to be relatively rare even among habitual cannabis users, has been reported and is characterized by recurrent vomiting, nausea, and abdominal pain. In extreme cases, it has led to kidney failure.[195] Finally, cannabis use has also been associated with impaired cognitive development in adolescents and acute psychosis in both adolescents and adults, as well as schizophrenia.[196] At this time, the nature of the link between cannabis use and schizophrenia is inconclusive, though a meta-analysis by Murrie et al. has found that 25% of individuals with first-episode substance-induced psychosis were later diagnosed with schizophrenia or schizoaffective disorder, which was higher than the previously reported meta-analytic estimate of 21%, and that the transition to schizophrenia was highest (34%) among individuals who had experienced cannabis-induced psychosis.[197]

More will be said about these matters in Chapter 22 (Adverse Side Effects and Health Risks of Cannabis).

7.8 Drug Interactions

As noted in the Drug Interactions sections for Dronabinol, Nabilone, and Cannabidiol above, drugs that affect the CNS may produce an additive effect when taken in conjunction with cannabis, particularly if it is high in THC. These include alcohol, antihistamines, barbiturates, benzodiazepines, buspirone, lithium, muscle relaxants, opioids, scopolamine, tricyclic antidepressants, and other anticholinergic agents.[198] Concomitant CBD and alcohol use, meanwhile, may cause increased somnolence. For an overview of drug/drug interactions, see Table 7.6.

Dronabinol and THC have been known to cause hypertension, hypotension, tachycardia, and syncope. Concomitant use with drugs that produce similar cardiac effects, such as amphetamines and other sympathomimetic agents, atropine, amoxapine, scopolamine, antihistamines and other anticholinergic agents, amitriptyline, and desipramine and other tricyclic antidepressants should be avoided.[198]

Because THC is highly bound to plasma proteins, it may displace or augment the free fraction of concomitantly administered protein-bound drugs.

Both THC and CBD are primarily metabolized by CYP2C9, CYP2C19, and CYP3A4 enzymes and may interact adversely with inhibitors and inducers. Additionally, CBD may interact with UGT1A9, UGT2B7, CYP1A2, CYP2B6, CYP2C8, CYP2C9, and CYP2C19 substrates.[123]

As noted above, concomitant use of CBD and clobazam, a benzodiazepine, has also been shown to produce a threefold increase in plasma concentrations of the active metabolite in clobazam (*N*-desmethylclobazam), and concomitant use of CBD with valproate often resulted in elevated levels of serum transaminase.[123]

7.9 Warnings and Precautions

Small to moderate dosages of THC (2.5-10 mg) typically produce relatively mild psychotropic effects, but they can still alter one's perception of time and interfere with judgment. Consequently, *it is recommended that patients do not drive or operate heavy machinery while experiencing either acute or the lingering effects of cannabis intoxication*. Furthermore, patients should not consume edible THC prior to driving, even if they believe that they will arrive to their destination prior to the onset of intoxication.

Moderate to large doses of THC (10-25 mg) can lead to anxiety, tachycardia at rest, and significantly impaired judgment.[5] Extremely high doses of THC may also precipitate an acute period of paranoid psychosis, and, as noted above, prolonged and excessive usage may possibly lead individuals who are genetically prone to schizophrenia to their first psychotic break.[196]

CBD does not produce intoxication, but it has been known to have a sedating effect. Consequently, it is not recommended that patients drive or operate heavy machinery until they have sufficient experience taking a specific formulation containing CBD.

As mentioned above, it is not recommended that pregnant or nursing women consume any cannabinoid.

7.9.1 Smoking and Vaping

Smoking cannabis does pose certain health risks, even though smoking flower cannabis may be perceived as the most natural way to consume the drug. Many of the same deleterious compounds found in tobacco smoke are found in the smoke of cannabis.[199] Additionally, the dynamics of cannabis smoking are distinct from tobacco smoking, and these inhalation volume, depth, and length only augment the harmful effects of smoking, particularly with regard to PAHs.

When compared to tobacco smokers, cannabis smokers tend to inhale a volume of smoke up to two-thirds larger, they tend to inhale as much as one-third deeper, and they tend to hold the smoke for as much as 4 times longer.[200] ElSohly and ElSohly concluded that smoking cannabis increased blood carboxyhemoglobin levels by a nearly fivefold increment when compared with smoking tobacco, that the amount of tar inhaled was approximately a threefold increase, and that cannabis smokers retained ~33% more inhaled tar than tobacco smokers ($P < .001$).[200] The writers reasoned that such proclivities among cannabis smokers were the reason why it has been reported that smoking only a few cigarettes of pure cannabis can lead to similar chronic respiratory issues and tracheobronchial epithelial histopathology as found in individuals who smoke upward of 20 tobacco cigarettes per day.[200]

Smoking cannabis poses additional hazards due to possible contamination from molds, heavy metals, and chemicals applied to the plant prior to harvest (pesticides, herbicides, fungicides, etc.). Pathogens, such as *Aspergillus* and *Salmonella*, may proliferate in herbal cannabis that has been poorly stored and can be delivered to users in the inhaled smoke.[192] Properly placing cannabis in airtight containers that are then stored in a cool, dark place can prevent contamination and potency degradation. For patients with compromised immune systems, smoking is not recommended, as raw cannabis may contain *Aspergillus*. If a patient is adamant, however, herbal cannabis can be sterilized by baking it in the oven for 5 minutes at 300°F (150°C), which is sufficient to kill *Aspergillus*.[201] Baking should not extend any longer, as this may vaporize many of the beneficial cannabinoids, including THC.

The consumption of agricultural chemicals or heavy metals can be avoided by recommending that patients only purchase flower cannabis that has been produced by a trusted grower or company that regularly tests its products for foreign contaminants. It should be noted that cannabis is not eligible for USDA organic certification because cannabis remains a controlled substance under federal law. Any company claiming to produce "organic" cannabis has not been inspected by the USDA and may have only received such certification from a private organization that may or may not be entirely trustworthy.

Vaporizing flower cannabis appears to be preferable to smoking flower cannabis, particularly if the cannabis is stored under ideal conditions and the cannabis is grown in a manner that upholds the ethos of organic agriculture. Vaporizing cannabis distillates or oils appears to be far less safe, as the long-term effects on the body, particularly the lungs, are not known. As noted above, patients appear unlikely to develop e-cigarette, or vaping, product use associated lung injury (EVALI), which can be fatal, if they avoid all vaping products obtained through illicit or even informal sources or use a device that vaporizes flower cannabis only.

7.10 Toxicity

In 1988, Francis L. Young, the chief administrative law judge of the Drug Enforcement Administration, wrote an opinion in which he claimed that, despite being used by humans for thousands of years, "There is no record in the extensive medical literature describing a proven, documented cannabis-induced fatality." Additionally, the judge placed the ratio between therapeutic dosage and LD-50 (lethality in 50% of administered animals) at between 1:20 000 and 1:40 000, which would require an individual consume nearly 1500 lb of cannabis to induce a lethal response. The judge concluded: "Marijuana, in its natural form, is one of the safest therapeutically active substances known to man. By any measure of rational analysis marijuana can safely be used within a supervised routine of medical care."[202]

As Hon. Young makes clear, cannabis can be toxic, but it seems safe to say that it would be impossible to ever accidentally consume such a massive amount of cannabis in its raw, herbal state to die from a technical overdose. In the vast majority of cases, when one ingests far more THC than they are accustomed to, they experience a very unpleasant level of intoxication, but these effects typically wear off after a night of sleep, though individual variables may influence such effects from being benign to acute psychoses.

That being said, cases of death due to complications arising from acute cannabis intoxication have been reported. Hartung et al. concluded that two men (ages 23 and 28) in Germany appear to have died due to arrhythmias evoked by consuming relatively small amounts of cannabis.[203] Grigoriadis et al. found that cannabis may produce myocardial dysfunction and cardiogenic shock in some patients.[204] Brucato also reports that several adverse cannabis-related cardiovascular events, including stroke and aneurysm, have led to serious and even fatal outcomes.[205] Additionally, chronic cannabis use can lead to cannabis hyperemesis syndrome, which can be fatal, and individuals who are allergic to cannabis can suffer anaphylaxis or other complications due to an allergic reaction. Cannabis can also lead to significant side effects and health risks that will be explored at length in Chapter 22 (Adverse Side Effects and Health Risks of Cannabis).

7.10.1 Lethal Dosages of THC and CBD

While it seems reasonable to assume that the increase in potency or the use of concentrated cannabis could be responsible for the increase in adverse cardiovascular events, data suggest that this is not a determining factor. The acute toxicity of individual cannabinoids for humans has not been substantiated, and LD50 estimates of the two major cannabinoids that have been discussed in this chapter, THC and CBD, vary widely depending on species and/or route of administration, but they are far too high to account for these phenomena.

Rosenkrantz et al. found that the LD50 for THC among Fischer rats was 800 mg/kg when an oral emulsion containing THC was administered, but that the LD50 for THC jumped to 1270 mg/kg when administered in sesame oil.[206] Nahas reported an even greater disparity when THC was administered intravenously, intraperitoneally, or intragastrically to rats and mice. Following intravenous administration for rats, LD50 was reported to be 29 mg/kg (range: 27-30 mg/kg), while the LD50 was 43 mg/kg (range: 37-49 mg/kg) for mice. In both species, death occurred within 15 minutes of administration. The reported LD50 for intraperitoneal and intragastric administrations was more in line with those of Rosenkrantz et al. For rats, the LD50 was 373 mg/kg (range: 305-454 mg/kg) or 666 mg/kg (range: 604-734 mg/kg) when administered intraperitoneally or intragastrically, respectively. For mice, the LD50 for intraperitoneal administration was 455 mg/kg (range: 419-493 mg/kg) and 482 mg/kg (451-515 mg/kg) for intragastric administration. All toxic signs disappeared within 1 day for surviving animals.[207] Nahas concluded that it is unlikely that humans could ingest enough cannabis to elevate THC plasma concentrations to a toxic level but did note that Indian literature available at the time (1972) recorded two fatalities following the consumption of large amounts of charas, as well as one speculative fatality that occurred after a 23-year-old student was found deceased in their room and all other causes of death were deemed ruled out.[207]

The LD50 of CBD in rhesus monkeys was found to be 212 mg/kg when administered intravenously, with cause of death typically being cardiac failure or respiratory arrest.[208] Intravenous administration was found to be far more lethal in monkeys than oral administration, with the same researchers being able to administer 300 mg/kg oral doses for 90 consecutive days without reported fatalities. Adverse effects noted by the researchers included significant increases in kidney and liver weights, decreases in testicular size, and inhibition of spermatogenesis.[208]

In summation, the existing literature indicates that cannabis is a potent intoxicant and that its use does present significant health risks, but it is not lethal in everyday use. Death as a direct result of cannabis ingestion is exceedingly rare, but cannabis intoxication can lead to potentially fatal complications (such as cardiac events or allergic reactions), and cannabis intoxication can significantly impair one's ability to drive, thereby leading to potentially fatal motor vehicle accidents whether one is experiencing the acute effects of cannabis intoxication or its lingering aftereffects.

Finally, it is also important to remember that there are significant differences in the way cannabis is used recreationally compared to when it is used as a medicine. Patients who use cannabis as a means for relief from pain or nausea typically want to avoid the side effects of intoxication and often want to find a balance where they can experience the therapeutic effects of cannabis without feeling "high." Consequently, it is important for medical professionals to recommend patients to start low and go slow, to explain the different effects as well as routes of administration, and to advise against the use of cannabis that has been obtained through illicit channels, as these products may pose significant health risks to patients.

REFERENCES

[1]Booth M. *Cannabis: A History*. New York, NY: Picador; 2003:118-119.

[2]Pertwee RG. Cannabinoid pharmacology: the first 66 years. *Br J Pharmacol.* 2006;147:S163-S171. doi: 10.1038/sj.bjp.0706406.

[3]ElSohly M, Gul W. Constituents of *Cannabis sativa*. In: Pertwee RG, ed. *Handbook on Cannabis*. New York, NY: Oxford University Press; 2014:3-22.

[4]Martin A, Rashidian N. *A New Leaf: The End of Cannabis Prohibition*. New York, NY: The New Press; 2014:16-17.

[5]Mechoulam R, Carlini EA. Toward drugs derived from *Cannabis*. *Naturwissenschaften*. 1978;65(4):174-179. doi: 10.1007/bf00450585.

[6]Mechoulam R, Gaoni Y. A total synthesis of *dl*-Δ[1]-tetrahydrocannabinol, the active constituent of hashish. *J Am Chem Soc*. 1965;67(14):3273-3275. doi: 10.1021/ja01092a065.

[7]Davis JP, Ramsey HH. Anti-epileptic action of marijuana-active substances. In: Belenko SR, ed. *Drugs and Drug Policy in America: A Documentary History*. Westport, CT: Greenwood Press; 2000:167.

[8]Perucca E. Cannabinoids in the treatment of epilepsy: hard evidence at last? *J Epilepsy Res*. 2017;7(2):61-76. doi: 10.14581/jer.17012.

[9]Gieringer D, Rosenthal E, Carter GT. *Marijuana Medical Handbook: Practical Guide to the Therapeutic Uses of Marijuana*. Oakland, CA: Quick American; 2008:33-35.

[10]FDA Regulation of Cannabis and Cannabis-Derived Products, Including Cannabidiol (CBD). United States Food and Drug Administration website. https://www.fda.gov/news-events/public-health-focus/fda-regulation-cannabis-and-cannabis-derived-products-including-cannabidiol-cbd. Updated September 30, 2019. Accessed October 15, 2019.

[11]Greenwich Biosciences, Inc. Epidiolex (cannabidiol) [package insert]. U.S. Food and Drug Administration website. https://www.epidiolex.com/sites/default/files/EPIDIOLEX_Full_Prescribing_Information.pdf#page=8. Revised June 2018. Accessed October 15, 2019.

[12]HB61. Alabama State Legislature website. http://alisondb.legislature.state.al.us/ALISON/SearchableInstruments/2016RS/PrintFiles/HB61-int.pdf. Accessed November 21, 2019.

[13]Medical Marijuana Registry Application Instructions. Alaska Department of Health and Social Services website. http://dhss.alaska.gov/dph/VitalStats/Documents/PDFs/MedicalMarijuana.pdf. Accessed November 21, 2019.

[14]Court says CBD oil is illegal. Talanei website. https://www.talanei.com/2019/07/12/court-says-cbd-oil-is-illegal/. July 12, 2019. Accessed November 21, 2019.

[15]FAQs—qualifying patients. Arizona Department of Health Services website. https://www.azdhs.gov/licensing/medical-marijuana/index.php#faqs-patients. Accessed November 21, 2019.

[16]Medical marijuana FAQ's. Arkansas Department of Health website. https://www.healthy.arkansas.gov/programs-services/topics/medical-marijuana-faqs#Questions%20about%20Medical%20Conditions. Accessed November 21, 2019.

[17]California medical marijuana law. NORML website. https://norml.org/legal/item/california-medical-marijuana. Accessed November 21, 2019.

[18]Recommend medical marijuana. Colorado Department of Public Health & Environment website. https://norml.org/legal/item/colorado-medical-marijuana. Accessed November 21, 2019.

[19]Connecticut medical marijuana law. NORML website. https://norml.org/legal/item/connecticut-medical-marijuana. Accessed November 21, 2019.

[20]Delaware medical marijuana law. NORML website. https://norml.org/legal/item/delaware-medical-marijuana. Accessed November 22, 2019.

[21]District of Columbia medical marijuana law. NORML website. https://norml.org/legal/item/district-of-columbia-medical-marijuana. Accessed November 22, 2019.

[22]Florida medical marijuana law. NORML website. https://norml.org/legal/item/florida-medical-marijuana-law. Accessed November 22, 2019.

[23]Low THC oil—FAQ for general public. Georgia Department of Public Health website. https://dph.georgia.gov/low-thc-oil-faq-general-public. Accessed November 26, 2019.

[24]Guam medical marijuana law. NORML website. https://norml.org/legal/item/guam-medical-marijuana-law. Accessed November 26, 2019.

[25]Hawaii medical marijuana law. NORML website. https://norml.org/legal/item/hawaii-medical-marijuana. Accessed November 26, 2019.

[26]Cannabidiol. Idaho Office of Drug Policy website. https://odp.idaho.gov/cannibidiol/. Accessed November 26, 2019.

[27]Debilitating conditions. Illinois Department of Public Health website. http://www.dph. illinois.gov/topics-services/prevention-wellness/medical-cannabis/debilitating-conditions. Accessed November 26, 2019.

[28]Indiana CBD-specific law. NORML website. https://norml.org/legal/item/indiana-cbd-specific-law. Accessed November 26, 2019.

[29]Iowa CBD-specific marijuana law. NORML website. https://norml.org/legal/item/iowa-cbd-marijuana-law. Accessed November 26, 2019.

[30]Senate Bill No. 28. Kansas State Legislature website. http://www.kslegislature.org/li/ b2019_20/measures/documents/sb28_enrolled.pdf. Accessed November 26, 2019.

[31]Senate Bill 124. Kentucky State Legislature website. https://apps.legislature.ky.gov/ record/14rs/sb124.html. Accessed November 26, 2019.

[32]Medical marijuana. Department of Agriculture & Forestry, State of Louisiana, website. http://www.ldaf.state.la.us/medical-marijuana/. Updated March 22, 2019. Accessed November 26, 2019.

[33]LD 1539, an act to amend Maine's medical marijuana law. Maine Statue Legislature website. https://legislature.maine.gov/legis/bills/bills_128th/billtexts/HP106001.asp. Accessed November 26, 2019.

[34]General information. Maryland Medical Cannabis Commission. https://mmcc.maryland. gov/Pages/general-information.aspx. Accessed November 26, 2019.

[35]Massachusetts medical marijuana law. NORML website. https://norml.org/legal/item/ massachusetts-medical-marijuana. Accessed November 26, 2019.

[36]Michigan medical marijuana law. NORML website. https://norml.org/legal/item/michigan-medical-marijuana. Accessed November 26, 2019.

[37]Chapter 311—S.F.No. 2470. Minnesota State Legislature website. https://www.revisor. mn.gov/laws/2014/0/Session+Law/Chapter/311/. Accessed November 26, 2019.

[38]Mississippi CBD-specific marijuana law. NORML website. https://norml.org/legal/item/ mississippi-cbd-marijuana-law. Accessed November 26, 2019.

[39]Missouri medical marijuana law. NORML website. https://norml.org/legal/item/missouri-medical-marijuana-law. Accessed November 26, 2019.

[40]Montana medical marijuana law. NORML website. https://norml.org/legal/item/montana-medical-marijuana. Accessed November 26, 2019.

[41]Nevada medical marijuana law. NORML website. https://norml.org/legal/item/nevada-medical-marijuana. Accessed November 26, 2019.

[42]New Hampshire medical marijuana law. NORML website. https://norml.org/legal/item/ new-hampshire-medical-marijuana. Accessed November 26, 2019.

[43]New Jersey medical marijuana law. NORML website. https://norml.org/legal/item/new-jersey-medical-marijuana. Accessed November 26, 2019.

[44]Healthcare Providers & Patients. New Mexico Department of Health website. https:// nmhealth.org/about/mcp/svcs/hpp/. Accessed November 27, 2019.

[45]New York medical marijuana law. NORML website. https://norml.org/legal/item/new-york-medical-marijuana-law. Accessed November 27, 2019.

[46]North Carolina CBD specific marijuana law. NORML website. https://norml.org/legal/item/ north-carolina-cbd-specific-marijuana-law. Accessed November 27, 2019.

[47]North Dakota medical marijuana law. NORML website. https://norml.org/legal/item/north-dakota-medical-marijuana. Accessed November 27, 2019.

[48]Ohio medical marijuana law. NORML website. https://norml.org/legal/item/ohio-medical-marijuana-law. Accessed November 27, 2019.

[49]Title 310. Oklahoma State Department of Health, Chapter 681. Medical Marijuana Control Program. Oklahoma Medical Marijuana Authority website. http://omma.ok.gov/Websites/

ddeer/images/Final%20November%20Emergency%20MM%20Rules-Website%20(002).pdf. Accessed November 21, 2019.

[50]Senate Bill 161. Oregon Legislature website. https://olis.leg.state.or.us/liz/2007R1/Downloads/MeasureDocument/SB161. Accessed November 27, 2019.

[51]Pennsylvania medical marijuana law. NORML website. https://norml.org/pa-2/item/pennsylvania-medical-marijuana-law. Accessed November 27, 2019.

[52]Puerto Rico medical marijuana law. NORML website. https://norml.org/legal/item/puerto-rico-medical-marijuana-law. Accessed November 27, 2019.

[53]Rhode Island medical marijuana law. NORML website. https://norml.org/legal/item/rhode-island-medical-marijuana. Accessed November 27, 2019.

[54]South Carolina medical marijuana law. NORML website. https://norml.org/legal/item/south-carolina-cbd-marijuana-law. Accessed November 27, 2019.

[55]Tennessee medical marijuana law. NORML website. https://norml.org/legal/item/tennessee-cbd-marijuana-law. Accessed November 27, 2019.

[56]Texas medical marijuana law. NORML website. https://norml.org/legal/item/texas-cbd-specific-marijuana-law. Accessed November 27, 2019.

[57]Virginia Islands medical marijuana law. NORML website. https://norml.org/legal/item/virgin-islands-medical-marijuana-law. Accessed November 27, 2019.

[58]Utah CBD-specific law. NORML website. https://norml.org/legal/item/utah-cbd-marijuana-law. Accessed November 27, 2019.

[59]Vermont medical marijuana law. NORML website. https://norml.org/legal/item/vermont-medical-marijuana. Accessed November 27, 2019.

[60]SB 1557 Pharmacy, Board of; cannabidiol and tetrahydrocannabinol oil, regulation of pharmaceutical. Virginia State Legislature website. https://lis.virginia.gov/cgi-bin/legp604.exe?191+sum+SB1557. Accessed November 22, 2019.

[61]Washington medical marijuana law. NORML website. https://norml.org/legal/item/washington-medical-marijuana. Accessed November 21, 2019.

[62]West Virginia medical marijuana law. NORML website. https://norml.org/legal/item/west-virginia-medical-marijuana-law. Accessed November 27, 2019.

[63]2017 Senate Bill 10. Wisconsin State Legislature website. http://docs.legis.wisconsin.gov/2017/related/acts/4. Accessed November 27, 2019.

[64]Wyoming CBD-specific marijuana law. NORML website. https://norml.org/legal/item/wyoming-cbd-specific-marijuana-law. Accessed November 27, 2019.

[65]Russo EB. Taming THC: potential cannabis synergy and phytocannabinoid-terpenoid entourage effects. *Br J Pharmacol.* 2011;163(7):1344-1364. doi: 10.1111/j.1476-5381.2011.01238.x.

[66]Santiago M, Sachdev S, Arnold JC, McGregor IS, Connor M. Absence of entourage: terpenoids commonly found in *Cannabis sativa* do not modulate the functional activity of Δ^9-THC at human CB_1 and CB_2 receptors. *Cannabis Cannabinoid Res.* 2019;4(3):165-176. doi: 10.1089/can.2019.0016.

[67]Gertsch J, Leonti M, Raduner S, et al. Beta-caryophyllene is a dietary cannabinoid. *Proc Natl Acad Sci U S A.* 2008;105(26):9099-9104. doi: 10.1073/pnas.0803601105.

[68]Lidicker G. Exploring the 'entourage effect' with Dr. Ethan Russo. CannabisMD website. https://cannabismd.com/basics/cannabis/exploring-the-entourage-effect-with-dr-ethan-russo/. Published October 14, 2019. Accessed November 21, 2019.

[69]AbbVie Inc. Marinol (dronabinol) [package insert]. U.S. Food and Drug Administration website. https://www.accessdata.fda.gov/drugsatfda_docs/label/2017/018651s029lbl.pdf. Revised August 2017. Accessed December 2, 2019.

[70]Carley DW, Prasad B, Reid KJ, et al. Pharmacotherapy of apnea by cannabimimetic enhancement, the PACE clinical trial: effects of dronabinol in obstructive sleep apnea. *Sleep.* 2018;41(1):zsx184. doi: 10.1093/sleep/zsx184.

[71]Valeant Pharmaceuticals International. Cesamet (nabilone) [package insert]. U.S. Food and Drug Administration website. https://www.accessdata.fda.gov/drugsatfda_docs/label/2006/018677s011lbl.pdf. Revised May 2006. Accessed December 2, 2019.

[72]Valeant Pharmaceuticals International. Cesamet (nabilone) [package insert]. U.S. Food and Drug Administration website. https://www.accessdata.fda.gov/drugsatfda_docs/label/2006/018677s011lbl.pdf. Revised May 2006. Accessed October 31, 2019.

[73]Greenwich Biosciences, Inc. Epidiolex (cannabidiol) [package insert]. U.S. Food and Drug Administration website. https://www.epidiolex.com/sites/default/files/EPIDIOLEX_Full_Prescribing_Information.pdf#page=8. Revised June 2018. Accessed December 2, 2019.

[74]McPartland JM, MacDonald C, Young M, Grant PS, Furkert DP, Glass M. Affinity and efficacy studies of tetrahydrocannabinolic acid A at cannabinoid receptor types one and two. *Cannabis Cannabinoid Res*. 2017;2(1):87–95. doi:10.1089/can.2016.0032.

[75]Grotenhermen F. Clinical pharmacokinetics of cannabinoids. In: Russo EM, Grotenhermen F, eds. *Handbook of Cannabis Therapeutics: From Bench to Bedside*. Binghamton, NY: Hawthorn Press, Inc; 2010:69-116. https://saltonverde.com/wp-content/uploads/2017/09/17-Handbook_cannabis_therapeutics_from_bench_to_bedside.pdf#page=190. Accessed October 8, 2019.

[76]Smith RN, Vaughan CG. The decomposition of acidic and neutral cannabinoids in organic solvents. *J Pharm Pharmacol*. 1977;29(5):286-290. doi: 10.1111/j.2042-7158.1977.tb11313.x.

[77]Grotenhermen F. Pharmacokinetics and pharmacodynamics of cannabinoids. *Clin Pharmacokinet*. 2003;42(4):327-360. doi: 10.2165/00003088-200342040-00003.

[78]ElSohly MA, Slade D. Chemical constituents of marijuana: the complex mixture of natural cannabinoids. *Life Sci*. 2005;78:539-548. doi: 10.1016/j.lfs.2005.09.011.

[79]Barrus DG, Capogrossi KL, Cates SC, et al. Tasty THC: promises and challenges of cannabis edibles. *Methods Rep RTI Press*. 2016;2016. doi: 10.3768/rtipress.2016.op.0035.1611.

[80]Scuderi C, De Filippis D, Iuvone T, Blasio A, Steardo A, Esposito G. Cannabidiol as medicine: a review of its therapeutic potential in CNS disorders. *Phytother Res*. 2009;23(5):597-602. doi: 10.1002/ptr.2625.

[81]Gieringer D, St. Laurent J, Goodrich S. Cannabis vaporizer combines efficient delivery of THC with effective suppression of pyrolytic compounds. *J Cannabis Therap*. 2004;4(1):7-27. doi: 10.1300/j175v04n01_02.

[82]Stockburger S. Forms of administration of cannabis and their efficacy. *J Pain Manage*. 2016;9(4):381-386.

[83]Sharma P, Murthy P, Srinivas Bharath MM. Chemistry, metabolism, and toxicology of cannabis: clinical implications. *Iran J Psychiatry*. 2012;7(4):149-156.

[84]Outbreak of lung injury associated with the use of e-cigarette, or vaping, products. Centers for Disease Control and Prevention website. https://www.cdc.gov/tobacco/basic_information/e-cigarettes/severe-lung-disease.html. Updated November 19, 2019. Accessed November 21, 2019.

[85]ElSohly MA, Mehmedic Z, Foster S, et al. Changes in cannabis potency over the last two decades (1995-2014)—analysis of current data in the United States. *Biol Psychiatry*. 2016;79(7):613-619. doi: 10.1016/j.biopsych.2016.01.004.

[86]Canada Parliament. *Cannabis: Report of the Senate Special Committee on Illegal Drugs Abridged version*. Toronto: University of Toronto Press; 2003:40.

[87]Neavyn MJ, Blohm E, Babu KM, Bird SB. Medical marijuana and driving: a review. *J Med Toxicol*. 2014;10(3):269-279. doi: 10.1007/s13181-014-0393-4.

[88]Huestis MA, Smith ML. Human cannabinoid pharmacokinetics and interpretation of cannabinoid concentrations in biological fluids and tissues. In: ElSohly MA, ed. *Marijuana and the Cannabinoids*. Totowa, NJ: Humana Press Inc; 2007:205-235.

[89]Grotenhermen F. Clinical pharmacokinetics of cannabinoids. In: Russo EM, Grotenhermen F, eds. *Handbook of Cannabis Therapeutics: From Bench to Bedside.* Binghamton, NY: Hawthorn Press, Inc; 2010:69-116. https://saltonverde.com/wp-content/uploads/2017/09/17-Handbook_cannabis_therapeutics_from_bench_to_bedside.pdf#page=190. Accessed October 9, 2019.

[90]Toennes SW, Ramaekers JG, Theunissen EL, Moeller MR, Kauert GF. Comparison of cannabinoid pharmacokinetic properties in occasional and heavy users smoking a marijuana or placebo joint. *J Anal Toxicol.* 2008;32(7):470-477. doi: 10.1093/jat/32.7.470.

[91]Spindle TR, Cone EJ, Schlienz NJ, et al. Acute effects of smoked and vaporized cannabis in healthy adults who infrequently use cannabis: a crossover trial. *JAMA Netw Open.* 2018;1(7):e184841. doi: 10.1001/jamanetworkopen.2018.4841.

[92]Ohlsson A, Lindgren JE, Andersson S, et al. Single-dose kinetics of deuterium-labelled cannabidiol in man after smoking and intravenous administration. *Biomed Environ Mass Spectrom.* 1986;13(2):77-83.

[93]Bonn-Miller MC, Loflin MJE, Thomas BF. Label accuracy of cannabidiol extracts sold online. *JAMA.* 2017;318(17):1708-1709. doi: 10.1001/jama/2017.11909.

[94]Warning Letters and Test Results for Cannabidiol-Related Products. United States Food & Drug Administration website. https://www.fda.gov/news-events/public-health-focus/warning-letters-and-test-results-cannabidiol-related-products. Accessed October 14, 2019.

[95]Grotenhermen F. Clinical pharmacokinetics of cannabinoids. In: Russo EM, Grotenhermen F, eds. *Handbook of Cannabis Therapeutics: From Bench to Bedside.* Binghamton, NY: Hawthorn Press, Inc; 2010:69-116. https://saltonverde.com/wp-content/uploads/2017/09/17-Handbook_cannabis_therapeutics_from_bench_to_bedside.pdf#page=190. Accessed October 11, 2019.

[96]Millar SA, Stone NL, Yates AS, O'Sullivan SE. A systematic review on the pharmacokinetics of cannabidiol in humans. *Front Pharmacol.* 2018;9:1365. doi: 10.3389/fphar.2018.01365.

[97]Manini AF, Yiannoulos G, Bergamaschi MM, et al. Safety and pharmacokinetics of oral cannabidiol when administered concomitantly with intravenous fentanyl in humans. *J Addict Med.* 2015;9(3):204-210. doi: 10.1097/ADM.0000000000000118.

[98]Russo EB. Cannabidiol claims and misconceptions. *Trends Pharmacol Sci.* 2017;38(3):198-201. doi: 10.1016/j.tips.2016.12.004.

[99]Huestis MA, Smith ML. Cannabinoid pharmacokinetics and dispositions in alternative matrices. In: Pertwee RG, ed. *Handbook on Cannabis.* New York, NY: Oxford University Press; 2014:296-316.

[100]Valiveti S, Hammell DC, Earles DC, Stinchcomb AL. In vitro/in vivo correlation studies for transdermal delta 8-THC development. *J Pharm Sci.* 2004;93(5):1154-1164. doi: 10.1002/jps.20036.

[101]Stinchcomb AL, Valiveti S, Hammell DC, Ramsey DR. Human skin permeation of delta8-tetrahydrocannabinol, cannabidiol, and cannabinol. *J Pharm Pharmacol.* 2004;56(3):291-297. doi: 10.1211/0022357022791.

[102]Bruni N, Della Pepa C, Oliaro-Bosso S, Pessione E, Gastaldi D, Dosio F. Cannabinoid delivery systems for pain and inflammation treatment. *Molecules.* 2018;23(10):2478. doi: 10.3390/molecules23102478.

[103]Touw M. The religious and medicinal uses of *Cannabis* in China, India and Tibet. *J Psychoactive Drugs.* 1981;13(1):23-34. doi: 10.1080/02791072.1981.10471447.

[104]Brenneisen R, Elgi A, ElSohly MA, Henn V. The effect of orally and rectally administered Δ9-tetrahydrocannabinol on spasticity: a pilot study with 2 patients. *Int J Clin Pharmacol Ther.* 1996;34(10):446-452.

[105]Ujváry I, Hanuš L. Human metabolites of cannabidiol: a review of their formation, biological activity, and relevance in therapy. *Cannabis Cannabinoid Res.* 2016;1(1):90-101. doi: 10.1089/can.2015.0012.

[106]Hazekamp A, Pappas G. Self-medication with cannabis. In: Pertwee RG, ed. *Handbook on Cannabis*. New York, NY: Oxford University Press; 2014:319-338.

[107]Rock EM, Kopstick RL, Limebeer CL, Parker LA. Tetrahydrocannabinolic acid reduces nausea-induced conditioned gaping in rats and vomiting in *Suncus murinus*. *Br J Pharmacol*. 2013;170(3):641-648. doi: 10.1111/bph.12316.

[108]Hunt CA, Jones RT. Tolerance and disposition of tetrahydrocannabinol in man. *J Pharmacol Exp Ther*. 1980;215(1):35-44.

[109]Grotenhermen F. Clinical pharmacokinetics of cannabinoids. In: Russo EM, Grotenhermen F, eds. *Handbook of Cannabis Therapeutics: From Bench to Bedside*. Binghamton, NY: Hawthorn Press, Inc; 2010:69-116. https://saltonverde.com/wp-content/uploads/2017/09/17-Handbook_cannabis_therapeutics_from_bench_to_bedside.pdf#page=190. Accessed October 9, 2019.

[110]Brunet B, Doucet C, Venisse N, et al. Validation of large white pig as an animal model for the study of cannabinoids metabolism: application of the study of THC distribution in tissues. *Forensic Sci Int*. 2006;161(2-3):169-174. doi: 10.1016/j.forsciint.2006.04.018.

[111]Kreuz DS, Axelrod J. Delta-9-tetrahydrocannabinol: localization in body fat. *Science*. 1973;179(4071):391-393. doi: 10.1126/science.179.4071.391.

[112]Grant KS, Petroff R, Isoherranen N, Stella N, Burbacher TM. Cannabis use during pregnancy: pharmacokinetics and effects on child development. *Pharmacol Ther*. 2018;182:133-151. doi: 10.1016/j.pharmthera.2017.08.014.

[113]Bertrand KA, Hanan NJ, Honerkamp-Smith G, Best BM, Chambers CD. Marijuana use by breastfeeding mothers and cannabinoid concentrations in breast milk. *Pediatrics*. 2018;142(3):e20181076. doi: https://doi.org/10.1542/peds.2018-1076.

[114]Perez-Reyes M, Wall ME. Presence of delta9-tetrahydrocannabinol in human milk. *N Engl J Med*. 1982;307(13):819-820. doi: 10.1056/NEJM198209233071311.

[115]Huestis MA. Human cannabinoid pharmacokinetics. *Chem Biodivers*. 2007;4(8):1770-1804. doi: 10.1002/cbdv.200790152.

[116]Zhornitsky S, Potvin S. Cannabidiol in humans—the quest for therapeutic targets. *Pharmaceuticals (Basel)*. 2012;5(5):529-552. doi: 10.3390/ph5050529.

[117]Agurell S, Halldin M, Lindgren J E, et al. Pharmacokinetics and metabolism of Δ^1-tetrahydrocannabinol and other cannabinoids with emphasis on man. *Pharmacol Rev*. 1986;38(1):21-43.

[118]Ellis GM Jr, Mann MA, Judson BA, Schramm NT, Tashchian A. Excretion patterns of cannabinoid metabolites after last use in a group of chronic users. *Clin Pharmacol Ther*. 1985;38(5):572-578. doi: 10.1038/clpt.1985.226.

[119]Feinshtein V, Erez O, Ben-Zvi Z, et al. Cannabidiol enhances xenobiotic permeability through the human placental barrier by direct inhibition of breast cancer resistance protein: an ex vivo study. *Am J Obstet Gynecol*. 2013;209(6):573.e1-573.e15. doi: 10.1016/j.ajog.2013.08.005.

[120]Jiang R, Yamaori S, Takeda S, Yamamoto I, Watanabe K. Identification of cytochrome P450 enzymes responsible for metabolism of cannabidiol in human liver microsomes. *Life Sci*. 2011;89(5-6):165-170. doi: 10.1016/j.lfs.2011.05.018.

[121]United States Food and Drug Administration. FDA briefing document. Peripheral and Central Nervous System Drugs Advisory Committee Meeting, NDA 210365, Cannabidiol. April 19, 2018. https://www.fda.gov/media/112565/download. Accessed October 31, 2019.

[122]AbbVie Inc. Marinol (dronabinol) [package insert]. U.S. Food and Drug Administration website. https://www.accessdata.fda.gov/drugsatfda_docs/label/2017/018651s029lbl.pdf. Revised August 2017. Accessed October 31, 2019.

[123]Greenwich Biosciences, Inc. Epidiolex (cannabidiol) [package insert]. U.S. Food and Drug Administration website. https://www.epidiolex.com/sites/default/files/EPIDIOLEX_Full_Prescribing_Information.pdf#page=8. Revised June 2018. Accessed October 31, 2019.

[124]Pisanti S, Malfitano AM, Ciaglia E, et al. Cannabidiol: state of the art and new challenges for therapeutic applications. *Pharmacol Ther.* 2017;175:133-150. doi: 10.1016/j.pharmthera.2017.02.041.

[125]Cheng D, Spiro AS, Jenner AM, Garner B, Karl T. Long-term cannabidiol treatment prevents the development of social recognition memory deficits in Alzheimer's disease transgenic mice. *J Alzheimers Dis.* 2014;42(4):1383-1396. doi: 10.3233/JAD-140921.

[126]Esposito G, De Filippis D, Maiuri MC, et al. Cannabidiol inhibits inducible nitric oxide synthase protein expression and nitric oxide production in ß-amyloid stimulated PC12 neurons through p38 MAP kinase and NF-κB involvement. *Neurosci Lett.* 2006;399(1-2):91-95. doi: 10.1016/j.neulet.2006.01.047.

[127]Esposito G, De Filippis D, Carnuccio R, Izzo AI, Iuvone T. The marijuana component cannabidiol inhibits ß-amyloid-induced tau protein hyperphosphorylation through Wnt/ß-catenin pathway rescue in PC12 cells. *J Mol Med.* 2006;84(3):253-258. doi: 10.1007/s00109-005-0025-1.

[128]Martin-Moreno AM, Reigada D, Belen G, et al. Cannabidiol and other cannabinoids reduce microglial activation in vitro and in vivo: relevance to Alzheimer's disease. *Mol Pharmacol.* 2011;76(6):964-973. doi: 10.1124/mol.111.071290.

[129]Scuderi C, Steardo L, Esposito G. Cannabidiol promotes amyloid precursor protein ubiquitination and reduction of beta amyloid expression in SHSY5Y^{APP+} cells through PPARY involvement. *Phytother Res.* 2014;28(7):1007-1013. doi: 10.1002/ptr.5095.

[130]Almeida V, Levin R, Peres FF, et al. Cannabidiol exhibits anxiolytic but not antipsychotic property evaluated in the social interaction test. *Prog Neuropsychopharmacol Biol Psychiatry.* 2013;41(5):30-35. doi: 10.1016/j.pnpbp.2012.10.024.

[131]Bergamaschi MM, Costa Queiroz RH, Nisihara Chagas MH, et al. Cannabidiol reduces the anxiety induced by simulated public speaking in treatment-naïve social phobia patients. *Neuropsychopharmacology.* 2011;36(6):1219-1226. doi: 10.1038/npp.2011.6.

[132]de Mello Schier AR, Oliveira Ribeiro NP, Coutinho DS, et al. Antidepressant-like and anxiolytic-like effects of cannabidiol: a chemical compound in *Cannabis sativa*. *CNS Neurol Disord Drug Targets.* 2014;13(6):953-960. doi: 10.2174/1871527313666140612114838.

[133]Lemos JI, Resstel LB, Guimarães FS. Involvement of the prelimbic prefrontal cortex on cannabidiol-induced attenuation of contextual conditional fear in rats. *Behav Brain Res.* 2010;207(1):105-111. doi: 10.1016/j.bbr.2009.09.045.

[134]Marinho ALZ, Vila-Verde C, Fogaça MV, Guimarães FS. Effects of intra-infralimbic prefrontal cortex injections of cannabidiol in the modulation of emotional behaviors in rats: contribution of 5HT$_{1A}$ receptors and stressful experiences. *Behav Brain Res.* 2015;286:49-56. doi: 10.1016/j.bbr.2015.02.023.

[135]Moreira FA, Aguiar DC, Guimarães FS. Anxiolytic-like effect of cannabidiol in the rat Vogel conflict test. *Prog Neuropsychopharmacol Biol Psychiatry.* 2006;30(8):1466-1471. doi: 10.1016/j.pnpbp.2006.06.004.

[136]Ligresti A, Moriello AS, Starowicz K, et al. Antitumor activity of plant cannabinoids with emphasis on the effect of cannabidiol on human breast carcinoma. *J Pharmacol Exp Ther.* 2006;318(3):1375-1387. doi: 10.1124/jpet.106.105247.

[137]McAllister SD, Murase R, Christian RT, et al. Pathways mediating the effects of cannabidiol on the reduction of breast cancer cell proliferation, invasion, and metastasis. *Breast Cancer Res Treat.* 2011;129(1):37-47. doi: 10.1007/s10549-010-1177-4.

[138]Pisanti S, Picardi P, D'Alessandro A, Laezza C, Bifulco M. The endocannabinoid signaling system in cancer. *Trends Pharmacol Sci.* 2013;34(5):273-282. doi: 10.1016/j.tips.2013.03.003.

[139]Ramer R, Fischer S, Haustein M, Manda K, Hinz B. Cannabinoids inhibit angiogenic capacities of endothelial cells via release of tissue inhibitor of matrix metalloproteinases-1 from lung cancer cells. *Biochem Pharmacol.* 2014;91(2):202-216. doi: 10.1016/j.bcp.2014.06.017.

[140]Rocha FCM, Dos Santos Júnior JG, Stefano SC, de Silveira DX. Systematic review of the literature on clinical and experimental trials on the antitumor effects of cannabinoids in gliomas. *J Neurooncol*. 2014;116(1):11-24. doi: 10.1007/s11060-013-1277-1.

[141]Scott KA, Dalgleish AG, Liu WM. The combination of cannabidiol and Δ9-tetrahydrocannabinol enhances the anticancer effects of radiation in an orthotopic murine glioma model. *Mol Cancer Ther*. 2014;13(12):2955-2967. doi: 10.1158/1535-7163. MCT-14-0402.

[142]Shrivastava A, Kuzontkoski PM, Groopman JE, Prasad A. Cannabidiol induces programmed cell death in breast cancer cells by coordinating the cross-talk between apoptosis and autophagy. *Mol Cancer Ther*. 2011;10(7):1161-1172. doi: 10.1158/1535-7163.MCT-10-1100.

[143]Booz GW. Cannabidiol as an emergent therapeutic strategy for lessening the impact of inflammation on oxidative stress. *Free Radic Biol Med*. 2011;51(5):1054-1061. doi: 10.1016/j. freeradbiomed.2011.01.007.

[144]Durst R, Danenberg H, Gallily R, et al. Cannabidiol, a nonpsychoactive cannabis constituent, protects against myocardial ischemic reperfusion injury. *Am J Physiol Heart Circ Physiol*. 2007;293(6):H3602-H3607. doi: 10.1152/ajpheart.00098.2007.

[145]Stanley CP, Hind WH, O'Sullivan SE. Is the cardiovascular system a therapeutic target for cannabidiol? *Br J Clin Pharmacol*. 2013;75(2):313-322. doi: 10.1111/j.1365-2125.2012.043.351.x.

[146]El-Alfy AT, Ivey K, Robinson K, et al. Antidepressant-like effect Δ9-tetrahydrocannabinol and other cannabinoids isolated from *Cannabis sativa L*. *Pharmacol Biochem Behav*. 2010;95(4):434-442. doi: 10.1016/j.pbb.2010.03.004.

[147]Hsiao YT, Yi PL, Li CL, Chang FC. Effect of cannabidiol on sleep disruption induced by the repeated combination tests consisting of open field and elevated plus-maze in rats. *Neuropharmacology*. 2012;62(1):373-384. doi: 10.1016/j.neuropharm.2011.08.013.

[148]Shoval G, Shbiro L, Hershkovitz L, et al. Prohedonic effect of cannabidiol in a rat model of depression. *Neuropsychobiology*. 2016;73(2):123-129. doi: 10.1159/000443890.

[149]Kozela E, Pietr M, Juknat A, et al. Cannabinoids Delta(9)-tetrahydrocannabinol and cannabidiol differentially inhibit the lipopolysaccharide-activated NF-kappaB and interferon-beta/STAT proinflammatory pathways in BV-2 microglial cells. *J Biol Chem*. 2010;285(3):1616-1626. doi: 10.1074/jbc.M109.069294.

[150]Rajesh M, Mukhopadhyay P, Bátkai S, et al. Cannabidiol attenuates cardiac dysfuction, oxidative stress, fibrosis, and inflammatory and cell death signaling pathways in diabetic cardiomyopathy. *J Am Coll Cardiol*. 2010;56(25):2115-2125. doi: 10.1016/j.jacc.2010.07.033.

[151]Weiss L, Zeira M, Reich S, et al. Cannabidiol lowers incidence of diabetes in non-obese diabetic mice. *Autoimmunity*. 2006;39(2):143-151. doi: 10.1080/08916930500356674.

[152]Consroe P, Laguna J, Allender J, et al. Controlled clinical trial of cannabidiol in Huntington's disease. *Pharmacol Biochem Behav*. 1991;40(3):701-708. doi: 10.1016/0091-3057(91)90386-g.

[153]Iuvone T, Esposito G, De Filippis D, Scuderi C, Steardo L. Cannabidiol: a promising drug for neurodegenerative disorders? *CNS Neurosci Ther*. 2009;15(1):65-75. doi: 10.1111/j. 1755-5949.2008.00065.x

[154]Sagredo O, Pazos MR, Satta V, et al. Neuroprotective effects of phytocannabinoid-based medicines in experimental modes of Huntington's disease. *J Neurosci Res*. 2011;89(9): 1509-1518. doi: 10.1002/jnr.22682.

[155]Hayakawa K, Mishima K, Nozako M, et al. Delayed treatment with cannabidiol has a cerebroprotective action via a cannabinoid receptor-independent myeloperoxidase-inhibiting mechanism. *J Neurochem*. 2007;102(5):1488-1496. doi: 10.1111/j.1471-4159. 2007.04565.x.

[156]Hayakawa K, Irie K, Sano K, et al. Therapeutic time window of cannabidiol treatment on delayed ischemic damage via high-morbidity group box1-inhibited mechanism. *Biol Pharm Bull*. 2009;32(9):1538-1544. doi: 10.1248/bpb.32.1538.

[157]Pazos MR, Cinquina V, Gómez A, et al. Cannabidiol administration after hypoxia-ischemia to newborn rats reduced long-term brain injury and restores neurobehavioral function. *Neuropharmacology*. 2012;63(5):776-783. doi: 10.1016/j.neuropharm.2012.05.034.

[158]Pazos MR, Mohammed N, Lafuente H, et al. Mechanisms of cannabidiol neuroprotection in hypoxic-ischemic newborn pigs: role of $5HT_{1A}$ and CB_2 receptors. *Neuropharmacology*. 2013;71:282-291. doi: 10.1016/j.neuropharm.2013.03.027.

[159]Ruiz-Valdepeñas L, Martinez-Orgado JA, Beníto C, et al. Cannabidiol reduces lipopoly-saccharide-induced vascular changes and inflammation in the mouse brain: an intravital microscopic study. *J Neuroinflammation*. 2011;8(1):5. doi: 10.1186/1742-2094-8-5.

[160]Appendino G, Gibbons S, Giana A, et al. Antibacterial cannabinoids from *Cannabis sativa*: a structure-activity study. *J Nat Prod*. 2008;71(8):1427-1430. doi: 10.1021/np8002673.

[161]Kozela E, Lev N, Kaushansky N, et al. Cannabidiol inhibits pathogenic T cells, decreases spinal microglial activation and ameliorates multiple sclerosis-like disease in C57BL/6 mice. *Br J Pharmacol*. 2011;163(7):1507-1519. doi: 10.1111/j.1476-5381.2011.01379.x.

[162]Mecha M, Torrao AS, Mestre L, et al. Cannabidiol protects oligodendrocyte progenitor cells from inflammation-induced apoptosis by attenuating endoplasmic reticulum stress. *Cell Death Dis*. 2012;3(6):e331. doi: 10.1038/cddis.2012.71.

[163]Mecha M, Feliú A, Iñigo PM, et al. Cannabidiol provides long-lasting protection against the deleterious effects of inflammation in a viral model of multiple sclerosis: a role for A2A receptors. *Neurobiol Dis*. 2013;59:141-150. doi: 10.1016/j.nbd.2013.06.016.

[164]Ribeiro A, Ferraz-de-Paula V, Pinheiro ML, et al. Cannabidiol, a non-psychoactive plant-derived cannabinoid, decreases inflammation in a murine model of acute lung injury: role for the adenosine A_{2A} receptor. *Eur J Pharmacol*. 2012;678(1-3):78-85. doi: 10.1016/j.ejphar.2011.12.043.

[165]Ribeiro A, Almeida VI, Costola-de-Souza C, et al. Cannabidiol improves lung function and inflammation in mice submitted to LPS-induced acute lung injury. *Immunopharmacol Immunotoxicol*. 2015;37(1):35-41. doi: 10.3109/08923973.2014.976794.

[166]De Filippis D, Esposito G, Cirillo C, et al. Cannabidiol reduces intestinal inflammation through the control of neuroimmune axis. *PLoS One*. 2011;6(12):e28159. doi: 10.1371/journal.pone.0028159.

[167]Naftali T, Lev LB, Yablecovitch D, Half E, Konikoff FM. Treatment of Crohn's disease with cannabis: an observational study. *Isr Med Assoc J*. 2011;13(8):455-458. PMID: 21910367.

[168]Sacerdote P, Martucci C, Vaccani A, et al. The nonpsychotropic component of marijuana cannabidiol modulates chemotaxis and IL-10 and IL-12 production of murine macrophages both in vivo and in vitro. *J Neuroimmunol*. 2005;159(1-2):97-105. doi: 10.1016/j.neuroim.2004.10.003.

[169]Buccellato E, Carretta D, Utan A, et al. Acute and chronic cannabinoid extracts administration affects motor function in a CREAE model of multiple sclerosis. *J Ethnopharmacol*. 2011;133(3):1033-1038. doi: 10.1016/j.jep.2010.11.035.

[170]Giacoppo S, SoundaraRajan T, Galuppo M, et al. Purified cannabidiol, the main non-psychotropic component of *Cannabis sativa*, alone, counteracts neuronal apoptosis in experimental multiple sclerosis. *Eur Rev Med Pharmacol Sci*. 2015;19(24):4906-4919. PMID: 26744883.

[171]Kozela E, Juknat A, Kaushansky N, et al. Cannabidiol, a non-psychoactive cannabinoid, leads to EGR2-dependent anergy in activated encephalitogenic T cells. *J Neuroinflammation*. 2015;12:52. doi: 10.1186/s12974-015-0273-0.

[172]Parker LA, Mechoulam R, Schlievert C. Cannabidiol, a non-psychoactive component of cannabis and its synthesis dimethylheptyl homolog suppress nausea in an experimental model with rats. *Neuroreport*. 2002;13(5):567-570. doi: 10.1097/00001756-200204160-00006.

[173]Rock EM, Limebeer CL, Mechoulam R, Piomelli D, Parker LA. The effect of cannabidiol and URB597 on conditioned gaping (a model of nausea) elicited by a lithium-paired context in the rat. *Psychopharmacology (Berl)*. 2008;196(3):389-395. doi: 10.1007/s00213-007-0970-1.

[174]Boychuk DG, Goddard G, Mauro G, Orellana MF. The effectiveness of cannabinoids in the management of chronic nonmalignant neuropathic pain: a systematic review. *J Oral Facial Pain Headache*. 2015;29(1):7-14. doi: 10.11607/ofph.1274.

[175]Chagas MHN, Eckeli AL, Zuardi AW, et al. Cannabidiol can improve complex sleep-related behaviours associated with rapid eye movement sleep behaviour disorder in Parkinson's disease patients: a case series. *J Clin Pharm Ther*. 2014;39(5):564-566. doi: 10.1111/jcpt.12179.

[176]Lastres-Becker I, Molina-Holgado F, Ramos JA, Mechoulam R, Fernández-Ruiz J. Cannabinoids provide neuroprotection against 6-hydroxydopamine toxicity in vivo and in vitro: relevance to Parkinson's disease. *Neurobiol Dis*. 2005;19(1-2):96-107. doi: 10.1016/j.nbd.2004.11.009.

[177]Zuardi AW, Crippa JAS, Hallak JEC, et al. Cannabidiol for the treatment of psychosis in Parkinson's disease. *J Psychopharmacol*. 2009;23(8):979-983. doi: 10.1177/0269881108096519.

[178]Crippa JA, Hallak JEC, Abilio VC, Tavares de Lacerda AL, Zuardi AW. Cannabidiol and sodium nitroprusside: two novel neuromodulatory pharmacological interventions to treat and prevent psychosis. *CNS Neurol Disord Drug Targets*. 2015;14(8):970-978. doi: 10.2174/1871527314666150909113930.

[179]Gomes FV, Llorente R, Del Bel EA, et al. Decreased glial reactivity could be involved in the antipsychotic-like effect of cannabidiol. *Schizophr Res*. 2015;164(1-3):155-163. doi: 10.1016/j.schres.2015.01.015.

[180]Zuardi AW, Crippa JAS, Hallak JEC, Moreira FA, Guimarães FS. Cannabidiol, a *Cannabis sativa* constituent, as an antipsychotic drug. *Braz J Med Biol Res*. 2006;39(4):421-429. doi: 10.1590/s0100-879x2006000400001.

[181]Zuardi AW, Crippa JAS, Hallak JEC, et al. A critical review of the antipsychotic effects of cannabidiol: 30 years of a translational investigation. *Curr Pharm Des*. 2012;18(32):5131-5140. doi: 10.2174/138161212802884681.

[182]Malfait AM, Gallily R, Sumariwalla PF, et al. The nonpsychoactive cannabis constituent cannabidiol is an oral anti-arthritic therapeutic in murine collagen-induced arthritis. *Proc Natl Acad Sci U S A*. 2000;97(17):9561-9566. doi: 10.1073/pnas.160105897.

[183]Gieringer D, Rosenthal E, Carter GT. *Marijuana Medical Handbook: Practical Guide to the Therapeutic Uses of Marijuana*. Oakland, CA: Quick American; 2008:11-12.

[184]Gieringer D, Rosenthal E, Carter GT. *Marijuana Medical Handbook: Practical Guide to the Therapeutic Uses of Marijuana*. Oakland, CA: Quick American; 2008:12.

[185]Erkelens JL, Hazekamp A. That which we call *Indica*, by any other name would smell as sweet. *Cannabinoids*. 2014;9(1):9-15. https://www.cannabis-med.org/data/pdf/en_2014_01_2_0.pdf. Accessed October 31, 2019.

[186]Bergamaschi MM, Costa Queiroz RH, Crippa JAS, Zuardi AW. Safety and side effects of cannabidiol, a *Cannabis sativa* constituent. *Curr Drug Saf*. 2011;6(4):237-249.

[187]Weil AT, Zinberg NE, Nelsen JM. Clinical and psychological effects of marijuana in man. In: Mikuriya TH, ed. *Cannabis: Collected Clinical Papers Volume 1: Marijuana: Medical Papers 1839-1972*. Nevada City, CA: Symposium Publishing; 2007:263.

[188]ElSohly MA, Ross SA, Mehmedic Z, Arafat R, Yi B, Banahan BF III. Potency trends of delta9-THC and other cannabinoids in confiscated marijuana from 1980-1997. *J Forensic Sci*. 2000;45(1):24-30.

[189]Mehmedic Z, Chandra S, Slade D, et al. Potency trends of Δ9-THC and other cannabinoids in confiscated cannabis preparations from 1993-2008. *J Forensic Sci.* 2010;55(5):1209-1217. doi: 10.1111/j.1556-4029.2010.01441.x.

[190]Monico N. Alcohol by Volume: Beer, Wine, & Liquor. Alcohol.org website. https://www.alcohol.org/statistics-information/abv/. Updated October 11, 2019. Accessed October 15, 2019.

[191]Ramos Barreda A, De Leon K, Urmas S. A simple guide to pot, THC and how much is too much. Los Angeles Times [Internet]. 2018 April 20. https://www.latimes.com/projects/la-me-weed-101-thc-calculator/. Accessed October 31, 2019

[192]Petro DJ. Pharmacology and toxicity of cannabis. In: Mathre ML, ed. *Cannabis in Medical Practice: A Legal, Historical and Pharmacological Overview of the Therapeutic Use of Marijuana.* Jefferson, NC: McFarland & Company, Inc; 1997:56-66.

[193]Notcutt W, Clarke EL. Cannabinoids in clinical practice: a UK perspective. In: Pertwee RG, ed. *Handbook on Cannabis.* New York, NY: Oxford University Press; 2014:415-432.

[194]Marijuana cannabis allergy. American Academy of Allergy, Asthma & Immunology website. https://www.aaaai.org/conditions-and-treatments/library/allergy-library/marijuana-cannabis-allergy. Accessed November 1, 2019.

[195]Galli JA, Sawaya RA, Friedenberg FK. Cannabinoid hyperemesis syndrome. *Curr Drug Abuse Rev.* 2011;4(4):241-249. doi: 10.2174/1874473711104040241.

[196]Morrison PD, Bhattacharyya S, Murray RM. Recreational cannabis: the risk of schizophrenia. In: Pertwee RG, ed. *Handbook on Cannabis.* New York, NY: Oxford University Press; 2014:661-673.

[197]Murrie B, Lappin J, Large M, Grant S. Transition of substance-induced, brief, and atypical psychoses to schizophrenia: a systematic review and meta-analysis. *Schizophr Bull.* 2020;46(3):505-16. doi: 10.1093/schbul/szb102.

[198]AbbVie Inc. Marinol (dronabinol) [package insert]. U.S. Food and Drug Administration website. https://www.accessdata.fda.gov/drugsatfda_docs/label/2017/018651s029lbl.pdf. Revised August 2017. Accessed November 1, 2019.

[199]ElSohly HN, ElSohly MA. Marijuana smoke condensate. In: ElSohly MA, ed. *Marijuana and the Cannabinoids.* Totowa, NJ: Humana Press Inc; 2007:67-96.

[200]ElSohly HN, ElSohly MA. Marijuana smoke condensate. In: ElSohly MA, ed. *Marijuana and the Cannabinoids.* Totowa, NJ: Humana Press Inc; 2007:93.

[201]Gieringer D, Rosenthal E, Carter GT. *Marijuana Medical Handbook: Practical Guide to the Therapeutic Uses of Marijuana.* Oakland, CA: Quick American; 2008:167-168.

[202]Young FL [Drug Enforcement Administration, United States Department of Justice]. Marijuana rescheduling petition docket no. 86-22 [opinion and recommended ruling, findings of fact, conclusions of law and decision of administrative law judge Francis L. Young, dated September 6, 1988.] http://www.druglibrary.org/schaffer/Library/studies/YOUNG/index.html. Accessed November 2, 2019.

[203]Hartung B, Kauferstein S, Ritz-Timme S, Daldrup T. Sudden unexpected death under acute influence of cannabis. *Forensic Sci Int.* 2014;237:e11-e13. doi: 10.1016/j.forsciint.2014.02.001.

[204]Grigoriadis CE, Cork DP, Dembitsky W, et al. Recurrent cardiogenic shock associated with cannabis use: report of a case and review of the literature. *J Emerg Med.* 2019;56(3):319-322. doi: 10.1016/j.jemermed.2018.12.013.

[205]Brucato R. Recreational cannabis: toxicity, stroke, aneurysm and cardiovascular events. *MOJ Toxicol.* 2019;5(3):101-104. https://medcraveonline.com/MOJT/MOJT-05-00162.pdf. Published May 24, 2019. Accessed November 4, 2019.

[206]Rosenkrantz H, Heyman IA, Braude MC. Inhalation, parenteral and oral LD50 values of Δ9-tetrahydrocannabinol in Fischer rats. *Toxicol Appl Pharmacol.* 1974;28(1):18-27. doi: 10.1016/0041-008x(74)90126-4.

[207]Nahas GG. Toxicology and pharmacology of *Cannabis sativa* with special reference to Δ9-THC. *Bull Narc*. 1972;24(2):11-28. United Nations Office on Drugs and Crime website. https://www.unodc.org/unodc/en/data-and-analysis/bulletin/bulletin_1972-01-01_2_page003.html. Accessed November 4, 2019.

[208]Rosenkrantz H, Fleischman RW, Grant RJ. Toxicity of short-term administration of cannabinoids to rhesus monkeys. *Toxicol Appl Pharmacol*. 1981;58(1):118-131. doi: 10.1016/0041-008x(81)90122-8.

8

The Pharmacodynamics of Cannabis

8.1 Overview of Pharmacodynamics

This chapter examines how cannabis produces its intoxicating as well as therapeutic effects, and it is recommended that readers familiarize themselves and have an understanding of the endocannabinoid system (ECS), which is described in Chapter 6 (The Endocannabinoid System). Pharmacodynamics is defined as the study of biochemical, molecular, and physiologic effects of a drug on the body or simply put what the drug does to the body. While the majority of these effects are produced when phytocannabinoids, particularly Δ^9-tetrahydrocannabinol (THC), interact with the two cannabinoid receptors (CBRs), CB_1 and CB_2, there is evidence that additional therapeutic effects are produced through other receptor-independent mechanisms. Emerging data suggest that phytocannabinoids and terpenic compounds found in *Cannabis sativa* can modulate the effects of THC through a process known as the entourage effect and that they may also interact with receptor systems that transcend the strict definition of the ECS, which currently only includes CB_1 and CB_2 receptors. Data also suggest that the effects of cannabidiol (CBD), which appears to have a very weak affinity for CBRs, are produced through indirect action upon CBRs.[1] As will be discussed later, some controversy has evolved around entourage effect based on a limited number of studies that challenge this concept and offer contradictory data.[2]

The wide variation of subjective effects reported from different cultivars of cannabis (and even specific chemotypes within this group) is indicative of the fact that different phytocannabinoid and terpenic profiles produce different experiences. Exactly how important these distinctions are from a clinical perspective is unclear. Cultivars with high levels of CBD and low levels of THC or cultivars with high levels of THC and low levels of CBD will undoubtedly have distinct therapeutic properties. The same level of certainty is not warranted when one compares cultivars with similar THC and CBD concentrations but different levels of minor cannabinoids (eg, cannabigerol [CBG] or cannabichromene [CBC]) and terpenic compounds.

8.2 Mechanism of Action

To understand the mechanism of action of *C sativa*, one must comprehend the same of its various constituents. As mentioned before, cannabis should not be considered a single drug but rather a constellation of several drugs contained within a single plant. Each of these drugs appears to not only have its own unique mechanisms of action and pharmacological properties but they may also modulate the effects of the other compounds contained within cannabis.

Unfortunately, studies about the pharmacodynamics of each individual phytocannabinoid have not been conducted. Consequently, this chapter will focus primarily on THC and CBD and only briefly examine the pharmacological properties of other cannabinoids and terpenic compounds.

8.2.1 Δ^9-Tetrahydrocannabinol

THC is the most abundant phytocannabinoid in drug-type cannabis, as well as the most well-studied cannabinoid. It is a CB_1 partial agonist and can behave as either an agonist or antagonist at CB_2 receptors and has approximately an equal affinity for both CB_1 and CB_2 receptors.[3] Of the naturally occurring phytocannabinoids, THC has the greatest efficiency (produces the strongest effects) at both CB_1 (K_i = 5.05-80.3 nM) and CB_2 receptors (K_i = 1.73-75.3 nM) (see Table 8.1). It has a greater efficiency than endogenous CB_1 ligands, such as anandamide (K_i = 22 nM[4]) and 2-arachidonoylglycerol (2-AG), which were described in Chapter 6 (The Endocannabinoid System) and do not produce the kinds of subjective effects associated with THC or cannabis in general. Conversely, THC is less efficacious than synthetic cannabinoids like nabilone, CP55,940, and HU-210, as well as its active metabolite 11-hydroxy-Δ9-tetrahydrocannabinol (11-OH-THC).[5]

The effects on mood, perception, emotion, and cognition often associated with cannabis use are due to the activation of CB_1 receptors, which are located primarily in neuronal terminals throughout the central nervous system (CNS) and, to a lesser extent, the peripheral nervous system (PNS), as described in Chapter 6 (see Table 6.1). When activated by endocannabinoids or phytocannabinoids like THC, CB_1 receptors mediate the release of excitatory and inhibitory neurotransmitters and modulate ion channels.[6] As noted in Chapter 6 (The Endocannabinoid System), the stimulation of CB_1 receptors inhibits adenylate cyclase, as well as N-, Q-, and L-type calcium channels. Activation of CB_1 receptors also stimulates the activity of mitogen-activated protein (MAP) kinases.[6]

TABLE 8.1 K_i values of Δ^9-THC, Δ^8-THC, CBN, Δ^9-THCV, CBD, CBG, and β-caryophyllene

Displacing compound	CB$_1$ K$_i$ (nM)	CB$_2$ K$_i$ (nM)	Reference
β-Caryophyllene	>10 000	155	Gertsch et al.[7]
CBD (cannabidiol)	4350[a]	2860	Showalter et al.[8]
	4900[b]	4200	Thomas et al.[9]; Thomas et al.[10]
	27 542	2399	MacLennan et al.[11]
	>10 000[a,c]	>10 000[c]	Bisogno et al.[12]
CBG (cannabigerol)	439[b]	337	Gauson et al.[13]
CBN (cannabinol)	120.2	100	MacLennan et al.[11]
	129.3[a]	ND	Booker et al.[14]
	392.2,[a,c] 211.2[d,c]	126.4[c]	Rhee et al.[15]
	326	96.3	Showalter et al.[8]
	1130	301	Felder et al.[16]
Δ^8-THC (Δ^8-tetrahydrocannabinol)	44[a]	44	Huffman et al.[17]
	47.6[a]	39.3[b]	Busch-Petersen et al.[18]
Δ^9-THC (Δ^9-tetrahydrocannabinol)	5.05	3.13	Iwamura et al.[19]
	8.33[b]	1.73[e]	Iwamura et al.[19]
	13.5[a]	6.8[a]	Iwamura et al.[19]
	21; 40.7[a]	36.4	Showalter et al.[8]
	35.3[a]	3.9[a]	Rinaldi-Carmona et al.[20]
	39.5[d,c]	40[c]	Bayewitch et al.[21]
	47.7[a]	ND	Booker et al.[14]
	53.3	75.3	Felder et al.[16]
	66.5,[a,c] 80.3[d,c]	32.2[c]	Rhee et al.[15]

(Continued)

TABLE 8.1 Continued

Displacing compound	CB$_1$ K$_i$ (nM)	CB$_2$ K$_i$ (nM)	Reference
Δ^9-THCV (Δ^9-tetrahydrocannabivarin)	46.6[b]	ND	Pertwee et al.[22]
	75.4[b]	62.8	Thomas et al.[23]
	286[a,f]	ND	Hill et al.[24]
	ND	145	Bolognini et al.[25]
	ND	225	Bolognini et al.[26]

Unless otherwise noted, all data are from experiments performed on membranes from cultured cells transfected with CBRs from humans and measured the displacement of [^{3}H]CP55,940.
[a]Experiment performed with rat brain (CB$_1$) and rat spleen (CB$_2$) membranes.
[b]Experiment performed with mouse brain (CB$_1$) and mouse spleen (CB$_2$) membranes.
[c]Experiment measured the displacement of [^{3}H]HU-243.
[d]Experiment performed with membranes from cultured cells transfected with rat CBRs.
[e]Experiment performed with membranes from cultured cells transfected with mouse CBRs.
[f]Experiment measured the displacement of [^{3}H]SR141716A.
N, Not determined.

Apart from the subjective effects mentioned above, assays with laboratory animals have shown that the activation of CB$_1$ receptors in the CNS also leads to antinociception (tail flick test), catalepsy (ring test), suppression of locomotor activity, and hypothermia.[6] Additionally, CB$_1$ receptors are found in the nucleus of the solitary tract, which may partially account for THC's well-documented antiemetic effects,[6] though this phenomenon may also be induced by the inhibition of 5-hydroxytryptamine, as THC and other cannabinoids have been shown to be 5-HT$_3$ antagonists.[3] Low or moderate doses of THC can also stimulate appetite (hyperphagia) by suppressing glutamatergic conduction via CB$_1$ stimulation, while higher doses can reduce appetite (hypophagia) through a CB$_1$-mediated reduction in GABAergic transmission.[27] CB$_1$ antagonists such as rimonabant have been shown to be effective at suppressing appetite by blocking CB$_1$ receptors in the hypothalamic arcuate nucleus, but the reduction in CB$_1$ signaling in other parts of the CNS produced significant adverse psychological effects such as anxiety and depression, as noted in Chapter 6 (The Endocannabinoid System).[27]

Stimulation of CB$_2$ receptors by THC also leads to the inhibition of adenylate cyclase and the stimulation of MAP kinases but does not modulate ion channels.[6] CB$_2$ receptors are located mainly in the immune system (spleen, tonsils, thymus, bone marrow, T and

B lymphocytes, NK cells, polymorphonuclear neutrophils, and mast cells) and modulate immune cell migration and the release of cytokines.[28] Significant concentrations of CB_2 receptors are also found in the bone, lungs, uterus, microglia, some parts of the CNS (see Table 6.2), and the level of CB_2 receptors available for stimulation increases significantly during inflammation or injury.[6] This indicates that CB_2 receptors play an immunomodulatory role.

Despite its effect on the ECS, the mechanism of action of THC is also CBR independent. THC binds to several receptors beyond what is typically understood to constitute the ECS, but the therapeutic role of these receptors remains unclear. These receptors include orphan G-protein receptors (GPR18 and GPR55), 5-HT$_3$ receptors, and transient receptor potential (TRP) channels, including TRP vanilloid, TRP melastatin, and TRP ankyrin subfamilies (TRPV2, TRPV3, TRPV4, TRPM8, TRPA1, and TRPA8). Of note, the TRPV1, the capsaicin receptor, does not appear to be modulated by THC.[29]

8.2.2 Cannabidiol

CBD is the most abundant phytocannabinoid in fiber-type cannabis and, though nonintoxicating, it is technically psychoactive and is known to counteract some of the psychological effects of THC, including anxiety, tachycardia, sedation, and hunger.[6] CBD has a very low affinity for CB_1 and CB_2 receptors (see Table 8.1) but in the presence of agonists like THC can antagonize CB_1 receptors—by acting as a negative allosteric modulator, and this could explain, in part, how CBD counteracts some of the effects of THC.[30] Additionally, CBD counteracts the potent psychological effects of the THC metabolite 11-OH-THC by interfering with its production through inhibiting THC metabolism in the liver (see 7.4.4 [Metabolism of THC] in Chapter 7 [The Pharmacokinetics of Cannabis]). Though CBD has a low binding affinity for CB_2 receptors, it may act as an antagonist or inverse agonist, which could be one of the mechanisms behind its anti-inflammatory effects.[30]

Beyond the traditional ECS, CBD has been shown to be active at TRPs, particularly TRPV1 (as an agonist) and TRPM8 (as an antagonist), and is also an agonist at TRPA1, TRPV2, and TRPV3 receptors.[29] This could potentially explain some of therapeutic properties of CBD, as the dysfunction of TRP channels has been observed in association with respiratory disorders, neuropathic pain, and inflammation.[29] CBD is also an agonist at 5-HT$_{1A}$ receptors and has been shown to enhance the signaling of adenosine receptors, which could possibly provide an explanation for its anxiolytic effects.[6] It has also been reported to be an antagonist at GPR55 at nanomolar to micromolar concentrations.[30]

8.3 The Entourage Effect

The entourage effect has been described elsewhere but deserves special attention here. Proponents of the entourage effect maintain that the many phytocannabinoids, terpenes, and terpenoids found within cannabis produce a synergistic effect when taken together and that many of the pharmacological properties of cannabis are altered or degraded when one isolates and administers only one or two phytocannabinoids at a time. The idea has gained significant traction and has upended the once commonly held belief that cannabis is merely a vehicle for THC. This is most certainly not the case, and there is a wealth of evidence to support the belief that THC and CBD operate in a synergistic manner, but the extent to which the entourage effect extends to other phytocannabinoids and terpenic compounds continues to be a matter of debate.

There are conflicting studies about the impact that terpenic compounds have on the ECS when used in conjunction with CBD and THC, and, in some cases, the effects these compounds have on the ECS appears to be virtually nonexistent.[2] (One major exception to this is β-caryophyllene, which is a CB_2 receptor ligand.[6]) Similarly, many phytocannabinoids that appear in cannabis in relatively small concentrations do not seem to be potent enough to exert any notable effects on the ECS (see Table 8.1). This suggests that the science does not support the existence of the entourage effect, even if many cannabis users express a belief that they experience different therapeutic and subjective effects when using cannabis preparations that contain the "full spectrum" of minor cannabinoids, terpenes, terpenoids, flavonoids, and other compounds compared to preparations that contain THC and CBD or only one of these phytocannabinoids.[31]

Proponents of the entourage effect counter that despite there being very few phytocannabinoids that are CBR ligands (see Table 8.1), there is a preponderance of anecdotal evidence to support claims about the existence of this effect. Moreover, they argue, its failure to directly interact with CBR does not preclude its existence. Instead of acting directly through the ECS, they affect it through other means, such as by inhibiting serotonin receptors or activating TRP channels (specifically TRPA1, TRPM8, VRPV1, TRPV2, TRPV3, TRPV4, and TRPV8). (An overview of the various receptors affected by the minor phytocannabinoids can be found in Table 8.2.[29]) The same can be said of terpenes and terpenoids; they also appear to indirectly affect the ECS or produce similar therapeutic effects as that of THC or CBD through other channels.

TABLE 8.2 Phytocannabinoid Receptor Activity

Phytocannabinoid	Receptor	Activity
THC (Δ^9-tetrahydrocannabinol)	CB_1	Agonist
	CB_2	Agonist
	GPR18	Agonist
	GPR55	Agonist/antagonist
	PPARγ	Agonist
	TRPA1	Agonist
	TRPA8	Agonist
	TRPM8	Antagonist
	TRPV2	Agonist
	TRPV3	Agonist
	TRPV4	Agonist
	5-HT_{3A}	Antagonist
	β-Adrenoceptor	Potentiator
	μ-Opioid	Negative allosteric modulator
	δ-Opioid	Negative allosteric modulator
CBD (cannabidiol)	CB_1	Antagonist/allosteric modulator
	CB_2	Inverse agonist/antagonist
	GPR55	Antagonist
	TRPA1	Agonist
	TRPM8	Antagonist
	TRPV1	Agonist
	TRPV2	Agonist
	TRPV3	Agonist
	5-HT_{1A}	Agonist

(Continued)

TABLE 8.2 Continued

Phytocannabinoid	Receptor	Activity
CBG (cannabigerol)	CB_1	Agonist/antagonist
	CB_2	Agonist
	TRPA1	Agonist
	TRPM8	Antagonist
	TRPV1	Agonist
	TRPV2	Agonist
	TRPV3	Agonist
	TRPV4	Agonist
	TRPV8	Antagonist
	$5\text{-}HT_{1A}$	Antagonist
	α-Adrenoceptor	Agonist
CBC (cannabichromene)	CB_1	Agonist
	CB_2	Agonist
	TRPA1	Agonist
	TRPM8	Antagonist
CBN (cannabinol)	CB_1	Agonist
	CB_2	Agonist
	TRPA1	Agonist
	TRPM8	Antagonist
	TRPV2	Agonist
	TRPV4	Agonist

TABLE 8.2 Continued

Phytocannabinoid	Receptor	Activity
THCV (tetrahydrocannabivarin)	CB_1	Agonist/antagonist
	CB_2	Agonist
	TRPA1	Agonist
	TRPM8	Antagonist
	TRPV1	Agonist
	TRPV2	Agonist
	TRPV3	Agonist
	TRPV4	Agonist
THCA-A (tetrahydrocannabinol acid A)	CB1	Agonist
	CB2	Agonist
	TRPA1	Agonist
	TRPM8	Antagonist
	TRPV2	Agonist
CBDV (cannabidivarin)	TRPA1	Agonist
	TRPM8	Antagonist
	TRPV1	Agonist
	TRPV2	Agonist
	TRPV4	Agonist
CBDA (cannabidiolic acid)	GPR55	Agonist
	TRPA1	Agonist
	TRPM8	Antagonist
	TRPV1	Agonist
	$5\text{-}HT_{1A}$	Agonist

TABLE 8.4 Observed Therapeutic Effects of Terpenic Compounds[a]

Terpenic Compound	Observed Effect
β-Myrcene	Analgesic
	Anticancer
	Anti-inflammatory
	Antiosteoarthritic
	Antiulcer
	Neuroprotective
	Sedative, muscle relaxant
Limonene	Acne treatment
	Antibiotic
	Anticancer
	Anti-inflammatory
	Anxiolytic
	Dermatophytosis treatment
	Gastroesophageal reflux
	Hyperalgesia treatment
	Immunostimulant
Linalool	Analgesic
	Anticancer
	Anticonvulsant
	Antidepressant
	Antileishmanial
	Antinociceptive
	Anxiolytic
	Burn treatment
	Local anesthetic
	Sedative

TABLE 8.4 Continued

Terpenic Compound	Observed Effect
α-Pinene	Antibiotic
	Anti-inflammatory
	Anxiolytic
	Bronchodilator
	Memory booster
β-Pinene	Antibiotic
β-Caryophyllene	Anti-inflammatory
	Antimalarial
	Antinociceptive
	Gastric cytoprotective
Humulene (α-humulene/ α-caryophyllene)	Anticancer
Nerolidol	Antileishmanial
	Antimalarial
	Dermatophytosis treatment
	Sedative
	Skin penetrant
Geraniol	Anticancer[34]
	Diabetic neuropathy treatment[35]
	Skin penetrant[36]
Borneol	Anti-inflammatory[37]
	Antinociceptive[37]
Δ-3-Carene	Osteoporosis treatment

(Continued)

TABLE 8.4 Continued

Terpenic Compound	Observed Effect
Terpinolene	Anticancer
	Antioxidant
	Sedative
α-Bisabolene	Anticancer[38]

[a]Unless otherwise noted, this table represents a summation of the following work:
Russo EB, Marcu J. Cannabis pharmacology: the usual suspects and a few promising leads. In: Kendall D, Alexander S, eds. *Advances in Pharmacology: Cannabinoid Pharmacology*. Cambridge, MA: Academic Press; 2017:67-134.

More research will be needed to conclusively demonstrate that the entourage effect exists and, more importantly, to reveal how relevant it is for clinicians to understand the nuances of the possible synergies between THC, CBD, minor cannabinoids, and terpenic compounds. At the very least, this seems like a plausible theory to explain why so many cannabis users prefer the therapeutic effects of "full-spectrum" cannabis as opposed to preparations that contain only THC or CBD.

8.4 Pharmacological Effects of THC and CBD

The pharmacological effects of THC and CBD are extensive and will constitute most of the remaining subject matter in this book. For a more in-depth analysis on a specific area, please consult the corresponding chapter. For an overview of the observed pharmacological effects of THC and CBD, please refer to Tables 8.5 and 8.6, respectively. Many of these effects have also already been described in previous chapters, particularly Chapter 4 (Constituents of Cannabis), Chapter 6 (The Endocannabinoid System), and Chapter 7 (The Pharmacology of Cannabis).

8.5 Hierarchy of Therapeutic Effects

Establishing a hierarchy of therapeutic effects for cannabis has been difficult because of regulatory hurdles that have been discussed in Chapter 5 (U.S. Regulations From Past to Present).

TABLE 8.5 Selected Therapeutic Applications of THC[a]

Analgesic[39]

Antibacterial/antiviral[40]

Antinociceptive[41]

Antipruritic agent

Antispasmodic[42]

Bronchodilator

Graft versus host disease treatment

Muscle relaxant

Neuropathic pain treatment[41]

Neuroprotective antioxidant

Reduces interocular pressure

[a]Unless otherwise noted, this table represents a summation of the following work:
Russo EB, Marcu J. Cannabis pharmacology: the usual suspects and a few promising leads. In: Kendall D, Alexander S, eds. *Advances in Pharmacology: Cannabinoid Pharmacology*. Cambridge, MA: Academic Press; 2017:67-134.

TABLE 8.6 Selected Therapeutic Applications of CBD

Addiction treatment[31]

Analgesic[43]

Anticancer[44]

Anticonvulsant[45]

Antidepressant[46]

Anti-inflammatory[47]

Antinausea[48]

Antioxidant[49]

Anxiolytic[50]

Graft versus host disease treatment[51]

Neuroprotective[52]

Perhaps more importantly, proper research has struggled to keep up with reports about the putative benefits of cannabis that frequently appear in media outlets dedicated to the celebration of cannabis and the promotion of its use to treat virtually all conditions without serious scrutiny. The data about these putative benefits are still wanting and very few established effects have been documented.

8.5.1 Established Effects

As discussed in Chapter 7 (The Pharmacology of Cannabis), only three preparations of cannabis have been approved by the Food and Drug Administration (FDA) for use in the United States: dronabinol/THC (Marinol), nabilone (Cesamet), and CBD (Epidiolex). THC (dronabinol) and nabilone have been approved as antiemetics and to treat cachexia, anorexia, weight loss, and nausea associated with chemotherapy or HIV/AIDS. CBD has been approved as an antiepileptic for patients with Lennox-Gastaut syndrome and Dravet syndrome.

8.5.2 Well-Confirmed Effects

Cannabis has also been shown anecdotally to be an effective treatment for several other disorders even if there are no FDA-approved medications to treat these conditions. THC shows promise as an anti-inflammatory and immunomodulator via the activation of the CB_2 receptors. CBD, meanwhile, appears to have anti-inflammatory effects that could treat a wide variety of conditions. Additionally, both THC and CBD may benefit hospice patients and others with terminal illnesses, who may obtain cannabis to mitigate pain, nausea, and other associated symptoms, regardless of condition.

Depending on the state, cannabis can also be recommended for:

- Alzheimer disease
- Amyotrophic lateral sclerosis (ALS)
- Anorexia nervosa
- Anxiety
- Arnold-Chiari malformation
- Arthritis
- Autism spectrum disorder
- Bulimia
- Causalgia
- Cerebral palsy

- Chronic inflammatory demyelinating polyneuropathy
- Chronic pancreatitis
- Chronic traumatic encephalopathy
- Cirrhosis
- Colitis
- Complex regional pain syndrome
- Crohn disease
- Cystic fibrosis
- Diabetes
- Dysmenorrhea
- Dystonia
- Ehlers-Danlos syndrome
- Elevated intraocular pressure
- Endometriosis
- Epidermolysis bullosa
- Epilepsy
- Fibromyalgia
- Fibrous dysplasia
- Friedrich ataxia
- Glaucoma
- Hepatitis C
- Huntington disease
- Hydrocephalus
- Hydromyelia
- Inclusion body myositis
- Interstitial cystitis
- Inflammatory bowel disease
- Intractable headache syndromes
- Irreversible spinal cord injury
- Lewy body disease (LBD)
- Lupus
- Medial arcuate ligament syndrome (MALS)
- Migraines
- Mitochondrial disease
- Muscular dystrophy
- Multiple sclerosis
- Myasthenia gravis
- Myoclonus
- Nail-patella syndrome
- Neuralgia
- Neuro-Behçet autoimmune disease
- Neurodegenerative disorders
- Neurofibromatosis
- Neuropathic pain

- Obstructive sleep apnea
- Obsessive-compulsive disorder (OCD)
- Opioid dependency
- Opioid substitution
- Osteoarthritis
- Osteogenesis imperfecta
- Parkinson disease
- Peripheral neuropathy
- Polycystic kidney disease (PKD)
- Post-concussion syndrome
- Post laminectomy syndrome
- Posttraumatic stress disorder (PTSD)
- Psoriasis
- Psoriatic arthritis
- Reflex sympathetic dystrophy
- Residual limb pain
- Rheumatoid arthritis
- Seizures
- Severe or chronic nausea
- Severe or chronic pain
- Severe and persistent muscle spasms
- Sickle cell diseases
- Sjögren syndrome
- Spasmodic torticollis
- Spinal cord diseases
- Spinal cord injury
- Spinal muscular atrophy
- Spinal stenosis
- Spinocerebellar ataxia syndrome
- Superior canal dehiscence syndrome
- Syringomyelia
- Tarlov cysts
- Tourette syndrome
- Traumatic brain injury
- Ulcerative colitis
- Vulvodynia

Table 7.1 contains a listing of the qualifying conditions for each state as of January 1, 2020. It is possible that some states may add or remove some of the conditions listing therein. Before recommending cannabis to a patient, clinicians should consult the Web sites of the appropriate state agencies to ensure compliance with all laws and regulations.

8.6 Conclusion

Research into the effects of cannabis is still ongoing, and a full understanding of how the many constituents within cannabis interact with the ECS and with systems independent of CBRs remains elusive due to a combination of regulatory obstacles and the difficulty of researching a plant that contains so many components. More clinical trials are needed to substantiate initial findings, and more studies are needed to better elucidate the interplay between terpenic compounds, phytocannabinoids, and the ECS. Additionally, more research must be conducted to better understand how other receptor systems interact with the ECS.

Despite a lack of data, evidence has emerged that reveals how integral the ECS is to regulation of numerous systems throughout the body and that many of the constituents found within cannabis have the ability to influence the ECS and, therefore, to be effective therapies for the treatment of myriad conditions. There is no longer a question of whether or not cannabis has any beneficial medical usage; the question is how to maximize the benefits of cannabis while minimizing the risks associated with cannabis use.

REFERENCES

[1]Cannabidiol (CBD) Critical Review Report. World Health Organization Expert Committee on Drug Dependence, Fortieth Meeting (Geneva, June 4-7, 2018). World Health Organization website. https://www.who.int/medicines/access/controlled-substances/Cannabidiol CriticalReview.pdf. Accessed December 4, 2019.

[2]Santiago M, Sachdev S, Arnold JC, McGregor IS, Connor M. Absence of entourage: terpenoids commonly found in *Cannabis sativa* do not modulate the functional activity of Δ^9-THC at human CB_1 and CB_2 receptors. *Cannabis Cannabinoid Res*. 2019;4(3):165-176. doi: 10.1089/can.2019.0016.

[3]Grotenhermen F. Pharmacokinetics and pharmacodynamics of cannabinoids. *Clin Pharmacokinet*. 2003;42(4):327-360. doi: 10.2165/00003088-200342040-00003.

[4]Reggio PH. Endocannabinoid binding to the cannabinoid receptors: what is known and what remains unknown. *Curr Med Chem*. 2010;17(14):1468-1486. PMID: 20166921.

[5]Pertwee RG, Cascio MG. Known pharmacological actions of delta-9-tetrahydrocannabinol and of four other chemical constituents of cannabis that activate cannabinoid receptors. In: Pertwee RG, ed. *Handbook on Cannabis*. New York: Oxford University Press; 2014:115-136.

[6]Russo EB, Marcu J. Cannabis pharmacology: the usual suspects and a few promising leads. In: Kendall D, Alexander S, eds. *Advances in Pharmacology: Cannabinoid Pharmacology*. Cambridge, MA: Academic Press; 2017:67-134.

[7]Gertsch J, Leonti M, Raduner S, et al. Beta-caryophyllene is a dietary cannabinoid. *Proc Natl Acad Sci U S A*. 2008;105(26):9099-9104. doi: 10.1073/pnas.0803601105.

[8]Showalter VM, Compton DR, Martin BR, Abood ME. Evaluation of binding in a transfected cell line expressing a peripheral cannabinoid receptor (CB_2): identification of cannabinoid receptor subtype selective ligands. *J Pharmacol Exp Ther*. 1996;278(3):989-999. PMID: 8819477.

[9]Thomas A, Ross RA, Saha B, et al. 6″-azidohex-2″-yne-cannabidiol: a potential neutral, competitive cannabinoid CB_1 receptor antagonist. *Eur J Pharmacol*. 2004;487(1-3):213-221. doi: 10.1016/j.ejphar.2004.01.023.

[10]Thomas A, Baillie GL, Phillips AM, et al. Cannabidiol displays unexpectedly high potency as an antagonist of CB_1 and CB_2 receptor agonists in vitro. *Br J Pharmacol*. 2007;150(5):613-623. doi: 10.1038/sj.bjp.0707133.

[11]MacLennan SJ, Reynen PH, Kwan J, Bonhaus DW. Evidence for inverse agonism in SR141716A at human recombinant cannabinoid CB_1 and CB_2 receptors. *Br J Pharmacol*. 1998;124(4):619-622. doi: 10.1038/sj.bjp.0701915.

[12]Bisogno T, Hanus L, De Petrocellis L, et al. Molecular targets for cannabidiol and its synthetic analogues: effect on vanilloid VR1 receptors and on the cellular uptake and enzymatic hydrolysis of anandamide. *Br J Pharmacol*. 2001;134(4):845-852. doi: 10.1038/sj.bjp.0704327.

[13]Guason LA, Stevenson LA, Thomas A, et al. Cannabigerol behaves as a partial agonist at both CB_1 and CB_2 receptors. In: Proceedings from the Symposium on the Cannabinoids; June 26-30, 2007; Saint-Sauveur, Québec. 206. https://icrs.co/SYMPOSIUM.2007/2007.ICRS. Program.and.Abstracts.pdf. Accessed April 21, 2020.

[14]Booker L, Naidu PS, Razdan RK, Mahadevan A, Lichtman AH. Evaluation of prevalent phytocannabinoids in the acetic acid model of visceral nociception. *Drug Alcohol Depend*. 2009;105(1-2):42-47. doi: 10.1016/j.drugalcdep.2009.06.009.

[15]Rhee MH, Vogel Z, Barg J, et al. Cannabinol derivatives: binding to cannabinoid receptors and inhibition of adenylylcyclase. *J Med Chem*. 1997;40(20):3228-3233. doi: 10.1021/jm970126f.

[16]Felder CC, Joyce KE, Briley EM, et al. Comparison of the pharmacology and signal transduction of the human cannabinoid CB_1 and CB_2 receptors. *Mol Pharmacol*. 1995;48(3):443-450. PMID: 7565624.

[17]Huffman JW, Liddle J, Yu S, et al. 3-(1′,1′-dimetheylbutyl)-1-deoxy-delta8-THC and related compounds: synthesis of selective ligands for the CB_2 receptor. *Bioorg Med Chem*. 1999;7(12):2905-2914. doi: 10.1016/s0968-0896(99)00219-9.

[18]Busch-Petersen J, Hill WA, Fan P, et al. Unsaturated side chain ß-11-hydroxyhexahydro-cannabinol analogs. *J Med Chem*. 1996;39(19):3790-3796. doi: 10.1021/jm950934b.

[19]Iwamura H, Suzuki H, Ueda Y, Kaya T, Inaba T. In vitro and in vivo pharmacological characterization of JTE-907, a novel selective ligand for cannabinoid CB_2 receptor. *J Pharmacol Exp Ther*. 2001;296(2):420-425. PMID: 11160626.

[20]Rinaldi-Carmona M, Barth F, Héaulme M, et al. SR141716A, a potent and selective antagonist of the brain cannabinoid receptor. *FEBS Lett*. 1994;350(2-3):240-244. doi: 10.1016/0014-5793(94)00773-x.

[21]Bayewitch M, Rhee MH, Avidor-Reiss T, et al. (-)-Δ^9-tetrahydrocannabinol antagonizes the peripheral cannabinoid receptor-mediated inhibition of adenylyl cyclase. *J Biol Chem*. 1996;271(17):9902-9905. doi: 10.1074/jbc.271.17.9902.

[22]Pertwee RG, Thomas A, Stevenson LA, et al. The psychoactive plant cannabinoid, Δ^9-tetrahydrocannabinol, is antagonized by Δ^8- and Δ^9-tetrahydrocannabivarin in mice in vivo. *Br J Pharmacol*. 2007;150(5):586-594. doi: 10.1038/sj.bpb.0707124.

[23]Thomas A, Stevenson LA, Wease KN, et al. Evidence that the plant cannabinoid Δ^9-tetrahydrocannabivarin is a cannabinoid CB_1 and CB_2 receptor antagonist. *Br J Pharmacol*. 2005;146(7):917-926. doi: 10.1038/sj.bjp.0706414.

[24]Hill AJ, Weston SE, Jones NA, et al. Δ^9-tetrahydrocannabivarin suppresses in vivo epileptic form and in vivo seizure activity in adult rats. *Epilepsia*. 2010;51(8):1522-1523. doi: 10.1111/j.1528-1167.2010.02523.x.

[25]Bolognini D, Cascio MG, Parolaro D, Pertwee RG. AM630 behaves as protean ligand at the human cannabinoid CB_2 receptor. *Br J Pharmacol*. 2012;165(8):2561-2574. doi: 10.1111/j.1476-5381.2011.01503.x.

[26]Bolognini D, Costa B, Maione S, et al. The plant cannabinoid Δ^9-tetrahydrocannabivarin can decrease signs of inflammation and inflammatory pain in mice. *Br J Pharmacol.* 2010;160(3):677-687. doi: 10.1111/j.1476-5381.2010.00756.x.

[27]Koch M. Cannabinoid receptor signaling in central regulation of feeding behavior: a mini-review. *Front Neurosci.* 2017;11:293.

[28]Pertwee RG. Endocannabinoids and their pharmacological action. In: Pertwee RG, ed. *Endocannabinoids.* Cham, Switzerland: Springer International Publishing AG; 2015:1-38.

[29]Muller C, Morales P, Reggio PH. Cannabinoid ligands targeting TRP channels. *Front Mol Neurosci.* 2018;11:487. doi: 10.3389/fnmol.2018.00487.

[30]Pisanti S, Malfitano AN, Ciaglia E, et al. Cannabidiol: state of the art and new challenges for therapeutic applications. *Pharmacol Ther.* 2017;175:133-150. doi: 10.1016/j.pharmthera.2017.02.041.

[31]Russo EB. Taming THC: potential cannabis synergy and phytocannabinoid-terpenoid entourage effects. *Br J Pharmacol.* 2011;163(7):1344-1364. doi: 10.1111/j.1476-5381.2011.01238.x.

[32]Paula-Freire LI, Andersen ML, Molska GR, Köhn DO, Carlini EL. Evaluation of the anti-nociceptive activity of *Ocimum gratissimum L.* (Lamiaceae) essential oil and its isolated activity principles in mice. *Phytother Res.* 2013;27(8):1220-1224. doi: 10.1002/ptr.4845.

[33]Costa CA, Cury TC, Cassettari BO, et al. *Citrus aurantium* L. essential oil exhibits anxio-lytic-like activity mediated by 5-HT$_{1A}$ receptors and reduces cholesterol after repeated oral treatment. *BMC Complement Altern Med.* 2013;13:42. doi: 10.1186/1472-6882-13-42.

[34]Wiseman DA, Werner SR, Crowell PL. Cell cycle arrest by the isoprenoids perillyl alcohol, geraniol, and farnesol is mediated by p21^{Cip1} and p27^{Kip1} in human pancreatic adenocarci-noma cells. *J Pharmacol Exp Ther.* 2007;320(3):1163-1170. doi: 10.1124/jpet.111666.

[35]Prasad SN, Muralidhara. Protective effects of geraniol (a monoterpene) in a diabetic neu-ropathy rat model: attenuation of behavioral impairments and biochemical perturbations. *J Neurosci Res.* 2014;92(9):1205-1216. doi: 10.1002/jnr.23393.

[36]Doan K, Bronaugh RL, Yourick JL. In vivo and in vitro skin absorption of lipophilic com-pounds, dibutyl phthalate, farnesol and geraniol in the hairless guinea pig. *Food Chem Toxicol.* 2010;48(1):18-23. doi: 10.1016/j.fct.2009.09.002.

[37]Almeida JR, Souza GR, Silva JC, et al. Borneol, a bicyclic monoterpene alcohol, reduces nociceptive behavior and inflammatory response in mice. *Scientific World Journal.* 2013;2013:808460. doi: 10.1155/2013/808460.

[38]Yeo SK, Ali AY, Hayward OA, et al. ß-Bisabolene, a sesquiterpene from the essential oil extract of opoponax (*Commiphora guidottii*), exhibits cytotoxicity in breast cancer cell lines. *Phytother Res.* 2015;30(3):418-425. doi: 10.1002/ptr.5543.

[39]Rahn EJ, Hohmann AG. Cannabinoids as pharmacotherapies for neuropathic pain: from the bench to the bedside. *Neurotherapeutics.* 2009;6(4):713-737. doi: 10.1016/j.nurt.2009.08.002.

[40]Van Klingeren B, Ten Ham M. Antibacterial activity of delta9-tetrahydrocannabinol and cannabidiol. *Antonie Van Leeuwenhoek.* 1976;42(1-2):9-12. doi: 10.1007/bf00399444.

[41]Hohmann AG, Suplita RL, Bolton NM, et al. An endocannabinoid mechanism for stress-induced analgesia. *Nature.* 2005;435(7045):1108-1112. doi: 10.1038/nature03658.

[42]Ungerleider JT, Andrysiak T, Fairbanks L, Ellison GW, Myers LW. Delta-9-THC in the treatment of spasticity associated with multiple sclerosis. *Adv Alcohol Subst Abuse.* 1987;7(1):39-50. doi: 10.1300/j251v07n01_04.

[43]Boychuk DG, Goddard G, Mauro G, Orellana MF. The effectiveness of cannabinoids in the management of chronic nonmalignant neuropathic pain: a systematic review. *J Oral Facial Pain Headache.* 2015;29(1):7-14. doi: 10.11607/ofph.1274.

[44]Pisanti S, Picardi P, D'Alessandro A, Laezza C, Bifulco M. The endocannabinoid signaling system in cancer. *Trends Pharmacol Sci.* 2013;34(5):273-282. doi: 10.1016/j.tips.2013.03.003.

[45]Jones NA, Hill AJ, Smith I, et al. Cannabidiol displays antiepileptiform and antiseizure properties in vitro and in vivo. *J Pharmacol Exp Ther*. 2010;332(2):569-577. doi: 10.1124/jpet.109.159145.

[46]El-Alfy AT, Ivey K, Robinson K, et al. Antidepressant-like effect Δ[9]-tetrahydrocannabinol and other cannabinoids isolated from *Cannabis sativa L. Pharmacol Biochem Behav*. 2010;95(4):434-442. doi: 10.1016/j.pbb.2010.03.004.

[47]Mecha M, Torrao AS, Mestre L, et al. Cannabidiol protects oligodendrocyte progenitor cells from inflammation-induced apoptosis by attenuating endoplasmic reticulum stress. *Cell Death Dis*. 2012;3(6):e331. doi: 10.1038/cddis.2012.71.

[48]Rock E M, Limebeer CL, Mechoulam R, Piomelli D, Parker LA. The effect of cannabidiol and URB597 on conditioned gaping (a model of nausea) elicited by a lithium-paired context in the rat. *Psychopharmacology (Berl)*. 2008;196(3):389-395. doi: 10.1007/s00213-007-0970-1.

[49]Hampson AJ, Grimaldi M, Axelrod J, Wink D. Cannabidiol and (-)Delta9-tetrahydrocannabinol are neuroprotective antioxidants. *Proc Natl Acad Sci U S A*. 1998;95(14):8268-8273. doi: 10.1073/pnas.95.14.8268.

[50]Almeida V, Levin R, Peres FF, et al. Cannabidiol exhibits anxiolytic but not antipsychotic property evaluated in the social interaction test. *Prog Neuropsychopharmacol Biol Psychiatry*. 2013;41(5):30-35. doi: 10.1016/j.pnpbp.2012.10.024.

[51]Yeshurun M, Shpilberg O, Herscovici C, et al. Cannabidiol for the prevention of graft-versus-host-disease after allogeneic hematopoietic cell transplantation: results of a phase II study. *Biol Blood Marrow Transplant*. 2015;21(10):1770-1775. doi: 10.1016/j.bbmt.2015.05.018.

[52]Martin-Moreno AM, Reigada D, Belen G, et al. Cannabidiol and other cannabinoids reduce microglial activation in vitro and in vivo: relevance to Alzheimer's disease. *Mol Pharmacol*. 2011;76(6):964-973. doi: 10.1124/mol.111.071290.

9

Commonly Encountered Preparations

9.1 Overview

Since the medicinal compounds available in cannabis plants can be consumed in so many ways, it may be intimidating for patients to walk into a dispensary without any knowledge of what they are likely to find there. Even perusing the available options for flower cannabis—which is cannabis that has undergone minimal processing—can be overwhelming, as there are numerous strengths and cultivars available in most dispensaries, and it can be difficult to make an educated decision about which to choose if one does not know what the values and indicators on the packaging mean. What is important to relay to patients is that the potency of cannabis is largely dependent upon Δ^9-tetrahydrocannabinol (THC) concentrations.

Furthermore, any questions about specific dosing amounts should focus on ensuring that patients "start low and go slow," meaning that they obtain cannabis that has a low THC concentration and titrate their dosage in a cautious and deliberate manner.

Most of the technical information about these different preparations, including bioavailability, absorption, distribution, and metabolization, was discussed in the Chapter 7 (The Classification of Cannabis, see specifically section 7.2 [Pharmacokinetics]). This chapter is meant only to elucidate, what patients will likely encounter in a dispensary.

9.2 The Budtender or Pharmacist

There are no current guidelines for dosing cannabis unless one is prescribing one of the three FDA-approved preparations discussed in Chapter 7 (The Pharmacology of Cannabis): dronabinol (Marinol), nabilone (Cesamet), or cannabidiol (Epidiolex). Any form of cannabis that is not one of these three preparations—excluding hemp-derived CBD products, which are available over the counter in virtually all states—cannot legally be prescribed. Though it may appear to be just a semantics, the use of the terms "prescribed" and "recommended" is important to differentiate. Medical professionals are barred from *prescribing* these preparations of cannabis because they are still regarded as Schedule I drugs by the federal government. Consequently, qualifying medical professionals (see Table 9.1) may only *recommend* that a patient obtain such products or authorize that patients use them, provided the medical professional and patient live in a state where a medical cannabis program exists. In many states, medical professionals must first be certified by the state to recommend or authorize the use of medicinal cannabis. In other states, no such special certification is necessary. In virtually all states with medical cannabis programs, medical professionals who recommend cannabis need to first conduct an in-person examination,

(*text continues on page 297*)

TABLE 9.1 Continued

State/Territory	Registration Required	Position
Washington	No	Properly licensed MDs, DOs, PAs, APRNs, and naturopaths who have a documented relationship with the patient.[49]
West Virginia	Yes	An MD or DO who is fully licensed by the state and who has passed a 4-hour training course on cannabis.[50] A training course and an electronic registry will be available in the near future.
Wisconsin	N/A	There is no medical cannabis program in Wisconsin. Physicians may recommend CBD preparations that are currently available over the counter.[51]
Wyoming	No	Any person licensed to practice medicine in the state of Wyoming who is also certified in neurology.[52]

have a bona fide physician-patient relationship, describe the potential health risks of cannabis use to the patient, and then fill out paperwork that allows patients entry into their state's program. For a brief overview of state-by-state regulations, see Table 9.1. For more details, please see this book's Web site: www.cannabistextbook.com.

Only after receiving a recommendation can patients go to a dispensary to obtain cannabis, provided the state has dispensaries. In states where adult-use has been legalized, they may choose an establishment that only caters to patients or one that caters to both patients and recreational users. If possible, it is best for patients to go to establishments that solely dispense medicinal cannabis. It should be noted that many states or territories have passed legislation allowing for medicinal cannabis dispensaries to operate, but this does not mean that one has opened to dispense THC-rich cannabis. Guam, as an example, has passed legislation to create a medical cannabis program and to legalize recreational cannabis, but no dispensaries of any kind are currently open in the territory.[53]

Depending on the state, the patient may encounter a pharmacist or a "budtender" when they arrive at the dispensary. It is far more likely that they will interact with a budtender, who is a specialist who has passed an online certification program but is not technically a pharmacist or a medical professional who is qualified to provide medical advice. In only six states (Arkansas, Connecticut, Minnesota, New York, Pennsylvania, and Virginia) a pharmacist is required to be onsite.[54,55] Those working at dispensaries will be responsible for helping patients decide upon a preparation and cultivar.

9.3 Indica vs Sativa

While the Indica/Sativa distinction has been touched upon in both Chapter 3 (The Constituents of Cannabis, see specifically section 3.5 [Vernacular Taxonomy—Sativa, Indica, and Ruderalis]) and Chapter 7 (The Pharmacology of Cannabis, see section 7.6 [Dosage]), it is worth mentioning again because many cultivar labels will describe the contents of their packaging as being "Indica dominant" or "Sativa dominant." While the science behind the Sativa/Indica divide is dubious, as decades of extensive interbreeding has made such distinctions largely meaningless, many users believe that it is an accurate depiction of how different cultivars of cannabis make them feel.[56]

Cultivars that are Sativa dominant are believed to offer a "head high," and cultivars that are Indica dominant are believed to produce a "body high."[57] The "head high" is characterized by what users describe as a more energetic experience, while the "body high" is characterized by a deeper sense of relaxation. Put another way, Sativa cultivars are for the daytime; Indica cultivars are for the night.

This is not due to any special compound that is unique to either Sativa or Indica, but rather because different cultivars contain different levels of minor cannabinoids (such as cannabigerol, cannabichromene, and cannabinol), flavonoids, and terpenic compounds, and the unique interplay between these compounds and the two major cannabinoids, THC and CBD, can affect the subjective effects of cannabis. A specific Indica cultivar should not be thought to produce a "body high" because it is an Indica *per se*, but, rather, because of how the cannabinoids, flavonoids, and terpenes interact with one another in the body. A very rough guide to the reputed effects of various terpenic compounds can be found in Table 9.2.

TABLE 9.2 Reputed Effects of Terpenes and Terpenoids

Terpene/Terpenoid	Subjective/Therapeutic Effects
Myrcene (a/k/a β-myrcene)	Anti-inflammatory, analgesic, sedative
Limonene	Antianxiety, mood booster
Linalool	Antianxiety, pain management
α-Pinene	Memory booster, THC attenuator
β-Pinene	Memory booster
β-Caryophyllene	CB_2 agonist, treatment for autoimmune disorders
Humulene (a/k/a α-humulene, α-caryophyllene)	Anti-inflammatory, appetite suppressant
Nerolidol	Sedative
Geraniol	Anti-inflammatory, relief from some forms of neuropathic pain
Borneol	Anti-inflammatory, antinociceptive
Δ-3-Carene	Anti-inflammatory, memory booster
Terpinolene	Sedative

9.4 Flower Cannabis

Flower cannabis is typically what one envisages upon thinking of cannabis. This preparation has been harvested, trimmed, dried, and cured, but it has otherwise not been processed. Some states, such as New York, have very tight regulations on the sale of flower cannabis through medical dispensaries. Other states, such as New Jersey, have tighter regulations on the sale of extracts. For a brief overview of state-by-state regulations on this subject, please see Table 9.1. For more information, please visit this book's Web site: www.cannabistextbook.com.

As discussed in Chapter 7 (The Pharmacology of Cannabis, specifically section 7.3 [Pharmacokinetics]), cannabis must be decarboxylated by introducing it to a heat source if one is to obtain the most valuable cannabinoids and terpenic compounds from flower cannabis. This process converts the phytocannabinoids cannabidiolic acid (CBDA) and Δ⁹-tetrahydrocannabinolic acids A and B (THCA-A and THCA-B) into cannabidiol (CBD) and Δ⁹-tetrahydrocannabinol (THC), respectively.

In most cases, patients who buy flower cannabis from the dispensary will opt to decarboxylate it by smoking it. They may choose to do so by rolling it into a cigarette (what is known as a joint), purchasing a pre-rolled cigarette, or smoking it in a pipe, a water pipe, a bong, or something more elaborate like a hookah. Water pipes, bongs, and hookahs filter particulate matter through the water and cool the smoke before it is inhaled.[58] Flower cannabis may also be vaporized by using a vaporizer that vaporizes the phytocannabinoids and terpenic compounds at heats below combustion (see Chapter 7 [The Pharmacology of Cannabis], section 7.4.2 [Routes of Administration and Absorption Overview]).

It is important to remind patients that cultivars that are high in THC (>15%) can produce more pronounced intoxicating effects with smaller doses. On the one hand, this means that patients can obtain a sufficient dose with a minimal amount of smoking, but the level of potency of these cultivars may make it difficult to self-titrate. Literature suggests that some of the effects of THC may be attenuated if a cultivar has a significant concentration of CBD, and patients who are new to cannabis may want to consider asking their budtender about cultivars (often referred to as "strains") that contain significant amounts of both THC and CBD (a range of 2.5%-10% and a range of 5%-15%, respectively). It is easier to self-titrate with cultivars that have lower levels of THC, but this may require several administrations before patients have inhaled a sufficient dosage to feel therapeutic effects. Ultimately, deciding on a cultivar and a THC concentration is a balancing act to which patients may need some time to fully adjust. Again, it is important to encourage them to start low and to go slow.

9.5 Concentrated Cannabis

As discussed in Chapter 1 (Cannabis: An Introduction, section 1.5 [Morphology]), the active compounds found in cannabis (phytocannabinoids, terpenes, and terpenoids) are found in trichomes, which may give cannabis a frosted look when seen with the naked eye. These small, mushroom-shaped glands can be separated from the vegetative matter either by hand or by use of solvents like carbon dioxide or butane.

9.5.1 Hashish and Kief

When separated out by hand, trichomes will look faintly like dust in small amounts. This resinous dust is known as *kief*. When kief is collected, slightly heated, and compressed into globules, it is known as either hashish or hash. The sole component of these preparations is trichomes, which means that they can be extremely potent.[59]

Kief is often separated from flower cannabis by accident or when breaking up a larger flower of cannabis to roll into a cigarette or place into a pipe. As the kief is potent, it is usually not discarded, but rather sprinkled on top of cannabis before it is smoked or rolled into a cigarette. Hash typically does burn if rolled into a cigarette on its own, so it is often broken up and mixed with tobacco or flower cannabis, and then smoked.

9.5.2 Vaporized Concentrates

More modern techniques accomplish the task of extracting the cannabinoids and terpenic compounds from the vegetative matter of cannabis by utilizing solvents like carbon dioxide or butane.[60] These preparations are typically known as either oil or distillate and have a wide range of potencies: they may be high in THC and low in CBD, high in THC and high in CBD, or low in THC and high in CBD. Oils or distillates may come in premade cartridges that are then inserted into devices ("vape pens") that heat the liquid to the point of vaporization. As is the case with smoking cannabis, the onset is very quick, allowing patients the ability to self-titrate dosages.[61]

As mentioned in the Inhalation section of Chapter 7 (The Pharmacology of Cannabis, section 7.4.2 [Routes of Administration and Absorption Overview]), patients should purchase these products only from licit sources to avoid inhaling potentially dangerous adulterants.

9.5.3 Dabbing

More concentrated forms of cannabis distillate are known as dabs, as a dose consists of only a "dab" of the concentrate. "Dabs" are an informal classification of cannabis concentrates but typically refer to products that contain substantial concentrations of THC (upwards of 90%), and they may look like wax, butter, honey, or even amber-colored rock candy.[60] Users heat the concentrate on a hot surface and then use what is known as a "dab rig" to inhale the resultant fumes.

This form of cannabis is far more common in the recreational market than the medicinal market, and only patients who require massive doses of THC should consider this method of administration, and even then only under extreme circumstances. While using such extremely concentrated forms of THC allows patients to obtain doses with a minimal amount of inhalation, they are extremely potent, and it may be difficult for even experienced patients to self-titrate when dabbing. It is virtually impossible for inexperienced patients to start low and go slow with products that contain such high concentrations of THC, and it is highly recommended that patients who are new to cannabis avoid these extreme forms of concentrates.

9.6 Edibles

Cannabis may be consumed in the form of edibles that are tablets, pills, or a host of confections ranging from chocolates to candies. As is the case with other forms of cannabis described above, patients should know that THC concentrations dictate the level of intoxication that they may experience after consumption and that the subjective effects of edibles are distinct from other routes of administration because a far greater amount of THC undergoes first-pass metabolism in the liver when cannabis is consumed by oral administration, which is then converted into 11-hydroxy-Δ^9-tetrahydrocannabinol (11-OH-THC), a molecule that is far more potent than its parent compound (see Oral Administration in 7.4.2, Routes of Administration and Absorption Overview).

Once again, it is stressed that patients start low and go slow with edible cannabis, particularly because onset can sometimes occur as long as an hour after the edible is ingested and the effects of the drug may persist for as long as 6 hours, depending on dosage. Patients who are inexperienced with cannabis should consume products that contain a balance of THC and CBD, and self-titrate in small increments, preferable 2.5 mg of THC.

9.7 Tinctures, Sublingual Lozenges, and Sprays

As an alternative to inhalation or oral administration, dispensaries will also typically have sublingual tinctures (oil- and alcohol-based), lozenges, or oromucosal sprays. As these preparations are introduced to the bloodstream through the mucous membrane lining the interior of the mouth, onset is more rapid than with oral administration, but slower than when cannabis is inhaled (see Sublingual Administration in 7.4.2, Routes of Administration and Absorption Overview). Additionally, this form of administration largely avoids first-pass metabolism by the liver, though some reflex swallowing is typical. Cannabis administered by this route allows patients to self-titrate more accurately than with inhalation or many forms of edible cannabis.

9.8 Topical Cannabis

Balms, creams, ointments, and other topical preparations containing hemp-derived CBD and zero THC are currently available at many pharmacies around the country. Claims that they treat conditions ranging from joint pain to eczema are common in gray literature, but very little scientific data have been produced to confirm the reputed benefits of this route of administration. Similarly, topical preparations containing THC, which should only be available at dispensaries, have not been subjected to rigorous enough studies at this time to corroborate preliminary claims of efficacy.

Conversely, transdermal patches may be a novel delivery mechanism for cannabinoids,[62] but more research is needed to confirm preliminary findings, and far more peer-reviewed studies need to be conducted before we understand how effective this route of administration is.

9.9 Conclusion

To conclude, recommending medicinal cannabis to treat a specific condition should be the beginning of a conversation, not the end. Patients should be advised about the multiple routes of administration and associated risks and benefits, as well as the benefits and risks of cannabis in general. They should also be endowed with the tools that allow them to start low and go slow, thereby granting them the ability to consume the proper dose of cannabis to appreciate its therapeutic benefits without experiencing adverse reactions or serious intoxication. As medical professionals, it is our duty to do our best to provide patients with enough knowledge so that they can make informed and responsible decisions about how they use cannabis as a medicine.

REFERENCES

[1]House Bill 61. Alabama Legislature. http://alisondb.legislature.state.al.us/ALISON/SearchableInstruments/2016RS/PrintFiles/HB61-int.pdf. Accessed November 21, 2019.

[2]Medical Marijuana Registry Application Instructions. Alaska Department of Health and Social Services website. http://dhss.alaska.gov/dph/VitalStats/Documents/PDFs/MedicalMarijuana.pdf. Accessed November 21, 2019.

[3]Court says CBD oil is illegal. Talanei website. https://www.talanei.com/2019/07/12/court-says-cbd-oil-is-illegal/. July 12, 2019. Accessed November 21, 2019.

[4]FAQs—qualifying patients. Arizona Department of Health Services website. https://www.azdhs.gov/licensing/medical-marijuana/index.php#faqs-patients. Accessed November 21, 2019.

[5]Information for physicians. Arkansas Department of Health website. https://www.healthy.arkansas.gov/programs-services/topics/information-for-physicians. Accessed November 21, 2019.

[6]Cannabis medical purposes. Medical Board of California website. https://www.mbc.ca.gov/Licensees/Prescribing/Cannabis.aspx. Accessed November 21, 2019.

[7]Recommend medical marijuana. Colorado Department of Public Health & Environment website. https://norml.org/legal/item/colorado-medical-marijuana. Accessed November 21, 2019.

[8]Physician/APRN requirements and eligibility. Connecticut Department of Consumer Protection website. https://portal.ct.gov/DCP/Medical-Marijuana-Program/Physician-Requirements-and-Eligibility. Accessed November 22, 2019.

[9]Chapter 49A. The Delaware Medical Marijuana Act. State of Delaware website. https://delcode.delaware.gov/title16/c049a/index.shtml. Accessed November 22, 2019.

[10]Legalization of Marijuana for Medical Treatment Initiative Amendment Act of 2010. City Council of the District of Columbia website. http://dcclims1.dccouncil.us/images/00001/20100120154529.pdf. Accessed November 22, 2019.

[11]Medical marijuana and integrative therapy. District of Columbia website. https://dchealth.dc.gov/service/medical-marijuana-and-integrative-therapy. Accessed November 22, 2019.

[12]Physicians. The Florida Department of Health Office of Medical Marijuana Use website. https://knowthefactsmmj.com/physicians/. Accessed November 22, 2019.

[13]House Bill 324/AP. Georgia Legislature website. http://www.legis.ga.gov/Legislation/20192020/187578.pdf. Accessed November 26, 2019.

[14]Draft Guam rules governing medical marijuana. Guam Department of Public Health and Social Services website. http://dphss.guam.gov/document/draft-guam-rules-governing-medical-marijuana/. Accessed November 26, 2019.

[15]Part IX. Medical use of cannabis. Hawaii Legislature website. https://www.capitol.hawaii.gov/hrscurrent/Vol06_Ch0321-0344/HRS0329/HRS_0329-0121.htm. Accessed November 26, 2019.

[16]Cannabidiol. Idaho Office of Drug Policy website. https://odp.idaho.gov/cannibidiol/. Accessed November 26, 2019.

[17]Public Act 098-0122. Illinois Legislature website. http://www.ilga.gov/legislation/publicacts/98/PDF/098-0122.pdf. Accessed November 26, 2019.

[18]Physician information. Illinois Department of Public Health website. dph.illinois.gov/topics-services/prevention-wellness/medical-cannabis/physician-information. Accessed November 26, 2019.

[19]Medical cannabidiol information for physicians. Iowa Department of Public Health website. https://idph.iowa.gov/omc/For-Physicians. Accessed November 26, 2019.

[20]Senate Bill No. 28. Kansas Legislature website. http://www.kslegislature.org/li/b2019_20/measures/documents/sb28_enrolled.pdf. Accessed November 26, 2019.

[21]Senate Bill 124. Kentucky Legislature website. https://apps.legislature.ky.gov/record/14rs/sb124.html. Accessed November 26, 2019.

[22]Senate Bill No. 271. Louisiana Legislature website. https://legiscan.com/LA/text/HB149/2015. Accessed November 26, 2019.

[23]LD 1539, an act to amend Maine's medical marijuana law. Maine Statue Legislature website. https://legislature.maine.gov/legis/bills/bills_128th/billtexts/HP106001.asp. Accessed November 26, 2019.

[24]Health-General Article Title 13. Miscellaneous health care programs, subtitle 33—Natalie M. LaPrade Medical Cannabis Commission. Maryland Medical Cannabis Commission website. https://mmcc.maryland.gov/Documents/09.21.2018%20Health-General%20Article,%20 13-3301-13-3316.pdf. Updated September 21, 2018. Accessed November 26, 2019.

[25]Guidance for healthcare providers regarding the medical use of marijuana. Commonwealth of Massachusetts website. https://www.mass.gov/doc/guidance-for-health-care-providers-on-the-medical-use-of-marijuana/download. Published December 1, 2017. Accessed November 26, 2019.

[26]Michigan medical marihuana act. Michigan Legislature website. legislature.mi.gov/(S(3tytotr5csepzr1zz5ycuno4))/mileg.aspx?page=getObject&objectName=mcl-333-26423. Accessed November 26, 2019.

[27]House Bill No. 1231. Mississippi Legislature website.

[28]Amendment 2. Missouri Secretary of State website. https://www.sos.mo.gov/CMSImages/Elections/Petitions/2018-051.pdf. Accessed November 26, 2019.

[29]Montana medical marijuana program physician statement for a debilitating medical condition. Montana Department of Public Health and Human Services website. https://dphhs.mt.gov/marijuana/physicians. Accessed November 21, 2019.

[30]Medical marijuana cardholder registry—FAQs. Nevada Division of Public and Behavioral Health website. http://dpbh.nv.gov/Reg/MM-Patient-Cardholder-Registry/dta/FAQs/Medical_Marijuana_Patient_Cardholder_Registry_-_FAQs/. Updated February 1, 2018. Accessed November 26, 2019.

[31]Qualifying patient application for the therapeutic use of cannabis. State of New Hampshire Department of Health and Human Services website. https://www.dhhs.nh.gov/oos/tcp/documents/applicationpatient.pdf. Accessed November 26, 2019.

[32]Medical cannabis program application form. New Mexico Department of Health website. https://nmhealth.org/publication/view/form/135/. Accessed November 27, 2019.

[33]Practitioner information. New York State Department of Health website. https://www.health.ny.gov/regulations/medical_marijuana/practitioner/. Accessed November 27, 2019.

[34]Session Law 2015-154. North Carolina Legislature website. https://www.ncleg.gov/Sessions/2015/Bills/House/PDF/H766v6.pdf. Accessed November 27, 2019.

[35]ND medical marijuana healthcare providers. North Dakota Department of Health website. https://www.health.nd.gov/mm/nd-medical-marijuana-healthcare-providers. Accessed November 27, 2019.

[36]House Bill 523. Ohio Legislature website. https://www.legislature.ohio.gov/legislation/legislation-summary?id=GA131-HB-523. Accessed November 27, 2019.

[37]Guidance for physicians. Oklahoma Medical Marijuana Authority website. http://omma.ok.gov/guidance-for-physicians. Accessed November 21, 2019.

[38]Physicians. Oregon Medical Marijuana Program website. https://olis.leg.state.or.us/liz/2007R1/Downloads/MeasureDocument/SB161. Accessed November 27, 2019.

[39]§ 1181.24 Physician registration. Pennsylvania Code website. http://www.pacodeandbulletin.gov/Display/pacode?file=/secure/pacode/data/028/chapter1181/s1181.24.html&d=reduce. Accessed November 27, 2019.

[40]Medical cannabis. Departmento de Salud, Gobierno de Puerto Rico website. http://www.salud.gov.pr/Dept-de-Salud/Pages/Cannabis-Medicinal.aspx. Accessed November 27, 2019.

10

Endocrinology

- Preliminary evidence supports favorable effects of cannabis and cannabinoids on insulin sensitivity.
- The role of the cannabinoid receptor type 1 (CB1) in feeding control and peripheral metabolic regulation makes it a possible target for obesity pharmacotherapies.
- The CB1 antagonist rimonabant was effective in treating obesity and improving cardiovascular risk factors, but its significant psychiatric side effects led to its removal from the European market in 2008.

10.1 Insulin Sensitivity and Type 1 Diabetes

There have not been trials of any sort to evaluate the effects of cannabinoids on insulin sensitivity in the type 1 diabetes population.

10.2 Insulin Sensitivity and Type 2 Diabetes

There is some evidence supporting favorable effects of cannabis and cannabinoids on insulin sensitivity. Chronic cannabis use appears to be inversely associated with body mass index and insulin resistance based upon results from cross-sectional observational studies.[1,2]

A small randomized trial of 12 participants with type 2 diabetes (T2D) examined the effects of 2 nonpsychoactive cannabinoids, cannabidiol (CBD) and delta-9-tetrahydrocannabivirin, alone and in combination, on glycemic and lipid parameters. At 13 weeks, the delta-9-tetrahydrocannabivirin group showed a slight reduction in fasting plasma glucose as well as improved insulin resistance. Eleven of 12 participants reported adverse events, most gastrointestinal, however.[3]

Large epidemiologic studies demonstrate an inverse association between self-reported cannabis use and T2D. A meta-analysis of National Health and Nutrition Examination Surveys data from 2005 to 2011 reported an odds ratio of 0.7 (95% CI, 0.5-0.97; adjusted for age, sex, ethnicity, body mass index, education, income-poverty ratio and past-year alcohol and tobacco use).[4]

10.3 Obesity

Many pharmacotherapies have aimed to address the growing obesity problem. Most of these medications have had significant side effects dampening enthusiasm for their use. The cannabinoid receptor type-1 (CB1) is involved in feeding control and peripheral metabolic regulation, making it a possible target for obesity pharmacotherapies.[5] CB1 has many functions, including the control of energy homeostasis. An increase in CB1 signaling stimulates feeding by inducing appetite, and a reduction in CB1 signaling induces hypophagia via an appetite suppressant effect.[6]

The CB1 antagonist rimonabant was introduced in Europe in 2006 with claims that it would decrease appetite and body weight. Rimonabant was effective in treating obesity, and it improved cardiovascular risk factors.[7,8] It was also associated with psychiatric side effects such as depression, anxiety, and suicidal ideation, which were predictable due to its mechanism of action. Rimonabant is a high-affinity CB1 blocker with full inverse agonist activity, blocking reward pathways leading to worsening depression.[9] These side effects led to the suspension of use in Europe in 2008.

Work has continued to try to develop CB1 antagonists that act solely on peripheral CB1 receptors located outside of the brain. Ruiz de Azua and colleagues (2017) designed a mouse model that could induce adipocyte-specific deletion of the CB1-encoding gene. Peripheral blockage of CB1 receptors in adult obese mice led to fat redistribution with decreased total adiposity and increased weight loss. The loss of CB1 receptors in adipocytes prevented diet-induced obesity and led to overall improvement in metabolic profile.[10] These results suggest a causal relationship between loss of CB1 receptors in adipocytes and systemic metabolic changes.

REFERENCES

[1]Le Strat Y, Le Foll B. Obesity and cannabis use: results from 2 representative national surveys. *Am J Epidemiol.* 2011;174:929-933.

[2]Penner EA, Buettner H, Mittelman MA. The impact of marijuana use on glucose, insulin, and insulin resistance among US adults. *Am J Med.* 2013;126:583-589.

[3]Jadoon KA, Ratcliffe SH, Barrett DA, et al. Efficacy and safety of cannabidiol and tetra-hydrocannabivarin on glycemic and lipid parameters in patients with type 2 diabetes: a randomized, double-blind, placebo-controlled, parallel group pilot study. *Diabetes Care.* 2016;39:1777-1786.

[4]Alshaarawy O, Anthony J. Cannabis smoking and diabetes mellitus: results from meta-analysis with eight independent replication samples. *Epidemiology.* 2015;26:597-600.

[5]Muller T, Demiziseux L, Troy-Fioramonti S. Overactivation of the endocannabinoid system alters the antilipolytic action of insulin in mouse adipose tissue. *Am J Physiol Endocrinol Metab.* 2017;313(1):E26-E36.

[6]Koch M. Cannabinoid receptor signaling in central regulation of feeding behavior: a mini-review. *Front Neurosci.* 2017;11:293.

[7]Aronne LJ, Pagotto U, Foster GD, et al. The endocannabinoid system as a target for obesity treatment. *Clin Cornerstone.* 2008;9(1):52-54.

[8]Andre A, Gonthier MP. The endocannabinoid system: its roles in energy balance and potential as a target for obesity management. *Int J Biochem Cell Biol.* 2010;42(11):1788-1801.

[9]Bermuda-Silva FJ, Viveros MP, McPartland JM, Rodriguez de Fonseca F. The endocannabinoid system, eating behavior and energy homeostasis: the end or a new beginning? *Pharmacol Biochem Behavior.* 2010;95(4):375-382.

[10]Ruiz de Azua I, Mancini G, Srivastava A. Adipocyte cannabinoid receptor CB1 regulates energy homeostasis and alternatively activated macrophages. *J Clin Invest.* 2017;127(11):4148-4162.

11

Oncology

- Numerous preclinical studies show that cannabinoids demonstrate anticancer activity, although randomized controlled trials (RCTs) of cannabinoids as pharmacotherapy for cancer are lacking.
- Based on the strength of multiple RCTs, dronabinol and nabilone earned FDA approval for the treatment of chemotherapy-induced nausea and vomiting (CINV). The National Academies of Science, Engineering, and Medicine note that there is "conclusive or substantial evidence" for cannabis or cannabinoids as treatment for CINV.
- Oncologists are uncomfortable with their lack of knowledge about medical cannabis, and they are interested in learning more on this topic.

11.1 Cancer

The initial evidence that cannabinoids may have anticancer activity was a 1975 report that demonstrated that Lewis lung carcinoma cells could be inhibited *in vitro* by Δ-9-THC, Δ-8-THC, and CBD.[1] A meta-analysis of 34 preclinical studies showed that cannabinoids selectively destroyed rodent glioma cells in all but one study while leaving normal cells unscathed.[2] Studies investigating the mechanism of action of cannabinoids illustrated antiproliferative effects via cell cycle arrest as well as cell death via toxicity, necrosis, and autophagy. Preclinical studies demonstrate that cannabinoids show specific cytotoxicity against tumor cells while protecting healthy tissue from apoptosis.[3] Cannabinoids also have potent anticancer activity against tumor xenografts, including tumors that have been shown to be highly resistant to standard chemotherapies.

These preclinical investigations have shown cannabinoids to have antitumoral effects in glioma, hepatocellular carcinoma, prostate cancer, lung cancer, cholangiocarcinoma, breast cancer, and melanoma.[2,4-9] Despite ample *in vitro* and animal studies demonstrating anticancer activity by cannabinoids, the National Academy of Science, Engineering, and Medicine report published in 2017 concluded that there was insufficient evidence that cannabinoids have anticancer effects in humans.[10] There are no randomized, double-blind, placebo-controlled trials of cannabis or cannabinoids as pharmacotherapy for cancer itself. One pilot study involved the application of topical THC to recurrent glioblastoma multiforme tumors in nine participants; no benefit beyond that of chemotherapy alone was demonstrated.[11] Other trials of cannabinoids for glioblastoma multiforme are ongoing, but results have yet to be published. Clinical trials of cannabinoids in cancer have been limited to investigations of their palliative properties during standard chemotherapy to prevent nausea, vomiting, and cachexia.[13]

11.2 Chemotherapy-Induced Nausea and Vomiting

A considerable evidence base shows that cannabis and specific cannabinoids are effective pharmacotherapy for nausea and vomiting due to chemotherapy. Two U.S. FDA–approved cannabinoids, dronabinol and nabilone, received indications for nausea and vomiting due to chemotherapy as a result of three RCTs of dronabinol (and four studies of levonantradol, a synthetic analog of dronabinol) and 14 RCTs of nabilone for this indication. There have been six studies of oral THC capsules as pharmacotherapy for this indication, five of which used the antiemetic prochlorperazine as a comparator and one that used the antihistamine hydroxyzine as a comparator.[12–18] All studies suggested a greater benefit of cannabinoids vs both placebo and active comparators, but these benefits did not reach statistical significance in all studies. Additional studies looking at cannabis with differing ratios of THC to CBD for nausea and vomiting due to chemotherapy are under way and use more contemporary antiemetic therapy as a control.[19]

In one study, the combination of dronabinol and ondansetron was not found to be superior to either drug alone as treatment for delayed emesis.[20]

In a randomized, double-blind, placebo-controlled trial of intravenous THC for postoperative nausea and vomiting in 40 participants, THC did not significantly lessen nausea and vomiting compared to placebo. Due to significant side effects—primarily sedation and confusion—and uncertain efficacy for postoperative nausea and vomiting, the study was discontinued after 40 participants.[21]

Smoked cannabis has been evaluated for CINV in two studies. In the first study, 15 participants receiving treatment with high-dose methotrexate were given both oral THC and smoked cannabis.[22] Both oral THC and smoked cannabis were effective in reducing nausea and vomiting in 14 of 15 participants compared to placebo. Higher plasma levels of cannabis were associated with greater antiemetic effect. In the second study, eight participants who received chemotherapy with doxorubicin and cyclophosphamide did not receive more benefit from oral THC or smoked cannabis vs placebo.[23]

Nabilone, one of three FDA-approved cannabinoids, has been evaluated for CINV in several studies. Nabilone was superior to placebo in treating CINV in three studies.[24–26] A number of studies compared nabilone to active controls. Six trials compared nabilone with prochlorperazine and others used metoclopramide, domperidone, and alizapride as comparators.[27–37] Nabilone was noted, however, to be associated with more central nervous system side effects such as light-headedness, drowsiness, postural dizziness and hypotension, euphoria, and even hallucinations than the comparator drugs.

[13]Duran M, Perez E, Abanades S, et al. Preliminary efficacy and safety of an oromucosal standardized cannabis extract in chemotherapy-induced nausea and vomiting. *Br J Clin Pharmacol*. 2010;70:656-663.

[14]Orr LE, McKernan JF, Bloome B. Antiemetic effect of tetrahydrocannabinol. Compared with placebo and prochlorperazine in chemotherapy-associated nausea and emesis. *Arch Intern Med*. 1980;140:1431-1433.

[15]Orr LE, McKernan JF. Antiemetic effect of delta 9-tetrahydrocannabinol in chemotherapy-associated nausea and emesis as compared to placebo and compazine. *J Clin Pharmacol*. 1981;21:80S.

[16]Ungerleider JT, Andrysiak T, Fairbanks L, Goodnight J, Sarna G, Jamison, K. Cannabis and cancer chemotherapy: a comparison of oral delta-9-THC and prochlorperazine. *Cancer*. 1982;50:636-645.

[17]Frytak S, Moertel CG, O'Fallon JR, et al. Delta-9-tetrahydrocannabinol as an antiemetic for patients receiving cancer chemotherapy. A comparison with prochlorperazine and a placebo. *Ann Intern Med*. 1979;91:825-830.

[18]Sallan SE, Cronin C, Zelen M, Zinberg NE. Antiemetics in patients receiving chemotherapy for cancer: a randomized comparison of delta-9-tetrahydrocannabinol and prochlorperazine. *N Engl J Med*. 1980;302:135-138.

[19]Mersiades A, Haber P, Stockler M, et al. Pilot and definitive randomized double-blind placebo-controlled trials evaluating anoral cannabinoid-rich THC/CBD cannabis extract for secondary prevention of chemotherapy-induced nausea and vomiting (CINV). *Asia-Pacific J Clin Oncol*. 2017;13:67-68.

[20]Meiri E, Jhangiani H, Vrendenburgh JJ, et al. Efficacy of dronabinol alone and in combination with ondansetron versus ondansetron alone for delayed chemotherapy-induced nausea and vomiting. *Curr Med Res Opin*. 2007;23:533-543.

[21]Kleine-Brueggeney M, Greif R, Brenneisen R, Urwyler N, Stueber F, Theiler LG. Intravenous delta-9-tetrahydrocannabinol to prevent postoperative nausea and vomiting: a randomized controlled trial. *Anesth Analg*. 2015;121:1157-1164.

[22]Chang AE, Shiling DJ, Stillman RC, et al. Delta-9-tetrahydrocannabinol as an antiemetic in cancer patients receiving high-dose methotrexate. A prospective, randomized evaluation. *Ann Intern Med*. 1979;91:819-824.

[23]Chang AE, Shiling DJ, Stillman RC, et al. A prospective evaluation of delta-9-tetrahydrocannabinol as an antiemetic in patients receiving adriamycin and cytotoxan chemotherapy. *Cancer*. 1981;47:1746-1751.

[24]Jones SE, Durant JR, Greco FA, Robertone A. A multi-institutional Phase III study of nabilone vs. placebo in chemotherapy-induced nausea and vomiting. *Br J Clin Pharmacol*. 2010;70:656-663.

[25]Levitt M. Nabilone vs. placebo in the treatment of chemotherapy-induced nausea and vomiting in cancer patients. *Cancer Treat Rev*. 1982;9(suppl B):49-53.

[26]Wada JK, Bogdon DL, Gunnell JC, Hum GJ, Gota CH, Rieth TE. Double-blind, randomized, crossover trial of nabilone vs. placebo in cancer chemotherapy. *Cancet Treat Rev*. 1982;9(suppl B):39-44.

[27]Crawford SM, Buckman R. Nabilone and metoclopramide in the treatment of nausea and vomiting due to cisplatinum: a double blind study. *Med Oncol Tumor Pharmacother*. 1986;3:39-42.

[28]Herman TS, Einhorn LH, Jones SE, et al. Superiority of nabilone over prochlorperazine as an antiemetic in patients receiving cancer chemotherapy. *N Engl J Med*. 1979;300:1295-1297.

[29]Steele N, Gralla RJ, Braun DW Jr, Young CW. Double-blind comparison of the anti-emetic effects of nabilone and prochlorperazine on chemotherapy-induced emesis. *Cancer Treat Rep*. 1980;64:219-224.

[30]Einhorn LH, Nagy C, Furnas B, Williams SD. Nabilone: an effective antiemetic in patients receiving cancer chemotherapy. *J Clin Pharmacol.* 1981;21(suppl B):25-33.

[31]Johansson R, Kilkku P, Groenroos M. A double-blind, controlled trial of nabilone vs. prochlorperazine for refractory emesis induced by cancer chemotherapy. *Cancer Treat Rev.* 1982;9(suppl B):25-33.

[32]Ahmedzai S, Carlyle DL, Calder IT, Moran F. Anti-emetic efficacy and toxicity of nabilone, a synthetic cannabinoid, in lung cancer chemotherapy. *Br J Cancer.* 1983;48:657-663.

[33]Chan HS, Correia JA, MacLeod SM. Nabilone versus prochloperazine for control of cancer chemotherapy-induced emesis in children: a double-blind, crossover trial. *Pediatrics.* 1987;79:946-952.

[34]Niiranen A, Mattson K. A cross-over comparison of nabilone and prochlorperazine for emesis induced by cancer chemotherapy. *Am J Clin Oncol.* 1985;8:336-340.

[35]Dalzell AM, Bartlett H, Lilleyman JS. Nabilone: an alternative antiemetic for cancer chemotherapy. *Arch Dis Child.* 1986;61:502-505.

[36]Pomeroy M, Fennelly JJ, Towers M. Prospective randomized double-blind trial of nabilone versus domperidone in the treatment of cytotoxic-induced emesis. *Cancer Chemother Pharmacol.* 1986;17:285-288.

[37]Niederle N, Schutte J, Schmidt CG. Cross-over comparison of the antiemetic efficacy of nabilone and alizapride in patients with nonseminomatous testicular cancer receiving cisplatin therapy. *Klin Wochenschr.* 1986;64:362-365.

[38]Niiranen A, Mattson K. Antiemetic efficacy of nabilone and dexamethasone: a randomized study of patients with lung cancer receiving chemotherapy. *Am J Clin Oncol.* 1987;10:325-329.

[39]Cunningham D, Forrest GJ, Soukop M, Gilchrist NL, Calder IT, McArdle CS. Nabilone and prochlorperazine: a useful combination for emesis induced by cytotoxic drugs. *Br J Med (Clin Res Ed).* 1985;291:864-865.

[40]Priestman SG, Priestman TJ, Canney PA. A double-blind randomised cross-over comparison of nabilone and metoclopramide in the control of radiation-induced nausea. *Clin Radiol.* 1987;38:543-544.

[41]Lewis IH, Campbell DN, Barrowcliffe MP. Effect of nabilone on nausea and vomiting after total abdominal hysterectomy. *Br J Anaesth.* 1994;73:244-246.

[42]Hesketh PJ, Kris MG, Basch E, et al. Antiemetics: American Society of Clinical Oncology clinical practice guideline update. *J Clin Oncol.* 2017;35(28):3240-3261.

[43]Braun IM, Wright A, Peteet J, et al. Medical oncologists' beliefs, practices and knowledge regarding marijuana used therapeutically: a nationally representative survey study. *J Clin Oncol.* 2018;36:1957-1962.

[44]Zylla D, Steele G, Eklund J, Mettner J, Arneson T. Oncology Clinicians and the Minnesota Medical Cannabis Program: a survey on the medical Cannabis practice patterns, barriers to enrollment, and educational needs. *Cannabis Cannabinoid Res.* 2018;3(1):195-202.

12

Gastroenterology

- The anti-inflammatory effects of cannabinoids suggest promise for this class of agents as pharmacotherapy for inflammatory bowel disease (IBD).
- Three randomized controlled trials (RCTs) of cannabinoids for Crohn's disease (CD) do not provide strong evidence for the effectiveness of cannabinoids for CD.
- Two RCTs of cannabinoids for ulcerative colitis demonstrate tolerability, but little evidence for efficacy.

As cannabis and cannabinoids have been explored as treatments for multiple medical problems, it has been noted that there is a high prevalence of cannabis use among patients with the

IBDs, CD, and ulcerative colitis (UC).[1] Patient-reported studies place the prevalence of cannabis use among patients with IBD at 6.8%-17.6%.[1,2] Underscoring the lack of acceptance of cannabinoid pharmacotherapy for medical conditions in general, studies in Spain and the United States show that only 33% and 12.8% of patients with IBD, respectively, who are using cannabis to address their symptoms IBD, tell their physicians about their use.[2,3]

IBD are chronic immune-mediated diseases of the gastrointestinal tract.[4] IBD is notable for periods of inflammatory flares, quiet stability, and relapse—this results in considerable psychological, emotional, and physical burdens on those with these disorders.[5] Cannabinoids have long been shown to demonstrate anti-inflammatory properties, and CB1 receptors are important in the control of gastrointestinal motility and gastric intestinal secretion.[6,7]

Patients with IBD often consider complementary medications to control symptoms of their disease. Patients with IBD have used cannabis to address symptoms of abdominal pain, nausea, diarrhea, anorexia, and to improve mood and functioning.[8,9] Despite the attributes of cannabinoids that would suggest promise in treating IBD, the first RCT of a cannabinoid for irritable bowel disease was not published until 2013.[10] A recent systematic review could not draw any firm conclusions about the safety and effectiveness of cannabis and cannabinoids as pharmacotherapy for IBD.[11]

12.1 Crohn's Disease

A small observational study was the first published report of cannabis as pharmacotherapy for CD.[12] Twenty-one of 30 patients interviewed demonstrated significant improvement in subjective disease symptomatology as measured by a ≥4-point reduction in the Harvey Bradshaw Index (HBI) following treatment with cannabis. Patients also reported less need for other medications following surgery. Three RCTs, all led by the same team of investigators, of cannabis and cannabinoids as pharmacotherapy for CD have been conducted. In a randomized, double-blind, placebo-controlled trial of 8 weeks of twice daily smoked cannabis (115 mg of tetrahydrocannabinol [THC]) for CD, no difference in remission, the primary outcome, was observed between cannabis and placebo, but the cannabis group had a significant response on the Crohn's Disease Activity Index (CDAI), with 90% of those treated with cannabis achieving a reduction in CDAI score of more than 100 points.[10] Higher rates of adverse events (AEs), albeit mild AEs like nausea, confusion, and dizziness, were observed in the cannabis group.

A second RCT by the same group evaluated cannabidiol (CBD) in active CD who were medically refractory to standard therapy (steroids, thiopurines, or tumor necrosis factor antagonists). Twenty-one participants were given 20 mg of CBD twice daily in an oil or placebo over 8 weeks.[13] At 8 weeks, 40% (4 of 10) of participants in the CBD group achieved remission while 33% (3 of 9) in the placebo group achieved remission. Thus, no difference in clinical remission rates was observed between the two groups. No difference in AEs was observed, either.

A third RCT from the same group randomized participants to either cannabis oil (15% CBD and 4% THC) or placebo oil over 8 weeks of treatment.[14] An abstract presented at an international meeting showed a significantly higher score on a quality of life score (SF-36) and the Crohn's Disease Activity Index in the cannabis oil group compared to placebo. This study did not report on AEs.

12.2 Ulcerative Colitis

Two RCTs of cannabis and cannabinoids for UC have been conducted. Irving et al. led a multicenter, placebo-controlled RCT that evaluated CBD up to 250 mg twice daily vs placebo in participants with mild to moderate UC over 10 weeks.[15] The primary outcome measure in this study was clinical remission defined as a Mayo score ≤2 with no subscore >1 after 10 weeks of treatment. There was no difference between the CBD group and the placebo group in clinical remission rates at 10 weeks. AEs such as dizziness, somnolence, headache, and fatigue were more common in the CBD group than the placebo group.

Another RCT of 32 participants with treatment-refractory UC evaluated 8 weeks of treatment with 2 cannabis cigarettes (11.5 mg THC and 23 mg THC/day) daily compared to placebo cigarettes.[16] Clinical remission and clinical response were not reported as outcomes for this RCT. Greater improvements in disease activity index (DAI) and Mayo endoscopic scores were seen in the active group compared to placebo. Details of AEs were not reported in this RCT.

12.3 IBD Combined

A small prospective observational study assessed the effects of smoked cannabis on quality of life and disease activity.[17] Thirteen participants with chronic IBD (11 CD and 2 UC) were prescribed 50 g of cannabis cigarettes per month and followed for 3 months. Patients reported improvements in health perception, social functioning, ability to work, physical pain, and depression. They also showed significant gains in disease activity in the patients with CD, as measured by the HBI, as well as weight.

REFERENCES

[1]Weiss A, Friedenberg F. Patterns of cannabis use in patients with inflammatory bowel disease: a population based analysis. *Drug Alcohol Depend.* 2015;156:84-89.

[2]Garcia-Planella E, Marin L, Domenech E, et al. Use of complementary and alternative medicine and drug abuse in patients with inflammatory bowel disease. *Med Clin (Barc).* 2007;128:45-48.

[3]Kerlin AM, Long M, Kappelman M, et al. Profiles of patients who use marijuana for inflammatory bowel disease. *Dig Dis Sci.* 2018;63:1600-1604.

[4]Mowat C, Cole A, Windsor A, et al. Guidelines for the management of inflammatory bowel disease in adults. *Gut.* 2011;60:571-607.

[5]Devlen J, Beusterien K, Yen L, et al. The burden of inflammatory bowel disease. *Inflamm Bowel Dis.* 2014;20:545-552.

[6]Pertwee RG, Ross RA. Cannabinoid receptors and their ligands. *Prostaglandins Leukot Essent Fat Acids.* 2002;66:101-121.

[7]Courts AA, Izzo AA. The gastrointestinal pharmacology of cannabinoids: an update. *Curr Opin Pharmacol.* 2004;4:572-579.

[8]Lal S, Prasad N, Ryan M, et al. Cannabis use amongst patients with inflammatory bowel disease. *Eur J Gastroenterol Hepatol.* 2011;23:891-896.

[9]Ravikoff Allegretti J, Courtwright A, Lucci M, et al. Marijuana use patterns among patients with inflammatory bowel disease. *Inflamm Bowel Dis.* 2013;19:2809-2814.

[10]Naftali T, Bar-Lev Schlieder L, Dotan I, et al. Cannabis induces a clinical response in patients with Crohn's disease: a prospective placebo-controlled study. *Clin Gastroenterol Hepatol.* 2013;11:1276-1280.e1.

[11]Kafil TS, Nguyen TM, MacDonald JK, Chande N. Cannabis for the treatment of Crohn's disease and ulcerative colitis: evidence from the Cochrane Reviews. *Inflamm Bowel Dis.* 2020;26(4):502-509.

[12]Naftali T, Lev LB, Yablecovitch D, et al. Treatment of Crohn's disease with cannabis: an observational study. *Isr Med Assoc J.* 2011;13:455-458.

[13]Naftali T, Mechulam R, Marii A, et al. Low-dose cannabidiol is safe but not effective in the treatment for Crohn's disease, a randomized controlled trial. *Dig Dis Sci.* 2017;62:1615-1620.

[14]Naftali T, Schlieder LBL, Konikoff FM. *The Effect of Cannabis on Crohn's Disease Patients.* Berlin, Germany: International Association of Cannabis Medicine (IACM); 2017.

[15]Irving PM, Iqbal T, Nwokolo C, et al. A randomized, double-blind, placebo-controlled, parallel-group, pilot study of cannabidiol-rich botanical extract in the symptomatic treatment of ulcerative colitis. *Inflamm Bowel Dis.* 2018;24:714-724.

[16]Naftali T, Bar Lev Schlieder L, Sklerovsky Benjaminov F, et al. Cannabis induces clinical and endoscopic improvement in moderately active ulcerative colitis (UC). *J Crohns Colitis.* 2018;12:S306.

[17]Lahat A, Lang A, Ben-Horin S. Impact of cannabis treatment on the quality of life, weight and clinical disease activity in inflammatory bowel disease patients: a pilot prospective study. *Digestion.* 2012;85:1-8.

13

Neurology

- There are more studies of cannabinoids for neurological disorders than most other areas of medicine in part due to the preponderance of cannabinoid receptors in the brain.
- Cannabidiol was FDA-approved for the pediatric epilepsies Dravet syndrome and Lennox-Gastaut syndrome in 2018.
- Promising work suggests that cannabinoids may be helpful in treating agitation associated with Alzheimer disease.
- Beyond conditions with FDA-approvals, spasticity associated with multiple sclerosis has perhaps the most evidence for effective cannabinoid pharmacotherapy.

Cannabinoids have been studied as pharmacotherapy for a host of neurological disorders. Cannabinoid receptors are located prominently throughout the brain; this is one reason for the extensive number of studies in this area. Epilepsy, agitation secondary to Alzheimer disease (AD), and muscle spasticity associated with multiple sclerosis are three conditions with at least moderate evidence supporting the use of cannabinoids as pharmacotherapy.

13.1 Epilepsy

A significant development in the advancement of cannabis and cannabinoids as medications was the depiction of families with children suffering from pediatric seizure disorders obtaining some measure of relief from cannabinoids. Faced with their children having dozens of seizures per day, these families often turned to preparations that contained higher concentrations of cannabidiol (CBD) vs delta-9-tetrahydrocannabinol (THC) or pure CBD. These miraculous accounts were shown widely on television shows such as Dr. Sanjay Gupta's cannabis specials on CNN. Their promising results played a prominent role in the further investigation of CBD and other cannabinoids as epilepsy medications.

Prior to the anecdotal success of CBD for limiting seizures, there were several preclinical studies demonstrating the antiseizure properties of THC and CBD in various animal models.[1,2] The 2000s also saw some case reports of THC proving useful as pharmacotherapy for seizures in German children with severe neurological conditions.[3,4] Another influential report describing CBD's anticonvulsant effects, coupled with its nonintoxicating characteristics, turned most of the attention to CBD as the cannabinoid with the most promise in treating seizures.[5] Despite concerns about biases in the anecdotal reporting of the success of CBD in treating young people with epilepsy, scientists pushed ahead with the evaluation of CBD as a pharmacotherapy for epilepsy.

In addition, GW Pharma was also moving forward with clinical trials aimed at earning an FDA approval for Epidiolex, its CBD preparation.

Raphael Mechoulam's group conducted one of the earliest studies of CBD for epilepsy, well ahead of most of the interest in CBD as a treatment for this medical condition. In a small pilot study of 9 participants, those taking 200 mg of CBD daily appeared to suffer fewer seizures over a 3-month period.[6] In a slightly larger study, 15 participants with secondarily generalized epilepsy with temporal focus were randomized to receive 200-300 mg of CBD daily in addition to their usual medication regimen. CBD was well-tolerated and 7 of 8 participants in the CBD group showed at least partial clinical improvement compared to those in the placebo group.[7] A larger open-label trial of 214 participants with severe, intractable, childhood-onset, treatment-resistant epilepsy showed that 25-50 mg/kg daily showed a reduction in monthly frequency of motor seizures from 30.0 to 15.8 in a 12-week treatment period.[8]

Devinsky's group also led one of the major RCTs that led to Epidiolex earning a FDA-approval. In a double-blind, placebo-controlled trial of 120 children and young adults with Dravet syndrome, a rare and complex childhood epilepsy associated with drug-resistant seizures and a high mortality rate, were randomized to receive either 20 mg/kg daily of CBD or placebo in addition to their standard medication regimen.[9] CBD decreased the median frequency of convulsive seizures per month from 12.4 to 5.9 vs a decrease of 14.9 to 14.1 in the placebo group. The CBD group did report more adverse events compared to the placebo group with respect to diarrhea (31% vs 10%), loss of appetite (28% vs 5%), and somnolence (36% vs 10%).

In an international, multicenter RCT of 171 participants with Lennox-Gastaut syndrome, a severe form of epileptic encephalopathy that leads to multiple type of seizures (including drop seizures) that often are treatment-resistant, CBD (200 mg/kg) or placebo was added to standard epilepsy medication regimens over 14 weeks.[10] CBD reduced drop seizure frequency by a median of 43.9% compared to a 21.8% reduction in the placebo group. The CBD group also had significantly more participants experiencing >50% reduction in drop seizure frequency vs placebo (44% vs 24%). The CBD group experienced an increased number of adverse events similar to the Devinsky Dravet syndrome study described above. Of note, the CBD group included 20 participants who experienced increases in liver function tests >3 times the upper limit of normal, while 1 participant in the placebo group had increased liver function tests.

On the basis of these RCTs, GW Pharma's Epidiolex was FDA-approved for the treatment of Dravet syndrome and Lennox-Gastaut syndrome in 2018.

13.2 Parkinson Disease

Parkinson disease (PD) has long been a therapeutic target for cannabinoids due to the density of cannabinoid receptors in the basal ganglia. Results have been mixed, however. An oral THC:CBD extract demonstrated no improvement on dyskinesia or other signs in 17 participants with PD.[11] In an open-label, uncontrolled, observational study of smoked or vaporized cannabis for pain in 20 patients with PD, cannabis significantly decreased motor disability and pain scores, and CBD was also helpful with respect to general symptoms of PD in a similar trial of 21 participants with PD.[12] In a second open-label, uncontrolled, observational study of smoked cannabis in 28 participants with PD, treatment with smoked cannabis yielded significant improvement on total motor disability scores.[13]

13.3 Alzheimer Disease

The endocannabinoid system plays a prominent role in many of the primary pathological processes involved in AD such as protein misfolding, excitotoxicity, neuroinflammation, mitochondrial dysfunction, and oxidative stress. CB2 receptor levels have been show to increase in AD especially in microglia located near senile plaques and the stimulation of the endocannabinoid system promotes beta-amyloid removal by macrophages. Acute effects of THC that include subjective feelings of euphoria, relaxation, and sedation have contributed to the investigation of cannabinoids as treatments for AD, especially the agitation that may result.

Given these subjective effects and relatively benign safety profile, investigators have studied THC preparations for the treatment of agitation in AD, and there have been several promising small studies. Volicer et al. administered dronabinol 2.5 mg twice daily to 15 participants with advanced AD and anorexia in a 6-week crossover RCT.[14] They observed a significant reduction in agitation as measured by the Cohen-Mansfield Agitation Inventory (CMAI) during dronabinol exposure. Patel et al. performed a retrospective chart review of 48 residents of an assisted living dementia unit who had AD and anorexia.[15] Following treatment with dronabinol 2.5 mg twice daily, agitation improved in 65% of these residents. Walther et al. reported decreased nocturnal motor activity and reduced agitation in six participants with dementia in an open-label trial of dronabinol 2.5 mg daily with no AEs attributed to drug exposure.[16] Woodward and colleagues published a case series of 40 inpatients AD agitation of advanced severity treated for 7 days with dronabinol (mean dose 7 mg daily) adjunctive to other psychotropics.[17] Pittsburgh Agitation Scale (PAS) scores decreased from a mean (SD) of 9.68 (3.91) to 5.25 (4.17) ($P < .0001$), for an effect size of 1.09. However, an RCT in 50 patients with AD and neuropsychiatric symptoms receiving 1.5 mg THC 3 times daily for 3 weeks vs placebo failed to produce a benefit.[18]

13.4 Dementia

Pure delta-9-tetrahydrocannabinol (THC) has been studied in four randomized controlled trials in participants with dementia. An initial safety crossover study in 10 participants with dementia found that treatment with THC was safe in this population; THC did not produce more adverse events than placebo.[19] Two studies evaluating the effects of THC treatment on neuropsychiatric symptoms in dementia found no difference between THC and placebo. In the first study by Van den Elsen et al., a crossover design of 22 participants receiving up to 3 mg of THC daily yielded no difference between THC and placebo in Neuropsychiatric Inventory (NPI) scores.[20] A second randomized, double-blind, placebo-controlled trial in 50 participants by the same group showed that 4.5 mg of THC daily also failed to produce a difference from placebo in NPI scores, nor were there differences in secondary outcome measures of agitation, quality of life, or activities of daily living.[18] A third trial by the same group, a randomized, placebo-controlled, crossover study of THC 3 mg daily in 18 participants with dementia showed that THC had no adverse effect upon balance, gait, and adverse events in this population.[21]

Cannabis oil containing THC as an add-on pharmacotherapy for dementia produced a significant reduction in Clinical Global Impression (CGI) and NPI scores in an open-label trial involving 11 patients, 10 of whom completed the study.[22]

13.5 Amyotrophic Lateral Sclerosis

There has been only one RCT evaluating a cannabinoid as pharmacotherapy for Amyotrophic Lateral Sclerosis. In a randomized, double-blind, placebo-controlled trial of dronabinol for amyotrophic lateral sclerosis, treatment with dronabinol yielded no reduction in cramps compared to placebo.[23]

13.6 Huntington Disease

A randomized, double-blind, placebo-controlled trial of nabiximols for Huntington disease failed to demonstrate any difference between nabiximols and placebo on motor, cognitive, behavioral, or functional scores in 26 patients (24 completed the study) treated over 12 weeks.[24] Other cannabinoids, namely nabilone and CBD, have been studied as pharmacotherapy for Huntington disease, yielding improvements in chorea and no difference from placebo, respectively.[25]

13.7 Multiple Sclerosis, Spasticity

Two meta-analyses addressed the literature of cannabis and cannabinoids for spasticity in multiple sclerosis. Whiting et al. reported that the pooled odds of patient-reported improvement on a global impression-of-change score was greater with nabiximols than with placebo (OR, 1.44; 95% CI, 1.07-1.94).[26] Meanwhile, Koppel et al. concluded that nabiximols is "probably effective" for reducing patient-reported spasticity scores.[27] Both meta-analyses stated that treatment with nabiximols does not produce differences in objective spasticity compared to placebo, although it was noted that the Ashworth Scale is not ideal to detect such differences.

Five randomized, double-blind, placebo-controlled trials of nabiximols for spasticity in multiple sclerosis have been conducted (one utilized a crossover design). Of these trials, three demonstrated that nabiximols treatment led to a significant difference in spasticity,[28–30] while nabiximols treatment failed to separate from placebo in the other two trials.[29,31] Further investigation of either secondary endpoints or of those previously in spasticity clinical trials showed decreases in subjective measures of spasticity and a recent observational study of patients with multiple sclerosis on nabiximols showed this as well.[31–33]

Dronabinol pharmacotherapy for multiple sclerosis has been studied in five randomized, double-blind, placebo-controlled trials. Three of these trials evaluated its effects upon spasticity in these participants, one assessed neuropathic pain, and one looked at its effects upon disease progression; one of the trials evaluated both spasticity and pain. Two of the spasticity trials, which enrolled 630, and 13 participants, respectively, found that treatment with dronabinol significantly reduced spasticity by self-report.[34,35] Killestein et al. found in 16 participants that dronabinol did not separate from placebo in its effects upon spasticity.[36] Dronabinol's effects upon neuropathic pain in MS patients has been mixed, with Svendsen et al. showing an effect in 24 participants while Schimrigk did not in 240 participants.[37,38] The CUPID trial of 493 participants with primary or secondary progressive MS found no evidence that dronabinol has an effect on MS progression.[39]

Van Amerongen et al. assessed the effects of a pure form of THC on spasticity and neuropathic pain in 24 participants with progressive MS and moderate spasticity. Treatment with THC decreased neuropathic pain immediately after administration but not when measured in daily diaries. A similar pattern was observed with subjective muscle spasticity; the THC group was also significantly more likely to experience adverse events than the placebo group.[40]

In a double-blind, randomized trial, patients with multiple sclerosis who received cosupplemented hemp seed and evening primrose oils had decreased extended disability status scores and lower liver transaminase levels compared to patients treated with a dietary intervention alone.[41]

13.8 Motor Neuron Disease

A preliminary report of results from a randomized, double-blind, placebo-controlled multicenter trial of cannabis sativa extract in patients with motor neuron disease, treatment with cannabis sativa extract produced no difference in the modified Ashworth Scale and pain scores. However, while there was a trend for improvement of all outcome measures, most outcomes were not significantly affected.[42]

13.9 Neurogenic Symptoms

Extracts containing THC, CBD, and THC and CBD in a 1:1 ratio produced a significant reduction in neurogenic symptoms including bladder control, muscle spasms, and spasticity in a series of randomized, double-blind, placebo-controlled crossover studies in 24 patients with chronic medical illnesses (18 were participants with multiple sclerosis) associated with neurogenic symptoms.[43]

13.10 Tourette Syndrome

Whiting et al. noted low-quality evidence for cannabis and cannabinoids improving outcomes in Tourette syndrome.[26] In two (n = 12 and 24) randomized, double-blind, placebo-controlled trials of dronabinol in participants with Tourette syndrome, dronabinol produced either significant improvement in tics or a trend toward such improvement, as well as a significant improvement in obsessive-compulsive behavior in one of the studies.[44,45]

13.11 Migraine and Cluster Headaches

In a preliminary investigation presented at a scientific conference in 2017, no difference was observed between cannabis and amitriptyline for prophylaxis of cluster or migraine headaches, although the control arm might not represent optimal control therapy. In a subset of participants with history of migraines when they were children, acute administration of cannabis as abortive therapy decreased attack pain for both migraines and cluster headaches.[46]

13.12 Traumatic Brain Injury

Traumatic brain injury involved glutamate excitotoxicity which may be counteracted by the neuroprotective antioxidant effects of cannabinoids.[47] Patients theorized to be suffering from chronic traumatic encephalopathy symptoms such as headache, nausea, insomnia, agitation, and psychosis have benefitted anecdotally from cannabis preparations. There is a considerable body of preclinical evidence demonstrating the neuroprotective effects of cannabinoids. Cannabis induces the expression of 2-arachidonoyl glycerol (2-AG), which reduced brain edema and infarct volume following severe closed head injury.[48] Similarly, the CB1 and CB2 receptor agonist Bay 38-7271 showed neuroprotective properties in traumatic brain injury and focal ischemic rat models.[48,49] Cannabinoid agonists have also been shown to protect hippocampal and cortical neurons from excitotoxicity.[50,51] Synthetic cannabinoids administered to rats increased hippocampal granule cell density and dendritic length in pyramidal cells.[52]

While the aforementioned preclinical studies are very promising, RCTs of cannabinoids for traumatic brain injury and chronic traumatic encephalopathy have yet to be conducted. Thus, expectations must be tempered and, unfortunately, this is another area where claims about the efficacy of cannabinoids has extended beyond the evidence, at times playing on the fears of those who worry that they may have chronic traumatic encephalopathy.

13.13 Obstructive Sleep Apnea

In the only randomized controlled trial of a cannabinoid as pharmacotherapy for obstructive sleep apnea, dronabinol produced lower scores on the apnea-hypopnea index, improved scores of self-report sleepiness, and greater treatment satisfaction than placebo. There was no difference between dronabinol and placebo in objective measures of sleepiness or incidence of adverse events.[53]

REFERENCES

[1]Wallace MJ, Blair RE, Falenski KW, Martin BR, DeLorenzo RJ. The endogenous cannabinoid system regulates seizure frequency and duration in a model of temporal lobe epilepsy. *J Pharmacol Exp Ther.* 2003;307:129-137.

[2]Do Val-da Silva RA, Peixoto-Santos JE, Kandratavicius L, et al. Protective effects of cannabidiol against seizures and neuronal death in a rat model of mesial temporal lobe epilepsy. *Front Pharmacol.* 2017;8:131.

[3]Lorenz R. On the application of cannabis in paediatrics and epileptology. *Neuro Endocrinol Lett.* 2004;25:40-44.

[4]Gottschling S. Cannabinoide bei kindern. Gute erfahrungen bei schmerzen, spastik und in der oncologic. *Ange Schmezth Palliat.* 2011;4:55-57.

[5]Jones NA, Hill AJ, Smith I, et al. Cannabidiol displays antiepilieptifom and antiseizure properties in vitro and in vivo. *J Pharmacol Exp Ther.* 2010;332:569-577.

[6]Mechoulam R, Carlini E. Toward drugs derived from cannabis. *Naturwissenschaften.* 1978;65(4):174-179.

[7]Cunha JM, et al. Chronic administration of cannabidiol to healthy volunteers and epileptic patients. *Pharmacology.* 1980;21(3):175-185.

[8]Devinsky O, Marsh E, Friedman D, et al. Cannabidiol in patients with treatment-resistant epilepsy: an open-label intervention trial. *Lancet Neurol.* 2016;15:270-278.

[9]Devinsky O, Cross JH, Laux L, et al. Trial of cannabidiol for drug-resistant seizures in the Dravet syndrome. *N Eng J Med.* 2017;376:2011-2020.

[10]Thiele EA, Marsh ED, French JA, et al. Cannabidiol in patients with seizures associated with Lennox-Gastaut syndrome (GWPCARE4): a randomised, double-blind, placebo-controlled phase 3 trial. *Lancet.* 2018;391:1085-1096.

[11]Carroll CB, Bain PG, Teare L, et al. Cannabis for dyskinesia in Parkinson disease: a randomized double-blind crossover study. *Neurology.* 2004;63:1245-1250.

[12]Chagas MH, Zuardi AW, Tumas V, et al. Effects of cannabidiol in the treatment of patients with Parkinson's disease: an exploratory double-blind trial. *J Psychopharmacol.* 2014;28:1088-1098.

[13]Lotan I, Treves TA, Roditi Y, Djaldetti R. Cannabis (medical marijuana) treatment for motor and non-motor symptoms of Parkinson disease: an open-label observational study. *Clin Neuropharmacol.* 2014;37:41-44.

[14]Volicer L, Stelly M, Morris J, McLaughlin J, Volicer B. Effects of dronabinol on anorexia and disturbed behavior in patients with Alzheimer's disease. *Int J Geriatr.* 1997;12:913-919.

[15]Patel S, Shua-Haim JR, Pass M. PC-037 Safety and efficacy of dronabinol in the treatment of agitation in patients with Alzheimer's disease with anorexia: a retrospective chart review. The Eleventh International Congress, 2003.

[16]Walther S, Mahlberg R, Eichmann U, Kunz D. Delta-9-tetrahydrocannabinol for night-time agitation in severe dementia. *Psychopharmacology (Berl).* 2006;185(4):524-528.

[17]Woodward MR, Harper DG, Stolyar A, Forester BP, Ellison JM. Dronabinol for the treatment of agitation and aggressive behavior in acutely hospitalized severely demented patients with noncognitive behavioral symptoms. *Am J Geriatr Psychiatry.* 2014;22(4):415-419.

[18]van den Elsen GA, Ahmed AI, Verkes RJ, et al. Tetrahydrocannabinol for neuropsychiatric symptoms in dementia: a randomized controlled trial. *Neurology.* 2015;84:2238-2346.

[19]Ahmed A, van der Marck MA, van den Elsen G, Olde Rikkert M. Cannabinoids in late-onset Alzheimer's disease. *Clin Pharmacol.* 2015;97:597-606.

[20]Van den Elsen GA, Ahmed AI, Verkes RJ, et al. Tetrahydrocannabinol in behavioral disturbances in dementia: a crossover randomized controlled trial. *Am J Geriatr Psychiatry.* 2015;23(12):1214-1224.

[21]Geke AH, van den Elsen GA, Tobben L, et al. Effects of tetrahydrocannabinol on balance and gait in patients with dementia: a randomised controlled crossover trial. *J Psychopharmacol.* 2017;31(2):184-191.

[22]Shelef A, Barak Y, Berger U, et al. Safety and efficacy of medical cannabis oil for behavioral and psychological symptoms of dementia: an-open label, add-on, pilot study. *J Alzheimers Dis.* 2016;51:15-19.

[23]Weber M, Goldman B, Truniger S. Tetrahydrocannabinol (THC) for cramps in amyotrophic lateral sclerosis: a randomised, double-blind crossover trial. *J Neurol Neurosurg Psychiatry.* 2010;81:1135-1140.

[24]Lopez-Sendon Moreno JL, Garcia Caldentey J, Trigo Cubillo P, et al. A double-blind, randomized, cross-over, placebo-controlled, pilot trial with Sativex in Huntington's disease. *J Neurol.* 2016;263:1390-4000.

[25]Saft C, von Hein SM, Lucke T, et al. Cannabinoids for the treatment of dystonia in Huntington's disease. *J Huntingtons Dis.* 2018;7(2):167-173.

[26]Whiting PF, Wolff RF, Deshpande S, et al. Cannabinoids for medical use: a systematic review and meta-analysis. *JAMA.* 2015;313(24):2456-2473.

[27]Koppel BS, Brust JC, Fife T, et al. Systematic review: efficacy and safety of medical marijuana in selected neurologic disorders. *Neurology.* 2014;82(17):1556-1563.

[28]Collin C, Davies P, Mutiboko IK, Ratcliffe S; Sativex in Spasticity in MS Study Group. Randomized controlled trial of cannabis-based medicine in spasticity caused by multiple sclerosis. *Eur J Neurol.* 2007;14:290-296.

[29]Aragona M, Onesti E, Tomassini V, et al. Psychopathological and cognitive effects of therapeutic cannabinoids in multiple sclerosis: a double-blind, placebo controlled, cross-over study. *Clin Neuropharmacol.* 2009;32:41-47.

[30]Novotna A, Mares J, Ratcliffe S, et al.; the Sativex Spasticity Study Group. A randomized, placebo-controlled, parallel-group, enriched-design study of nabiximols (Sativex), as add-on therapy, in subjects with refractory spasticity caused by multiple sclerosis. *Eur J Neurol.* 2011;18:1122-1131.

[31]Leocani L, Nuara A, Houdayer E, et al. Sativex and clinical-neurophysiological measures of spasticity in progressive multiple sclerosis. *J Neurol.* 2015;262(11):2520-2527.

[32]Haupts M, Vila C, Jonas A, Witte K, Alvarez-Ossorio L. Influence of previous failed antispasticity therapy on the efficacy and tolerability of THC:CBD oromucosal spray on multiple sclerosis spasticity. *Eur Neurol.* 2016;75(5-6):236-243.

[33]Vermersch P, Trojano M. Tetrahydrocannabinol:cannabidiol oromucosal spray for multiple sclerosis-related resistant spasticity in daily practice. *Eur Neurol.* 2016;76(5-6):216-226.

[34]Zajicek JP, Hobart JC, Slade A, Barnes D, Mattison PG; MUSEC Research Group. Multiple Sclerosis and extract of cannabis: results of the MUSEC trial. *J Neurol Neurosurg Psychiatry.* 2012;83:1125-1132.

[35]Ungerleider JT, Andyrsiak T, Fairbanks L, Ellison GW, Myers LW. Delta-9-THC in the treatment of spasticity associated with multiple sclerosis. *Adv Alcohol Subst Abuse.* 1987;7:39-50.

[36]Killestein J, Hoogervorst EL, Rief M, et al. Safety, tolerability and efficacy of orally administered cannabinoids in MS. *Neurology.* 2002;58:1404-1407.

[37]Schimrigk S, Marziniak M, Neubauer C, Kugler EM, Werner G, Abramov-Sommariva D. Dronabinol is a safe long-term treatment option for neuropathic pain patients. *Eur Neurol.* 2017;78(5-6):320-329.

[38]Svendsen KB, Jensen TS, Bach FW. Does the cannabinoid dronabinol reduce central pain in multiple sclerosis? Randomized double blind placebo controlled crossover trial. *BMJ.* 2004;329:253.

[39]Ball S, Vickery J, Hobart J, et al. The Cannabinoid Use in Progressive Inflammatory Brain Disease (CUPID) trial: a randomised double-blind placebo-controlled parallel-group multicenter trial and economic evaluation of cannabinoids to slow progression in multiple sclerosis. *Health Technol Assess.* 2015;19:1-187.

[40]Van Amerongen G, Kanhai K, Baakman AC, et al. Effects on spasticity and neuropathic pain of an oral formulation of delta-9-tetrahydrocannabinol in patients with progressive multiple sclerosis. *Clin Ther.* 2017;40:1467-1482.

[41]Rezapour-Firouzi S, Arefhosseini SR, Ebrahimi-Mamaghani M, et al. Activity of liver enzymes in multiple sclerosis patients with Hot-nature diet and co-supplemented hemp seed, evening primrose oils intervention. *Complement Ther Med.* 2014;22:986-993.

[42]Riva N, Mora G, Soraru G, et al. The canals study: a randomized, double-blind, placebo-controlled, multicentre study to assess the safety and efficacy on spasticity symptoms of a cannabis sativa extract in motor neuron disease patients. Amyotrophic lateral sclerosis and frontotemporal degeneration. Conference: 27th International Symposium on ALS/MND. Ireland. Conference start: December 7, 2016. Conference end: December 9, 2016, 17, 44.

[43]Wade DT, Robson P, House H, Makela P, Aram J. A preliminary controlled study to determine whether whole-plant cannabis extracts can improve intractable neurogenic symptoms. *Clin Rehabil.* 2003;17:21-29.

[44]Muller-Vahl KR, Schneider U, Koblenz A, et al. Treatment of Tourette's syndrome with delta 9-tetrahydrocannabinol (THC): a randomized crossover trial. *Pharmacopsychiatry.* 2002;35:57-61.

[45]Muller-Vahl KR, Schneider U, Prevedel H, et al. Delta 9-tetrahydrocannabinol (THC) is effective in the treatment of tics in Tourette syndrome: a 6-week randomized trial. *J Clin Psychiatry.* 2003;64:459-465.

[46]Nicolodi M, Sandoval V, Terrine A. Therapeutic use of cannabinoids-dose finding, effects and pilot data of effects in chronic migraine and cluster headache. *Eur J Neurol.* 2017;24:287. Conference: 3rd Congress of the European Academy of Neurology, Netherlands.

[47]Hampson RE, Deadwyler SA. Role of cannabinoid receptors in memory storage. *Neurobiol Dis.* 1998;5:474-482.

[48]Sarne Y, Asaf F, Fishbein M, Gafni M, Keren O. The dual neuroprotective-neurotoxic profile of cannabinoid drugs. *Br J Pharmacol.* 2011;163(7):1391-1401.

[49]Sarne Y, Keren O. Are cannabinoid drugs neurotoxic or neuroprotective? *Med Hypotheses.* 2004;63(2):187-192.

[50]Abood ME, Rivzi G, Sallapurdi N, McAllister SD. Activation of the CB1 cannabinoid receptor protects cultured mouse spinal neurons against excitotoxicity. *Neurosci Lett.* 2001;309(3):197-201.

[51]Hampson AJ, Grimaldi M. Cannabinoid receptor activation and elevated cyclic AMP reduce glutamate neurotoxicity. *Eur J Neurosci.* 2001;13(8):1529-1536.

[52]Chan GC, Sills RC, Braun AG, Haseman JK, Bucher JR. Toxicity and carcinogenicity of delta-9-tetrahydrocannabinol in Fischer rats and B6C3F1 mice. *Fund App Toxicol.* 1996;30(1):109-117.

[53]Carley DW, Prasad B, Reid KJ, et al. Pharmacotherapy of apnea by cannabimimetic enhancement, the PACE Clinical Trial: effects of dronabinol in obstructive sleep apnea. *Sleep.* 2018;41(1):zsx184.

14

Psychiatry

- Strong interest in cannabinoids as treatment for psychiatric disorders has led to numerous studies but few randomized, controlled trials.
- Cannabidiol (CBD) has promise as a pharmacotherapy for psychotic disorders as well as disorders on the anxiety spectrum.
- There are no randomized controlled trials (RCTs) of cannabinoids as pharmacotherapy for opioid use disorder, although CBD warrants further study.

Aside from chronic noncancer pain, psychiatric disorders are among the most common reasons that people use cannabis and cannabinoids medicinally.[1] Some think cannabinoids may be helpful based upon their previous experiences or because they have seen claims of efficacy on various media platforms. As a result, clinicians regularly field questions about the effects of cannabis and cannabinoids upon psychiatric disorders. As discussed in the Adverse Effects chapter, cannabis appears to have deleterious effects upon several psychiatric disorders, so clinicians must use extreme caution when entertaining the notion of using cannabinoids for psychiatric conditions.

14.1 Anxiety

Anxiety is one of the top reasons that many patients say they use cannabis. While many patients question the effectiveness of cannabis as pharmacotherapy for anxiety after an extended period of use, the complex relationship between cannabinoids and anxiety is confusing for many. A recent meta-analysis by Black et al. reviewed 31 studies that measured the effects of cannabinoids on anxiety.[2] Seventeen of these studies were randomized controlled trials. Seven studies of pharmaceutical tetrahydrocannabinol (THC) (with or without cannabidiol [CBD]), $n = 252$, improved anxiety symptoms among participants with other medical conditions (standardized mean difference −0.25 [95% CI −0.49 to −0.01]. Many of these trials were part of the FDA packages for dronabinol and nabilone, and the participants suffered from chronic noncancer pain and multiple sclerosis. The evidence GRADE, however, was very low.

Two studies examining the effects of CBD on social anxiety did not find a significant improvement in anxiety symptoms compared with placebo.[3,4] However, due to the preclinical studies that have demonstrated CBD to have anxiolytic properties, there are physicians who are utilizing CBD as pharmacotherapy for treatment-refractory anxiety.

14.2 Posttraumatic Stress Disorder

Several investigations have looked at the relationships of cannabis and cannabinoids and posttraumatic stress disorder (PTSD).

There is a hypothetical rationale for cannabis and cannabinoids as being effective pharmacotherapy for PTSD, but more so for CBD and its anxiolytic properties.[5] A retrospective chart review of patients with PTSD prescribed nabilone in addition to their usual medications noted that nabilone was associated with a significant improvement in duration of sleep, reduction of nightmares, and improvement in PTSD symptom severity.[6] Another chart review of patients with PTSD experiencing nightmares showed that adjunct nabilone led to reduced nightmares and improved overall sleep.[7] A double-blind, crossover study of 10 male soldiers with PTSD and nightmares showed that nabilone pharmacotherapy resulted in a significant reduction in nightmares but no change in PTSD symptoms.[8] Roitman et al. added oral THC to current medications in patients with chronic PTSD and reported mixed results in measures of sleep and PTSD symptoms but an overall improvement in functioning as measured by the Clinician Global Impressions scale.[9] Two observational studies associated increased cannabis use with increased PTSD symptom severity.[10,11] Another observational study of New Mexico residents who enrolled in the states' medical cannabis program to treat PTSD found that these residents generally found cannabis useful in reducing their symptoms.[12]

14.3 Depression

The meta-analysis of Black et al. (2019) found that pharmaceutical THC (with or without CBD) did not significantly affect mood.[2] This supported a previous meta-analysis in 2015 by Whiting et al.[13] There have not any interventional studies of cannabis or cannabinoids, including CBD, to treat depression. While the aforementioned meta-analyses do not show an overall effect of cannabis upon mood, there have been studies like a recent observational study of cancer patients that showed cannabis to reduce depressive symptoms during the course of the study.

14.4 Autism

Anecdotal evidence of cannabinoids, mostly CBD, benefitting those with autism spectrum disorders (ASD) has created a growing interest in cannabinoids as possible pharmacotherapy for ASD. Animal studies suggest that alteration of the endocannabinoid

sample sizes, duration of follow-up, and lack of uniformity of outcome measures, there is enough evidence to consider cannabis or cannabinoids as third-line treatments for chronic pain under the right circumstances. These circumstances involve a collaboration between the patient and a doctor that knows them well, resulting often in multiple medication trials of medications of different classes and modalities along with procedures where appropriate (usually injections).

We think it is critical to draw a distinction between those with chronic pain on prescribed opioids and those with opioid use disorder using illicit opioids like fentanyl. There are doctors, often specialty physicians whose physicians whose practices consist largely of writing for medical cannabis certifications, who will certify the use of medical cannabis as a treatment for opioid use disorder. They sometimes refer to cannabis as "an exit drug" for these patients. Relying on medical cannabis as the primary pharmacotherapy for opioid use disorder is a risky plan, especially considering that we have three effective medications for opioid use disorder, buprenorphine, methadone, and naltrexone. These are potentially life-saving medications, and every effort should be made to start patients with opioid use disorder on these medications as soon as possible. There are no interventional studies of cannabis as pharmacotherapy for patients with opioid use disorder.

Yasmin Hurd's group at Mount Sinai has done an interesting series of studies that suggest promise for CBD as a pharmacotherapy for cannabis use disorder. They showed that CBD reduces reinstatement of opioid-seeking behavior triggered by drug cues in animals with a history of heroin self-administration.[23] This reduction of heroin-seeking behavior lasted for weeks following CBD administration.[24] These preclinical findings translated to humans in a recent exploratory double-blind randomized placebo-controlled trial that assessed the effects of CBD administration on drug cue-induced craving and anxiety in patients with opioid use disorder.[25] Acute CBD administration significantly reduced both craving and anxiety in response to drug cues vs placebo. These effects were still evident 7 days after CBD exposure.

REFERENCES

[1]Lucas P, Walsh Z. Medical cannabis access, use, and substitution for prescription opioids and other substances: a survey of authorized medical cannabis patients. *Int J Drug Policy*. 2017;42:30-35.

[2]Black N, Stockings E, Campbell G, et al. Cannabinoids for the treatment of mental disorders and symptoms of mental disorders: a systematic review and meta-analysis. *Lancet Psychiatry*. 2019;6(12):995-1010. doi: 10.1016/S2215-0366(19)30401-8.

[3]Bergamaschi MM, Queriroz RHC, Chagas MHN, et al. Cannabidiol reduces the anxiety induced by simulated public speaking in treatment-naïve social phobia patients. *Neuropsychopharmacology*. 2011; 36:1219-26.

[4]Crippa JAS, Derenusson GN, Ferrari TB, et al. Neural basis of anxiolytic effects of cannabidiol (CBD) in generalized social anxiety disorder: a preliminary report. *J Psychopharmacol*. 2011;25:121-30.

[5]Haney M, Evins AE. Does cannabis cause, exacerbate or ameliorate psychiatric disorders? An oversimplified debate discussed. *Neuropsychopharmacology*. 2016;41(2):393-401.

[6]Cameron C, Watson D, Robinson J. Use of a synthetic cannabinoid in a correctional population for posttraumatic stress disorder-related insomnia and nightmares, chronic pain, harm reduction, and other indications: a retrospective evaluation. *J Clin Psychopharmacol*. 2014;34:559-564.

[7]Fraser GA. The use of synthetic cannabinoid in the management of treatment-resistant nightmares in posttraumatic stress disorder (PTSD). *CNS Neurosci Ther*. 2009;15:84-88.

[8]Jetly R, Heber A, Fraser G, et al. The efficacy of nabilone, a synthetic cannabinoid, in the treatment of PTSD-associated nightmares: a preliminary randomized, double-blind, placebo-controlled cross-over design study. *Psychoneuroendocrinology*. 2015;51:585-588.

[9]Roitman P, Mechoulam R, Cooper-Kazar R, et al. Preliminary, open-label, pilot study of add-on oral Δ^9-tetrahydrocannabinol in chronic post-traumatic stress disorder. *Clin Drug Investig*. 2014;34:587-591.

[10]Bonn-Miller MO, Vujanovic AA, Drescher KD. Cannabis use among military veterans after residential treatment for posttraumatic stress disorder. *Psychol Addict Behav*. 2011;25:485-491.

[11]Boden MT, Babson KA, Vujanovic AA, et al. Posttraumatic stress disorder and cannabis use characteristics among military veterans with cannabis dependence. *Am J Addict*. 2013;22:277-284.

[12]Greer GR, Grob CS, Halberstadt AL. PTSD symptom reports of patients evaluated for the New Mexico Medical Cannabis Program. *J Psychoactive Drugs*. 2014;46:73-77.

[13]Whiting PF, Wolff RF, Deshpande S, et al. Cannabinoids for medical use: a systematic review and meta-analysis. *JAMA*. 2015;313(24):2456-2473.

[14]Agarwal R, Burke SL, Maddux M. Current state of evidence of cannabis utilization for treatment of autism spectrum disorders. *BMC Psychiatry*. 2019;19:328.

[15]Fleury-Teixeira P, Caixeta FV, Ramires da Silva LC, Brasil-Neto JP, Malcher-Lopes R. Effect of CBD-enriched Cannabis sativa extract on autism spectrum disorder symptoms: an observational study of 18 participants undergoing compassionate use. *Front Neurol*. 2019;10:1145.

[16]Brandt A, Rehm J, Lev-Ran S. Clinical correlates of cannabis use among individuals with attention deficit hyperactivity disorder. *J Nerv Ment Dis*. 2018;206(9):726-732.

[17]Cooper RE, Williams E, Seegobin S, Tye C, Kunsti J, Asherson P. Cannabinoids in attention-deficit/hyperactivity disorder: a randomised-controlled trial. *Eur Neuropsychopharmacol*. 2017;27(8):795-808.

[18]Bhattacharyya S, Wilson R, Appiah-Kusi E, et al. Effect of cannabidiol on medial temporal, midbrain, and striatal dysfunction in people at clinical high risk of psychosis: a randomized clinical trial. *JAMA Psychiat*. 2018;75:1107-1117.

[19]Leweke FM, Piomelli D, Pahlisch F, et al. Cannabidiol enhances anandamide signaling and alleviates psychotic symptoms of schizophrenia. *Transl Psychiatry*. 2012;2:e94.

[20]Leweke FM, Hellmich M, Pahlisch F, et al. Modulation of the endocannabinoid system as a potential new target in the treatment of schizophrenia. *Schizophr Res*. 2014;153:S47.

[21]McGuire P, Robson P, Cubala WJ, et al. Cannabidiol (CBD) as an adjunctive therapy in schizophrenia: a multicenter randomized controlled trial. *Am J Psychiatry*. 2018;175:225-231.

[22]Boggs DL, Surti T, Gupta A, et al. The effects of cannabidiol (CBD) on cognition and symptoms in outpatients with chronic schizophrenia a randomized placebo controlled trial. *Psychopharmacology (Berl)*. 2018;235:1923-1932.

[23]Babalonis S, Haney M, Malcolm RJ, et al. Oral cannabidiol does not produce a signal for abuse liability in frequent marijuana smokers. *Drug Alcohol Depend.* 2017;172:9-13.

[24]Ren Y, Whittard J, Higeura-Matas A, et al. Cannabidiol, a non-psychotropic component of cannabis, inhibits cue-induced heroin seeking and normalizes discrete mesolimbic neuronal disturbances. *J Neurosci.* 2009;29:14764-146769.

[25]Hurd YL, Spriggs S, Alishayev J, et al. Cannabidiol for the reduction of cue-induced craving and anxiety in drug-abstinent individuals with heroin use disorder: a double-blind randomized placebo-controlled trial. *Am J Psychiatry.* 2019;176:911-922.

15

Gynecology

- Many, but not all, preclinical studies evaluating the effect of cannabinoids on sexual function suggest that cannabinoids enhance sexual function. No randomized controlled trials have been completed in this area.
- The endocannabinoid system has been shown to interact with specific mechanisms associated with endometriosis pain, including inflammation, cell proliferation, and cell survival.
- Five clinical trials have shown that treatment with N-palmitoylethanolamine (PEA), an endogenous fatty acid amide that binds to the peroxisome proliferator–activated receptor, produces a statistically-significant improvement in dysmenorrhea and chronic pelvic pain.

15.1 Sexual Function

Although results are not uniform, preclinical studies suggest that delta-9-tetrahydrocannabinol (THC) enhances sexual function. Multiple studies in mammals have shown THC to enhance female lordosis, a posture assumed by some female mammals in mating, in which the back of the animal is arched downward.[1-3] Lordosis represents sexual receptivity. Mani et al. also evaluated receptivity when progesterone and dopamine were blocked and showed that receptivity was inhibited.[3] This suggests that THC-induced receptivity is mediated by progesterone and dopamine. Memos et al. carried out a series of experiments in rats that showed anandamide (AEA) improved sexual function as measured by female rats making more visits to male rats for sexual activity and the endocannabinoid antagonist SR141716 inhibited this behavior.[4] Interestingly, they found that AEA and SR141716 did not affect lordosis. Similarly, multiple other preclinical studies showed that cannabinoid agonists did not enhance lordosis.[5-7]

The varied findings in the animal studies might be accounted for by a number of factors. Variation in animals, compounds, different behavioral models, route of administration, and hormonal milieu may have played a role in the variability seen in study results.

Few human studies have been done, and most have relied on self-report data. Several survey studies have supported the notion that adults feel that female sexual function is improved by moderate doses of cannabis.[8-10]

15.2 Endometriosis

The endocannabinoid system has been shown to interact with specific mechanisms associated with endometriosis pain, including inflammation, cell proliferation, and cell survival.[11-14] These processes are important in endometriosis-associated pain and in the establishment of the disease, its maintenance, and recurrence. CB1 receptors are expressed in great numbers in the uterus, and while CB2 receptors are expressed in abundance in the periphery, there are some in the uterus.[15,16] AEA has been shown to play an important role in folliculogenesis, preovulatory follicle maturation, oocyte maturation, and ovulation.[17] A study of women who had undergone IVF or intracytoplasmic sperm injection-embryo transfer showed higher plasma AEA levels at ovulation and lower levels of AEA during implantation for successful pregnancies.[18] Disruptions of endocannabinoid signaling are associated with miscarriage in early pregnancy.[19]

One human study showed a significant increase in endocannabinoid ligands and decreased CB1 expression in women with endometriosis vs those without. Endometriosis is another medical condition that some have hypothesized as an "endocannabinoid deficiency."[20] Lower ECS function may lead to growth of endometriosis tissue and a more severe pain experience.[20,21]

Five clinical studies, including two randomized controlled trials, have studied the relationship between the ECS and endometriosis-associated pain. All of the trials evaluated PEA, an endogenous fatty acid amide that binds to the peroxisome proliferator–activated receptor. PEA does not have a strong affinity for CB1 or CB2 but is thought to potentiate endocannabinoid actions. All of the trials, including the two randomized control trials (RCTs), demonstrated a statistically significant improvement in dysmenorrhea and chronic pelvic pain.[14,22–25] PEA was usually used in conjunction with polydatin, an antioxidant. These promising preliminary studies warrant additional RCTs in this area.

REFERENCES

[1] Gordon JH, Bromley BL, Gorski, et al. Delta—9-tetrahydrocannabinol enhancement of lordosis behavior in estrogen-treated female rats. *Pharmacol Biochem Behav*. 1978;8:603-608.

[2] Turley WA Jr, Floody OR. Delta-9-tetrahydrocannabinol stimulates receptive and proceptive sexual behaviors in female hamsters. *Pharmacol Biochem Behav*. 1981;14:745-747.

[3] Mani SK, Mitchell A, O'Malley BW. Progesterone receptor and dopamine receptors are required in delta-9-tetrahydrocannabinol modulation of sexual receptivity in female rats. *Proc Natl Acad Sci*. 2001;98:1249-1254.

[4] Memos NK, Vela R, Tabone C, et al. Endocannabinoid influence on partner preference in female rats. *Pharmacol Biochem Behav*. 2014;124:380-388.

[5] Ferrari F, Ottani A, Guiliani D. Inhibitory effects of the cannabinoid agonist HU 210 on rat sexual behaviour. *Physiol Behav*. 2000;69:547-554.

[6] Lopez HH, Webb SA, Nash S. Cannabinoid antagonism increases female sexual motivation. *Pharmacol Biochem Behav*. 2009;92:17-24.

[7] Chadwick B, Saylor AJ, Lopez HH. Adolescent cannabinoid exposure attenuates female sexual motivation but does not alter adulthood CB1R expression or estrous cyclicity. *Pharmacol Biochem Behav*. 2011;100:157-164.

[8] US Commission on Marihuana and Drug Abuse. Marihuana: a signal of misunderstanding. Appendix. The technical papers of the first report of the National Commission on Marihuana and Drug Abuse. Washington, DC: US Government Printing Office; 1972:434-439.

[9] Palamar JJ, Acosta P, Ompad DC, et al. A qualitative investigation comparing psychosocial and physical sexual experiences related to alcohol and marijuana use among adults. *Arch Sex Behav*. 2018;47:757-770.

[10]Lynn BK, Lopez JD, Miller C, et al. The relationship between marijuana use prior to sex and sexual function in women. *Sex Med.* 2019;7:192-197.

[11]Dmitrieva N, Nagabukuro H, Resuehr D, et al. Endocannabinoid involvement in endometriosis. *Pain.* 2010;151:703-710.

[12]Morotti M, Vincent K, Becker CM. Mechanisms of pain in endometriosis. *Eur J Obstet Gynecol Reprod Biol.* 2016;209:8-13. doi: 10.1016/j.ejogrb.2016.07.497.

[13]Kobayashi H, Yamada Y, Morioka S, et al. Mechanism of pain generation for endometriosis-associated pelvic pain. *Arch Gynecol Obstet.* 2014;289:13-21.

[14]Giugliano E, Cagnazzo E, Soave I, et al. The adjuvant use of N-palmitoylethanolamine and transpolydatin in the treatment of endometriotic pain. *Eur J Obstet Gynecol Reprod Biol.* 2013;168:209-213.

[15]Resuehr D, Glore DR, Taylor HS, et al. Progesterone-dependent regulation of endometrial cannabinoid receptor type 1 (CB1-R) expression is disrupted in women with endometriosis and in isolated stromal cells exposed to 2,3,7,8-tetrachlorodibenzo-p-dioxin (TCDD). *Fertil Steril.* 2012;98:948-956.e1.

[16]Sanchez AM, Vigano P, Mugione A, et al. The molecular connections between the cannabinoid system and endometriosis. *Mol Hum Reprod.* 2012;18:563-571.

[17]El-Talatini MR, Taylor AH, Elson JC, et al. Localisation and function of the endocannabinoid system in the human ovary. *PLoS One.* 2009;4:e4579.

[18]El-Talatini MR, Taylor AH, Konje JC. Fluctuation in anandamide levels from ovulation to early pregnancy in in-vitro fertilization embryo transfer women, and its hormonal regulation. *Hum Reprod.* 2009;24:1989-1998.

[19]Chan HW, McKirdy NC, Peiris HN, et al. The role of endocannabinoids in pregnancy. *Reproduction.* 2013;146,R101-R109.

[20]Russo EB. Clinical endocannabinoid deficiency (CECD). *Neuroendocrinol Lett.* 2008;25:31-39.

[21]Smith SC, Wagner MS. Clinical endocannabinoid deficiency (CECD) revisited: can this concept explain the therapeutic benefits of cannabis in migraine, fibromyalgia, irritable bowel syndrome and other treatment-resistant conditions? *Neuroendocrinol Lett.* 2014;35:198-201.

[22]Tartaglia E, Armentano M, Guigliano B, et al. Effectiveness of the association N-palmitoylethanolamine and transpolydatin in the treatment of primary dysmenorrhea. *J Pediatr Adolesc Gynecol.* 2015;28:447-450.

[23]Caruso S, Iraci Sareri M, Casella E, et al. Chronic pelvic pain, quality of life and sexual health of women treated with palmitoylethanolamide and alpha-lipoic acid. *Minerva Ginecol.* 2015;67:413-419.

[24]Cobellis L, Castaldi MA, Nocerino A, et al. Micronized *N*-palmitoylethanolamine and transpolydatin in the management of pelvic pain related to endometriosis. *Giornale Ital Ostetr Ginecol.* 2010;32:160-165.

[25]Lo Monte G, Soave I, Marci R. [Administration of micronized palmitoylethanolamide (PEA)-transpolydatin in the treatment of chronic pelvic pain in women affected by endometriosis: preliminary results]. *Minerva Ginecol.* 2013;65:453-463.

16

Rheumatology

- Considerable preclinical evidence demonstrates the anti-inflammatory properties of several cannabinoids, and the only randomized controlled trial (RCT) showed nabiximols to be a safe and effective treatment option for rheumatoid arthritis.
- Abstracts describing a RCT of the CB2 agonist lenabasum report initial efficacy for this agent as a medication for dermatomyositis.
- A prospective observational study of medical cannabis and a RCT of nabilone for fibromyalgia both show promising results in the treatment of pain associated with fibromyalgia.

16.1 Rheumatoid Arthritis

A number of preclinical studies suggest clinical utility of
cannabinoids as pharmacotherapy for rheumatoid arthritis
(RA) because of their anti-inflammatory effects. Cannabinoid
receptors are present in the synovial tissue of patients with RA or
osteoarthritis.[1] The synthetic cannabinoid WIN55, 212-2 mesylate
is able to decrease the production of inflammatory mediators in the
synovial fibroblasts of RA patients.[2] The classical murine collagen-
induced arthritis (CIA) model has been used for a number of
studies evaluating possible medications for RA. In the CIA model,
cannabidiol (CBD) has been shown to have an anti-inflammatory
effect, and activation of the CB2 receptor decreases joint
destruction.[3,4] Other cannabinoids shown to have anti-inflammatory
properties in the CIA model are JHW-133, HU-320, and THC.[5-7]
Overall, cannabinoids have been shown to have significant *in vitro*
anti-inflammatory effects on several different components of the
immune system related to the pathogenesis of RA, suggesting that
they could affect several key processes at the same time.[8]

As is the case with medical conditions as we have seen
throughout the book, RCTs have lagged behind promising
preclinical evidence. As of 2020, results from only one RCT
for cannabinoid pharmacotherapy for RA has been published.
Blake et al. compared nabiximols with placebo for the treatment
of pain in a randomized, double-blind, parallel group study in
58 participants with RA over a 5-week period.[9] Compared to
placebo, nabiximols produced statistically-significant improvements
in pain on movement, pain at rest, quality of sleep, disease activity,
and the pain at present component of the Short-form McGill Pain
Questionnaire. No effects on morning stiffness was observed,
although baseline scores were low. Nabiximols was well-tolerated,
with mostly mild or moderate adverse effects observed and no
adverse effect–related withdrawals or serious adverse effects in the
nabiximols group.

16.2 Dermatomyositis

Dermatomyositis (DM) is another systemic autoimmune disorder
for which cannabinoids are being investigated as pharmacotherapy.
The synthetic cannabinoid ajulemic acid in moderate to high

concentrations was shown to significantly reduce the production of TNF-α, IFN-α, and IFN-β, key cytokines in the pathogenesis of DM in peripheral blood mononuclear cells taken from patients with DM.[10]

Two abstracts presented at a national meeting describe the only randomized controlled trial (RCT) of cannabinoid pharmacotherapy for DM. A small RCT investigated the safety, tolerability, and efficacy of lenabasum, a nonimmunosuppressive, synthetic, oral preferential CB2 agonist that triggers resolution of innate immune responses, in 22 participants with treatment-refractory DM over 12 weeks.[11] Lenabasum separated from placebo on clinically meaningful improvement in Cutaneous Dermatomyositis Disease Area and Severity Index (CDASI) with mean reduction ≥5 points at the end of the study. Lenabasum also provided greater improvement than placebo in CDASI damage index, patient-reported global skin disease and overall disease assessments, skin symptoms including photosensitivity and itch, fatigue, sleep, pain interference with activities, and, finally, physical function. Participants could opt to continue on in a 28-week open-label extension trial. They showed improvements in CDASI activity score and physician Likert assessments of global disease activity, skin disease activity, and extramuscular disease activity. There were also improvements in multiple patient-reported outcomes, including visual analog scale scores of global disease activity, skin disease activity, itch and pain, as well as the Skin-dex-29 symptoms domain and the PROMIS-29 physical function, fatigue, pain interference, and anxiety domains.[12]

16.3 Fibromyalgia

Fibromyalgia is a chronic widespread pain condition marked by centralized pain.[13] Pain secondary to fibromyalgia is thought to result from an increase in the processing of pain or a decrease in the inhibition of pain. Ethan Russo, a international leader in the area of cannabinoid pharmacology, hypothesized that fibromyalgia may represent a state of "endocannabinoid deficiency."[14] With pain and insomnia as key issues related to fibromyalgia and no pharmacotherapy identified as being effective, some have turned to cannabinoids as a possible treatment.

A prospective observational study with a 6-month follow-up period tracked patients who received care for fibromyalgia in a

17

Internal Medicine/ Primary Care

- Dronabinol has been shown to stimulate appetite in patients with wasting conditions such as HIV.
- The relationship between cannabis and pain has gained attention in the context of the opioid epidemic.
- There is a solid rationale for cannabinoids as pain relievers that may reduce need for opioid medications.
- A small but growing literature suggests promise for cannabis and cannabinoids as effective treatments for chronic pain.
- The rate and scale of research into the efficacy of cannabis and cannabinoids for pain have not kept pace with the incredible level of public interest.

Primary care doctors must consider cannabis and cannabinoids daily. Their patients either are curious about cannabis and cannabinoids like cannabidiol (CBD) or they are already taking them to treat medical conditions. Thus, it is imperative that primary care doctors, perhaps even more so than other doctors, be aware of the evidence related to the use of cannabis and cannabinoids as pharmacotherapy for medical conditions.

17.1 Appetite Stimulation in Wasting Conditions Like HIV

Cannabinoids have been assessed for appetite stimulation in four studies. All of the studies evaluated dronabinol and one of those studies also evaluated cannabis in comparison to placebo (three studies) and megestrol acetate (one study).[1-4] There was some evidence that dronabinol pharmacotherapy led to increased weight gain in comparison to placebo. Limited evidence suggested that dronabinol may also be associated with increased appetite, greater percentage of body fat, reduced nausea, and improved functional status. The trial that assessed dronabinol and cannabis showed significantly greater weight gain in both compared to placebo.[3] The trial comparing dronabinol with megestrol acetate found that megestrol acetate was associated with greater weight gain and that the combination of dronabinol and megestrol acetate did not produce additional weight gain.[4] As a result of this evidence, dronabinol was FDA-approved for appetite stimulation in wasting conditions like HIV/AIDs in 1985.

17.2 Pain

The United States is in the midst of an opioid epidemic. People are dying every day as a result of their use of increasingly potent opioids like fentanyl. Many of the people who die as a result of fentanyl overdoses started using prescription opioids for pain. Individuals prescribed opioids, especially if they have other vulnerabilities such as a positive family history of a substance use disorder, may become addicted to these opioids and then turn to illicit opioids once they can no longer obtain prescription opioids either legitimately or illegally. These people may then buy heroin or fentanyl, placing them at increased risk of opioid overdose. This familiar scenario underscores the need for novel analgesics.

Cannabis and cannabinoids hold promise as effective analgesics. For many years, patients who are prescribed opioids have described needing fewer opioids for pain when they are using cannabis concurrently. As a result, pain relief is the most commonly-cited reason for the medical use of cannabis.[5,6] Interest in the use of cannabis for pain was bolstered by a recent report by the National Academies Committee on the Health Effects of Marijuana (2017), in which the authors, a collection of preclinical and clinical experts in the field of cannabinoids, concluded that there is "conclusive or substantial evidence" that cannabis is effective for the treatment of chronic pain in adults.[7]

These anecdotes have been supported by several of the papers examining the relationship between cannabis laws and opioid-related adverse effects and opioids prescribing. The most influential of these studies, by Bachhuber et al. in JAMA Internal Medicine in 2014, showed a 25% reduction in opioid overdose mortality in states with medical cannabis laws.[8] While another study published in 2019 appeared to show the chronological end of Bachhuber's data as an inflection point with opioid mortality increasing in states with medical cannabis laws after 2014,[9] there are additional studies showing the relationship between cannabis policies and decreased utilization of opioids. Shi studied cannabis- and opioid-related hospitalizations on a state level before and after enactment of medical cannabis laws and found that, while there was no change in cannabis-related hospitalizations during the study period, there was a 23% reduction in hospitalizations related to opioid use disorder (OUD) and a 13% reduction in opioid-related overdoses.[10] Bradford, Wen, and Hockenberry showed in two studies looking at Medicare and Medicaid data that fewer opioids were prescribed in medical cannabis states, and Livingston et al. extended this notion to states with legalized recreational cannabis.[11,12]

These studies, while important, have several important limitations. First, they are ecologic analyses, so we have limited clarity on cause and effect. We do not know whether patients actually avoided or reduced use of opioids because of increased access to cannabis as to many other factors such as racial composition, educational attainment, prevalence of disease, disability, and suicide rates. In addition, it is hard to know how generalizable the findings are. Conclusions drawn from Medicare Part D or Medicaid data, which include primarily disabled individuals, individuals aged 65 and over, and others with low income levels such as families, children, or pregnant women, may not be applicable to other demographic groups. Nevertheless, these results appear to support preclinical research showing that cannabinoid and opioid receptor systems mediate common signaling pathways central to clinical issues of tolerance, dependence, and addiction. There are enough data to prompt additional thought about how we should continue to study the relationship between cannabinoids and opioids in states with medical or recreational cannabis policies.

To be clear, the data demonstrating a relationship between cannabis policies and reduced opioid adverse effects and mortality are not overwhelming. However, given the fact that Americans are dying daily as a result of opioid overdoses, we should examine all possible solutions to this problem. Thus, we should set up the infrastructure necessary to study this relationship further through cannabis registries in states with medical cannabis policies, for example. We must move toward obtaining more definitive answers to these questions when lives are at stake. On a related note, if we are truly interested in finding the answers to questions like this, then more resources must be allocated to research in this area. To date, the U.S. Government, via the National Institutes of Health, has funded the overwhelming majority of research into questions like this. To advance public health at a rate and scale commensurate with public interest, additional funding sources must be identified. Two leading candidates are groups profiting directly from cannabis: states with cannabis policies who collect taxes related to the sale of cannabis and companies that sell cannabis. Unfortunately, these groups have not, for the most part, contributed to the advancement of cannabis science in a meaningful way yet. For example, states could mandate that a portion of all profits from the sale of cannabis should go toward research into important cannabis questions such as cannabis as a pain medication and the effects of cannabis upon driving.

17.3 The Endocannabinoid System and Mechanisms of Pain Reduction

In order to understand the hypothetical underpinnings of cannabis as a pain reliever, we must briefly discuss the endocannabinoid system. Neural and nonneural cells in injured tissues produce arachidonic acid derivatives called endocannabinoids,[13] which modulate neural conduction of pain signals by mitigating sensitization and inflammation via the activation of cannabinoid receptors that are also targeted by Δ^9-tetrahydrocannabinol.[14] CB1 receptors modulate the release of neurotransmitters in the brain and spinal cord.[15] CB1 receptors are also found in nociceptive and nonnociceptive sensory neurons of the dorsal root ganglion and trigeminal ganglion,[16] as well as in defense cells such as macrophages, mast cells, and epidermal keratinocytes.[17] CB2 receptors are expressed in cells of hematopoietic origin.[18] There are few CB2 located in the brain, spinal cord, and dorsal root ganglion, but they increase in response to peripheral nerve damage.[19] They regulate neuro-immune interactions and interfere with inflammatory hyperalgesia.

The endocannabinoids anandamide and 2-arachidonoyl-*sn*-glycerol (2-AG) are produced in injured tissues via distinct biochemical pathways to suppress sensitization and inflammation by activation of cannabinoid (CB) receptors. Anandamide can act as an autocrine or paracrine messenger and follows one of two pathways. In a reaction catalyzed by fatty acid amide hydrolase, it can be broken down to arachidonic acid and ethanolamine or,[20] alternatively, it can be directly catalyzed by COX-2 into proalgesic prostamides.[21] Anandamide mobilizes in response to inflammation and nerve injury and modulates nociceptive signals by activating local CB1 receptors. 2-AG is formed by the hydrolysis of phosphatidylinositol-4,5-biphosphate (PIP$_2$), a phospholipid at the center of a lipid pathway that produces several intracellular and transcellular messengers.[20] It plays a prominent role in the descending modulation of pain during acute stress.[22] Anandamide and 2-AG are activated during tissue injury to provide a first response to nociceptive signals. Thus, understanding how endogenous cannabinoids work helps explain the potential efficacy of exogenous cannabinoids, such as those found in the cannabis plant, in treating pain.

Preclinical and human laboratory studies of cannabis in pain models underscore the complexities of cannabis' analgesic effects. THC has been shown to produce analgesic and antihyperalgesic effects in animal models,[23,24] and experimental research examining the effects of cannabis on human pain response has focused either on healthy adults or clinical pain samples. For example, Wallace et al. evaluated the effects of smoked cannabis (low, medium, or high doses vs inactive placebo) on intradermal capsaicin-induced pain responses using a randomized, double-blind crossover trial in 15 healthy volunteers (mean age of 28.9; 58% male).[25] Interestingly, results indicated a significant decrease in pain with the medium cannabis dose and a significant increase in pain with the high dose. No differences were observed with the low cannabis dose, and there was no effect on the area of hyperalgesia at any dose. The authors concluded that there is likely a therapeutic window of modest analgesia for smoked cannabis, illustrating one of many challenges present when treating pain with cannabis.

17.4 Acute Pain

Despite significant interest in the development of novel analgesics to treat acute pain in the context of the opioid epidemic, there have been limited evaluations of the efficacy of cannabis or cannabinoids for acute pain. A recent systematic review concluded, "on the basis of the available randomized controlled trial evidence, cannabinoids have no role in the management of acute pain."[26] That may overstate the findings of their systematic review of six small RCTs and six crossover studies of various cannabinoids, mostly dronabinol and nabilone. The clinical trials appear to demonstrate treatment effect for cannabinoids vs placebo. The limitations of these studies are similar to those of other cannabinoid efficacy trials—small sample sizes, limited duration of treatment, and a lack of uniformity of measurement of pain outcomes.

17.5 Chronic Pain

A recent systematic review and meta-analysis of cannabinoids for medical use examined 28 randomized trials among 2454 patients with chronic pain and showed that, compared with placebo, cannabinoids were associated with greater reduction in pain (37% vs 31%; OR 1.41, 95% CI 0.99-2.00) and greater average reduction in numerical pain ratings (−0.46, 95% CI −0.80 to −0.11).[27] Whiting et al. concluded that there was moderate evidence supporting the use of cannabinoids for the treatment of chronic pain. In this review, neuropathy was the most commonly cited source of chronic pain. The majority of trials focused on testing the effects of plant-derived cannabinoids. Only 5 of the 28 studies assessed the effects of vaporized or smoked cannabis plant flower. Cannabinoids were associated with an increased risk for short-term adverse events, including serious adverse events, compared to placebo.

One study not included in Whiting's meta-analysis was a placebo-controlled trial of inhaled aerosolized cannabis that demonstrated a dose-dependent reduction in diabetic peripheral neuropathy spontaneous pain ratings among patients with treatment-refractory pain.[28] Similarly, Wilsey et al. conducted a randomized, placebo-controlled crossover trial of vaporized cannabis among 42 participants with central neuropathic pain related to spinal cord injury and disease.[29] The trial showed that vaporized cannabis flower reduced neuropathic pain scale ratings, but there was no evidence of dose-dependent effect. These authors concluded that additional research is necessary to examine how interactions among cannabinoids may influence analgesic response.

Collectively, the research on cannabis for chronic pain indicates that although the results of experimental studies with healthy adults are mixed, there is converging evidence to support the notion that cannabis can produce acute pain-inhibitory effects among individuals with chronic pain. This observation is consistent with the recent NASEM report on cannabis that concluded that there is "conclusive or substantial evidence" of benefit from cannabis or cannabinoids for chronic pain. However, it is important to also highlight the NASEM statement that more research is needed to better understand the efficacy, dose-response effects, routes of administration, and side effect profiles for cannabis products that are commonly used in the United States.[7]

17.6 CBD and Pain

Despite the intense interest in CBD as a pain reliever, as of November 2019, there are no published studies of a pure CBD product for pain. Even without such evidence, there are millions of Americans currently using CBD products from a variety of sources to treat pain. The aforementioned studies examined THC alone or THC in combination with CBD. Thus, it is important to point out that the widespread use of CBD for pain is yet another example of public use preceding rigorous science.

It is easy to understand why so many patients are trying CBD as a treatment for pain, though. There is a growing body of evidence suggesting that CBD has analgesic and anti-inflammatory properties. CBD appears to have a more favorable side effect profile than THC as well. CBD has been shown to have an ability to inhibit the production of inflammatory cytokines, including IL-1β, IL-6, and interferon-β in lipopolysaccharide-stimulated microglial cells.[30] CBD was also shown, in a viral model of multiple sclerosis, to down-regulate the expression of vascular cell adhesion molecules and chemokines, resulting in the reduction of motor deficits.[31] CBD also exerts an anti-inflammatory effect in the retina by inhibiting adenosine uptake, which in turn activates receptors in the retinal microglial cells.[32] This suggest promise for CBD in treating retinal inflammatory disorders. Similarly, CBD has been demonstrated to reduce intestinal inflammation through the control of the neuroimmune axis, making it a promising medication for inflammatory bowel disease. Finally, several preclinical studies show that CBD produces reductions in pain and inflammation in models of neuropathic pain and osteoarthritis.[33-35]

17.7 Distinction Between Cannabis and Cannabinoids for Chronic Pain vs Opioid Use Disorder

As we have discussed, there is evidence to suggest the possibility that cannabis and cannabinoids reduce the need for prescribed opioids. This reduction in opioid use may in turn lead to other positive outcomes, such as reduced opioid mortality. The evidence is not overwhelming, but it is enough to consider cannabis and cannabinoids as an option for patients with chronic pain who have, in collaboration with their doctor, worked down the list of first- and second-line treatments for chronic pain without much success. In those patients, especially in the context of the opioid epidemic where people are dying each day often as a result of fatal opioid overdoses, we should consider cannabis and cannabinoids. Similarly, on a larger scale, we must set up the infrastructure to study further the relationship between cannabinoids and opioids. For example, states with medical cannabis policies should have registries in place to monitor the impact of medical cannabis upon significant medical outcomes such as opioid overdoses, health care utilization, and hospitalizations. When people are dying each day, we should consider all possible options, no matter how polarizing that option might be.

It is critical to distinguish between people with chronic pain who are prescribed opioids by their doctors and people with OUD. The latter group, whether they are buying prescription opioids to use beyond what had been prescribed or if they are using a gram of fentanyl intravenously each day, are not groups that are appropriate for medical cannabis or cannabinoids. We have three medication for OUD—buprenorphine, methadone, and injectable naltrexone—that are FDA-approved for OUD with strong evidence supporting their use. These medications are among the best tools that we have in the treatment of substance use disorders. They improve outcomes and reduce the likelihood that patients will suffer from opioid overdoses. To eschew these medications for medical cannabis is a potentially deadly mistake. There are doctors who do this, though—there are some who talk about medical cannabis as "an exit strategy" from opioids without drawing a distinction between those with chronic pain on prescription opioids and those using illicit opioids. We do not recommend cannabis or cannabinoids as the primary treatment for those with OUD, and we caution against any treatment plans for OUD that do not include the FDA-approved medications for OUD.

REFERENCES

[1]Struwe M, Kaempfer SH, Geiger CJ, et al. Effect of dronabinol on nutritional status in HIV infection. *Ann Pharmacother*. 1993;27(7-8):827-831.

[2]Beal JE, Olson R, Laubenstein L, et al. Dronabinol as a treatment for anorexia associated with weight loss in patients with AIDS. *J Pain Symptom Manage*. 1995;10(2):89-97.

[3]Abrams DI, Hilton JF, Leiser RJ, et al. Short-term effects of cannabinoids in patients with HIV-1 infection: a randomized, placebo-controlled clinical trial. *Ann Intern Med*. 2003;139(4):258-266.

[4]Timpone JG, Wright DJ, Li N, et al. Division of AIDS Treatment Research Initiative. The safety and pharmacokinetics of single-agent and combination therapy with megestrol acetate and dronabinol for the treatment of HIV wasting syndrome: the DATRI 004 Study Group. *AIDS Res Hum Retroviruses*. 1997;13(4):305-315.

[5]Bestrashniy J, Winters KC. Variability in medical marijuana laws in the United States. *Psychol Addict Behav*. 2015;29(3):639-642.

[6]Ilgen MA, Bohnert K, Kleinberg F, et al. Characteristics of adults seeking medical marijuana certification. *Drug Alcohol Depend*. 2013;132(3):654-659.

[7]National Academies of Sciences, Engineering, and Medicine. *The Health Effects of Cannabis and Cannabinoids: The Current State of Evidence and Recommendations for Research*. Washington, DC: The National Academies Press; 2017. doi: 10.17226/24625.

[8]Bachhuber MA, Saloner B, Cunningham CO, et al. Medical cannabis laws and opioid analgesic overdose mortality in the United States, 1999-2010. *JAMA Intern Med*. 2014;174:1668-1673.

[9]Shover CL, Davis CS, Gordon SC, Humphreys K. Association between medical cannabis laws and opioid overdose mortality has reversed over time. *Proc Natl Acad Sci*. 2019;116(26):12624-12626. doi: 10.1073/pnas.1903434116.

[10]Shi Y. Medical marijuana policies and hospitalizations related to marijuana and opioid pain relievers. *Drug Alcohol Depend*. 2017;173:144-150.

[11]Bradford AC, Bradford WD, Abraham A, Adams GB. The impact of medical cannabis laws in opioid prescribing in Medicare Part D, 2010-2015. *JAMA Int Med*. 2018;178(5):667-672.

[12]Wen H, Hockenberry JM. The impact of recreational marijuana laws and medical marijuana laws on opioid prescribing for Medicaid enrollees. *JAMA Int Med*. 2018;178(5): 673-679.

[13]Piomelli D, Sasso O. Peripheral gating of pain signals by endogenous lipid mediators. *Nat Neurosci*. 2014;17:164-174.

[14]Rice AS. Cannabinoids and pain. *Curr Opin Investig Drugs*. 2001;2(3):399-414.

[15]Castillo PE, Younts TJ, Chavez AE, et al. Endocannabinoid signaling and synaptic function. *Neuron*. 2012;76(1):70-81.

[16]Price TJ, Helesic G, Parghi D, et al. The neuronal distribution of cannabinoid receptor type 1 in the trigeminal ganglion of the rat. *Neuroscience*. 2003;120(1):155-162.

[17]Sugawara K, Zakany N, Hudt T, et al. Cannabinoid receptor 1 controls human mucosal-type mast cell degranulation and maturation in situ. *J Allergy Clin Immunol*. 2013;132(1):182-193.

[18]Stander S, Schemlz M, Metze D, et al. Distribution of cannabinoid receptor 1 (CB1) and 2 (CB2) on sensory nerve fibers and adnexal structures in human skin. *J Dermatol Sci*. 2005;38(3):177-188.

[19]Guindon J, Hohmann AG. The endocannabinoid system and pain. *CNS Neurol Disord Drug Targets*. 2009;8(6):403-421.

[20]Piomelli D, Astarita G, Rapaka R. A neuroscientist's guide to lipidomics. *Nat Rev Neurosci*. 2007;8(10):743-754.

[21]Massaro M, Martinelli R, Gatta V, et al. Transcriptome-based identification of new anti-anti-inflammatory and vasodilating properties of the n-3 fatty acid docosahexaenoic acid in vascular endothelial cell under proinflammatory conditions. *PLoS One*. 2016;11(4):e0129652.

[22]Hohmann AG, Suplita RL, Bolton NM, et al. An endocannabinoid mechanism for stress-induced analgesia. *Nature*. 2005;435:1108-1112.

[23]Lim G, Sung B, Ji RR, et al. Upregulation of spinal cannabinoid-1-receptors following nerve injury enhances the effect of WIN55,212-2 on neuropathic pain behaviour in rats. *Pain*. 2003;105:275-283.

[24]Johanek LM, Heitmiller DR, Turner M, et al. Cannabinoids attenuate capsaicin-evoked hyperalgesia through spinal and peripheral mechanisms. *Pain*. 2001;93:303-315.

[25]Wallace M, Schulteis G, Atkinson JH, et al. Dose-dependent effects of smoked cannabis on capsaicin-induced pain and hyperalgesia in healthy volunteers. *Anesthesiology*. 2007;107:785-796.

[26]Stevens AJ, Higgins MD. A systematic review of the analgesic efficacy of cannabinoid medications in the management of acute pain. *Acta Anaesthesiol Scand*. 2017;61(3):268-280.

[27]Whiting PF, Wolff RF, Deshpande S, et al. Cannabinoids for medical use: a systematic review and meta-analysis. *JAMA*. 2015;313(24):2456-2473.

[28]Wallace MS, Marcotte TD, Umlauf A, et al. Efficacy of inhaled cannabis on painful diabetic neuropathy. *J Pain*. 2015;16(7):616-627.

[29]Wilsey BL, Deutsch R, Samara E, et al. A preliminary evaluation of the relationship of cannabinoid blood concentrations with the analgesic response to vaporized cannabis. *J Pain Res.* 2016;9:587-598.

[30]Kozela E, Pietr M, Juknat A, et al. Cannabinoids Delta(9)-tetrahydrocannabinol and cannabidiol differentially inhibit the lipopolysaccharide-activated NF-kappB and interferon-beta/STAT proinflammatory pathways in BV-2 microglial cells. *J Biol Chem.* 2010;285:1616-1626.

[31]Mecha M, Feliu A, Inigo PM, et al. Cannabidiol provides long-lasting protection against the deleterious effects of inflammation in a viral model of multiple sclerosis: a role for A2A receptors. *Neurobiol Dis.* 2013;59:141-150.

[32]Liou GI, Auchampach JA, Hillard CJ, et al. Mediation of cannabidiol anti-inflammation in the retina by equilibrative nucleoside transporter and A2A adenosine receptor. *Invest Ophthalmol Vis Sci.* 2008;49:5526-5531.

[33]Ward SJ, McAllister SD, Kawamura R, et al. Cannabidiol inhibits paclitaxel-induced neuropathic pain through 5-HT(1A) receptors without diminishing nervous system function or chemotherapy efficacy. *Br J Pharmacol.* 2014;171:636-645.

[34]Hammell D, Zhang L, Ma F, et al. Transdermal cannabidiol reduces inflammation and pain-related behaviours in a rat model of arthritis. *Eur J Pain.* 2016;936-948.

[35]Philpott HT, O'Brien M, McDougall JJ. Attenuation of early phase inflammation by cannabidiol prevents pain and nerve damage in rat osteoarthritis. *Pain.* 2017;158:2442.

18

Ophthalmology

- Multiple routes of administration have been studied after cannabis was initially shown to lower intraocular pressure (IOP).
- Each route of administration has challenges with effects, absorption, or side effects.
- Given the risk:benefit ratio of cannabis for glaucoma compared to other pharmacotherapies and surgical procedures for glaucoma, no major medical organization has endorsed the use of medical cannabis for glaucoma.
- In a small case series, medical cannabis showed some promise as an adjunct treatment to botulinum injections for benign essential blepharospasm.

18.1 Glaucoma

Glaucoma refers to a family of ocular disorders characterized by optic neuropathy and resulting visual field defects. It is commonly associated with elevated IOP and causes irreversible vision loss. Peripheral vision loss usually occurs first, but if left untreated, glaucoma can lead to blindness. Glaucoma affects more than 3 million Americans and is a leading cause of blindness in the United States.[1] Currently, the only known modifiable risk factor for glaucoma progression is increased IOP.

Smoked cannabis was first shown to lower IOP in 1971.[2] Multiple methods of THC administration in addition to smoking have been shown to lower IOP, including oral, intravenous, sublingual, and topical.[3-6] The sublingual investigation was a small randomized, double-blind, placebo-controlled crossover trial of oral THC extract, cannabidiol, and placebo in six participants with ocular hypertension or early-stage glaucoma. Oral THC extract (5 mg) produced a transient decrease in IOP, and cannabidiol did not separate from placebo on measures of IOP.[5]

There are problems with each of these routes of administration. Smoked cannabis lowers IOP by ~25% in 60%-65% of patients with and without glaucoma.[6-8] Greater change in IOP from baseline was associated with increasing doses of THC. Unfortunately, the effect from smoked cannabis lasts only 3-4 hours with no relationship between dose and duration of effect.[7] Thus, patients with glaucoma using medical cannabis would have to smoke at least 6-8 times a day in order to achieve a consistent decrease in IOP. This administration schedule would increase the potential for side effects such as the development of cannabis use disorder.

Topical application might appear to be an optimal route of administration, but penetration of the eye is difficult due to the high lipophilicity and low aqueous solubility of the cannabinoid extracts. Topical THC preparations have been shown to cause local irritation and corneal injury while also failing at times to produce the desired hypotensive effect.[8,9] Oral administration of THC has been limited by variable absorption.[3] While standard treatments for glaucoma are superior at this time compared to medical cannabis, there may be a place for medical cannabis in end-stage glaucoma patients who have failed maximal medical therapy and surgery or who are poor surgical candidates.[10]

The American Medical Association, the American Society of Addiction Medicine, the American Glaucoma Society, the Canadian Ophthalmology Society, and other organizations do not support the use of medical cannabis for glaucoma. Ultimately, these organizations have determined that the potential benefits of medical cannabis pharmacotherapy for glaucoma do not outweigh the challenges of various routes of administration or the limited efficacy compared to other medical and surgical interventions. Further studies of alternate routes of administration or greater refinement of cannabinoid molecule delivery for glaucoma pharmacotherapy are needed.

18.2 Blepharospasm

There has also been an initial evaluation of medical cannabis for benign essential blepharospasm (BEB), a common craniofacial movement disorder. BEB affects 32.2 per 1 million people and is characterized by excessive involuntary blinking, photophobia, and uncontrolled eyelid closure that can cause functional blindness.[11,12] One standard treatment for BEB is lifelong therapy with scheduled periocular botulinum toxin injections, which reduce symptoms of facial dystonia. A small retrospective study observed the effects of medical cannabis therapy as an adjunct treatment to maintenance botulinum toxin therapy in patients with BEB.[13] Five patients with BEB receiving maintenance botulinum toxin injections were certified for medical cannabis use as an adjunct treatment. Four of five patients tolerated medical cannabis well; three of five patients reported subjective improvement in symptoms of BEB. Three of five participants completed objective measures of BEB severity and only one of those patients demonstrated scores indicative of improvement on those measures. This observational case series may provide a foundation for future prospective double-blind studies of cannabinoids for BEB.

REFERENCES

[1]The Eye Diseases Prevalence Research Group. Prevalence of open-angle glaucoma among adults in the United States. *Arch Ophthalmol.* 2004;122:532-538.

[2]Hepler RS, Frank IR. Marihuana smoking and intraocular pressure. *JAMA.* 1971;217:1932.

[3]Merritt JC, Crawford WJ, Alexander PC, Anduze AL, Gelbart SS. Effect of marihuana on intraocular and blood pressure in glaucoma. *Ophthamology.* 1980;87:222-228.

[4]Purnell WD, Gregg JM. Delta(9)-tetrahydrocannabinol, euphoria and intraocular pressure in man. *Ann Ophthalmol.* 1975;7:921-923.

[5]Tomida I, Azuara-Blanco A, House H, Flint M, Pertwee RG, Robson PJ. Effect of sublingual application of cannabinoids on intraocular pressure: a pilot study. *J Glaucoma.* 2006;15:349-353.

[6]Merritt JC, Olsen JL, Armstrong JR, McKinnon SM. Topical delta 9-tetrahydrocannabinol in hypertensive glaucomas. *J Pharm Pharmacol.* 1981;33:40-41.

[7]Green K. Marijuana smoking vs. cannabinoids for glaucoma therapy. *Arch Ophthalmol.* 1998;116(11):1433-1437.

[8]Green K, Roth M. Ocular effects of topical administration of delta 9-tetrahydrocannabinol in man. *Arch Ophthalmol.* 1982;100:265-267.

[9]Jay WM, Green K. Multiple-drop study of topically applied 1% delta 9-tetrahydrocannabinol in human eyes. *Arch Ophthalmol.* 1983;101:591-593.

[10]Sun X, Xu CS, Chadha N, Chen A, Liu J. Marijuana for glaucoma: a recipe for disaster or treatment? *Yale J Biol Med.* 2015;88:265-269.

[11]Jankovic J, Kenny C. Botulinum toxin in the treatment of blepharospasm and hemifacial spasm. *J Neural Transm (Vienna).* 2008;115:585-591.

[12]Czyz CN, Burns JA, Petrie T, Watkins JR, Cahill KV, Foster JA. Long-term botulinum toxin treatment of benign essential blepharospasm, hemifacial spasm, and Meige syndrome. *Am J Ophthalmol.* 2013;156:173-177.

[13]Radke PM, Mokhtarzadeh A, Lee MS, Harrison AR. Medical cannabis, a beneficial high in treatment of blepharospasm? An early observation. *Neuroophthalmology.* 2017;41:253-258.

19

Hepatology

- Cannabinoid receptors may prove to be targets in the treatment of hepatic fibrosis, with the CB1 receptor promoting fibrosis while the CB2 receptor restricts it.
- Animal models show that CBD affects multiple aspects of alcohol use disorder, including ethanol intake, motivation for ethanol, relapse, reinstatement of ethanol consumption after extinction, as well as levels of anxiety and impulsivity associated with ethanol intake.
- CBD may be able to reduce liver steatosis and fibrosis that are induced by both binge and chronic ethanol administrations because of its antioxidant, immunomodulatory, and lipid metabolic regulation characteristics.

■ A body of literature supporting the role of the endocannabinoid system in hepatic encephalopathy points toward medications that affect CB1 and CB2 receptors, as well as CBD, as possible medications with possible roles in treating hepatic encephalopathy.

To date, there have been no clinical studies of cannabis or cannabinoids for the treatment of chronic liver diseases or complications stemming from chronic liver diseases. Cannabinoid receptors are rarely expressed in a normal liver, but up-regulation of CB1 and CB2 receptors and increased concentrations of endocannabinoids have been shown in the liver during the course of chronic progressive liver disease. Thus, there is a growing body of preclinical evidence suggesting a role for agents targeting cannabinoid receptors as well as cannabidiol (CBD) as possible pharmacotherapies for chronic liver disease and their complications.

19.1 Hepatic Fibrosis

The CB1 receptor is involved in regulation of hepatic fibrosis and the profibrogenic effect of CB1 signaling.[1] The antifibrogenic results were obtained either by pharmacological inactivation of CB1 with rimonabant, a selective antagonist of the CB1 receptor, and via genetic inactivation in homozygous CB1-deficient mice. While the CB1 receptor appears to have profibrogenic effects, studies evaluating the CB2 receptor show antifibrogenic effects in the liver. In a liver injury model, CB2 knockout mice developed augmented cirrhosis when exposed to CCl$_4$ compared to wild-type animals.[2] This series of investigations showed that stimulation of the CB2 receptor with THC or the selective CB agonist JWH-015 are dose dependent and expressed as growth inhibition or apoptosis. Siegmund et al. (2005) showed that anandamide (AEA) acts directly on hepatic stellate cells to induce cell death.[3]

19.2 Reduction of Drinking Levels

Four important studies have demonstrated the effects of CBD on alcohol consumption in animal models. CBD reduces ethanol intake, motivation for ethanol, relapse, reinstatement of ethanol consumption after extinction, as well as levels of anxiety and impulsivity associated with ethanol intake. CBD reduced the reinforcing properties, motivation for ethanol consumption, and ethanol relapse in a study of male C57BL/6J mice, an ethanol-preferring strain.[4] In the same strain of mice, the same group of investigators showed that combining CBD and the opioid antagonist naltrexone reduces ethanol consumption and motivation to drink ethanol more efficiently than either drug administered alone.[5] Transdermal CBD administered to male Wistar rats in an extinction paradigm showed that CBD reduced reinstatement induced by context, stress, and medication.[6] In this same series of experiments, CBD also reduced anxiety and impulsivity in these animals. The potential of CBD to affect multiple aspects of alcohol use disorder enhances the intrigue about CBD as a potential pharmacotherapy for this disorder.

19.3 Alcohol-Related Liver Inflammation

Preclinical studies have shown that CBD may be able to reduce liver steatosis and fibrosis that are induced by both binge and chronic ethanol administrations because of its antioxidant, immunomodulatory, and lipid metabolic regulation characteristics. CBD's potential impact upon steatosis was shown in a study of ethanol-fed rodents where CBD triggered the activation of an endoplasmic reticulum stress response, which led to the selective death of activated hepatic stellate cells via activation of the inositol-requiring enzyme 1/apoptosis signal–regulating kinase 1/c-Jun N-terminal kinase (IRE1/ASK1/JNK) pathway.[7] In another

20

Dermatology

- Preclinical studies of endocannabinoids and synthetic cannabinoids suggest multiple mechanisms by which these agents may be useful in the treatment of many dermatologic conditions.
- RCTs of cannabinoids as pharmacotherapy are limited, but they demonstrate the promise of cannabinoids in treating acne vulgaris, asteatotic dermatitis, and atopic dermatitis.
- Case reports and an open-label trial point to pruritis as another possible pharmacotherapeutic target for cannabinoids.

Recent studies describing the expression of both CB1 and CB2 receptors on cutaneous sensory nerve fibers, mast cells, and keratinocytes suggest a possible role for cannabinoids in the treatment of dermatologic conditions.[1] The current evidence on the use of cannabinoids for the treatment of dermatologic conditions supports a wide variety of potential applications. Most of the available data are preclinical, underscoring a need for randomized controlled trials (RCTs) of cannabinoids as pharmacotherapy for dermatologic conditions.[2]

20.1 Acne Vulgaris

A preclinical study of sebocytes with knocked out CB2 receptors demonstrated significant suppression of basal lipid production typical in the development of acne.[3] This provides a rationale for evaluating both CB2 agonists and antagonists as possible acne pharmacotherapy. Another study showed that several phytocannabinoids including cannabichromene (CBC), tetrahydrocannabivarin (THVC), and cannabidivarin (CBDV) reduced arachidonic-induced acnelike lipogenesis while demonstrating anti-inflammatory characteristics.[4] Ali et al. investigated the effects of a 3% cannabis extract cream on sebum level and erythema in 11 patients with acne in an open-label trial.[5] Use of the cannabis extract cream twice a day on the right cheek for 12 weeks led to a significant decrease in sebum level measured by a photometric device compared to a control cream. The cream also led to a significant decrease in erythema as measured by a reflectance spectrophotometer.

20.2 Allergic Contact Dermatitis

A series of preclinical studies utilizing a mouse model illustrated the ability of CB2 to mediate both the exaggeration and inhibition of inflammatory responses in allergic contact dermatitis.[6] A CB2 antagonist increased inflammatory response, while CB2-selective antagonists/inverse agonists decreased inflammation.

have been demonstrated to decrease expression of VEGF and other proangiogenic factors, inhibit melanoma progression, and limit metastatic spread.[23,24] Nabiximols inhibit melanoma variability, proliferation, and tumor growth while increasing autophagy and apoptosis compared to standard treatment with temozolomide, an oral chemotherapy drug.[25]

20.9 Systemic Sclerosis

In animal models of systemic sclerosis, the CB2-selective agonist JWH-133 significantly mitigated clinical disease. It was postulated that this agonist restricts immune responses that typically result in tissue damage.[6] Similarly, the synthetic cannabinoid receptor agonist WIN55,212-2 was shown to reduce extracellular matrix deposition and antagonize several other characteristics of scleroderma fibroblasts, including the ability to resist apoptosis and to transdifferentiate these cells into myofibroblasts.[26]

REFERENCES

[1]Stander S, Luger TA. Itch in atopic dermatitis-pathophysiology and treatment. *Acta Dermatovenerol Croat*. 2010;18(4):289-296.

[2]Eagelston LR, Yazd NK, Patel RR, et al. Cannabinoids in dermatology: a scoping review. *Dermatol Online J*. 2018;24(6):1-17.

[3]Dobrosi N, Toth BI, Nagy G, et al. Endocannabinoids enhance lipid synthesis and apoptosis of human sebocytes via cannabinoid receptor-2-mediated signaling. *FASEB J*. 2008;22(10):3685-3695.

[4]Olah A, Markovics A, Szabo-Papp J, et al. Differential effectiveness of selected non-psychotropic phytocannabinoids on human sebocyte functions implicates their introduction in dry/seborrheic skin and acne treatment. *Exp Dermatol*. 2016;25(9):701-707.

[5]Ali A, Akhtar N. The safety and efficacy of 3% cannabis seeds extract cream for reduction of human cheek skin sebum and erythema content. *Pak J Pharm Sci*. 2015;28(4):1389-1395.

[6]Basu S, Dittel BN. Unraveling the complexities of cannabinoid receptor 2 (CB2) immune regulation in health and disease. *Immunol Res*. 2011;51(1):26-38.

[7]Yuan C, Wang XM, Guichard A, et al. N-palmitoylethanolamine and N-acetylethanolamine are effective in asteatotic eczema: results of a randomized, double-blind, controlled study in 60 patients. *Clin Interv Aging*. 2014;9:1163-1169.

[8]Zhang H, Yang Y, Cui J, Zhang Y. Gaining a comprehensive understanding of pruritis. *Indian J Dermatol Venereol Leprol*. 2012;78(5):523-544.

[9]Tey HL, Yosipovitch G. Targeted treatment of pruritus: a look into the future. *Br J Dermatol*. 2011;165(1):5-17.

[10]Varothai S, Nitayavardhana S, Kulthanan K. Moisturizers for patients with atopic dermatitis. *Asian Pac J Allergy Immunol*. 2013;31(2):91-98.

[11]Mollanazar NK, Smith PK, Yosipovitch G. Advances in therapeutic strategies for the treatment of pruritis. *Expert Opin Pharmacother*. 2016;17(5):671-687.

[12]Stull C, Lavery MJ, Yosipovitch G. Advances in therapeutic strategies for the treatment of pruritis. *Expert Opin Pharmacother*. 2016;17(5):671-687.

[13]Eberlein B, Eicke C, Reinhardt HW, Ring J. Adjuvant treatment of atopic eczema: assessment of an emollient containing N-palmitoylethanolamine (ATOPA study). *J Eur Acad Dermatol Venereol*. 2008;22(1):73-82.

[14]Kircik L. A nonsteroidal lamellar matrix cream containing palmitoyethamolamide for the treatment of atopic dermatitis. *J Drugs Dermatol*. 2010;9(4):334-338.

[15]Luca T, Di Benedetto G, Scuderi MR, et al. The CB1/CB2 receptor agonist WIN-55,212-2 reduces viability of human Kaposi's sarcoma cells in vitro. *Eur J Pharmacol*. 2009;616(1-3):16-21.

[16]Maor Y, Yu J, Kuzontkoski PM, et al. Cannabidiol inihibits growth and induces programmed cell death in Kaposi Sarcoma-associated Herpesvirus-infected endothelium. *Genes Cancer*. 2012;3(7-8):512-520.

[17]Patel T, Yosipovitch G. The management of chronic pruritis in the elderly. *Skin Therapy Lett*. 2010;15(8):5-9.

[18]Brooks JP, Malic CC, Judkins KC. Scratching the surface-Managing the itch associated with burns: a review of current knowledge. *Burns*. 2008;34(6):751-760.

[19]Feramisco JD, Berger TG, Steinhoff M. Innovative management of pruritis. *Dermatol Clin*. 2010;28(3):467-478.

[20]Visse K, Blome C, Phan NQ, Augustin M, Stander S. Efficacy of body lotion containing N-palmitoylethanolamine in subjects with chronic pruritis due to dry skin: a dermatocosmetic study. *Acta Derm Venereol*. 2017;97(5):639-641.

[21]Derakhshan N, Kazemi M. Cannabis for refractory psoriasis-High hopes for a novel treatment and a literature review. *Curr Clin Pharmacol*. 2016;11(2):146-147.

[22]Wilkinson JD, Williamson EM. Cannabinoids inhibit human keratinocyte proliferation through a non-CB1/CB2 mechanism and have a potential therapeutic value in the treatment of psoriasis. *J Dermatol Sci*. 2007;45(2):87-92.

[23]Bowles DW, O'Bryant CL, Camidge DR, Jimeno A. The intersection between cannabis and cancer in the United States. *Crit Rev Oncol Hematol*. 2012;83(1):1-10.

[24]Kupczyk P, Reich A, Szepietowski JC. Pruritis in the elderly. *Clin Dermatol*. 2011;29(1):15-23.

[25]Armstrong JL, Hill DS, McKee CS, et al. Exploiting cannabinoid-induced cytotoxic autophagy to drive melanoma cell death. *J Invest Dermatol*. 2015;135(60):1629-1637.

[26]Garcia-Gonzalez E, Selvi E, Balistreri E, et al. Cannabinoids inhibit fibrogenesis in diffuse systemic sclerosis fibroblasts. *Rheumatology*. 2009;48(9):1050-1056.

21

Cannabis Use Disorder

- Although only a subset of cannabis users develop cannabis use disorder, the considerable number of users in the United States means that millions of Americans meet criteria for cannabis use disorder.
- Cannabis use disorder is marked by tolerance, withdrawal, and the use of cannabis despite its use contributing to significant problems in key areas like work, school, and relationships.
- A variety of medications, including all three FDA-approved cannabinoids, have been evaluated as medications for cannabis use disorder. More studies are needed, but the results of these studies have not led to the pursuit of cannabis use disorder as a FDA indication for these medications.

We have covered the therapeutic use of cannabis in the previous chapters. We have made it clear that there is a growing body of evidence supporting the therapeutic use of cannabis and cannabinoids for medical conditions. Given the limited number of cannabinoids that are FDA-approved (3 as of January 2020), it is understandable why patients may wonder if the combination of over 140 cannabinoids in the cannabis plant may outperform the three FDA-approved cannabinoids for a given medical condition. This rational is similar to that of "the entourage effect" whereby some believe that the cannabis plant and its hundreds of chemicals may prove more efficacious than isolated cannabinoids. We also have discussed previously the problems that result when patients are interested in utilizing medications that are not FDA-approved. Thus, we continue to advocate for rigorous clinical trials of cannabis and cannabinoids for medical conditions in order to demonstrate efficacy with more certainty and to perhaps increase the number of available FDA-approved cannabinoids.

There are people who use cannabis in a problematic way, and some of them meet criteria for cannabis use disorder. In an effort to be thorough, then, we will cover the use of cannabinoids to treat cannabis use disorder. A subset of adult patients who use cannabis, about 9%, develop problems in key areas of their lives such as work, school, and relationships. The percentages are higher in young people, with about 16% or one in six young people who use cannabis ultimately meeting criteria for cannabis use disorder. These individuals take their use of a substance that is less harmful on the whole than alcohol or opioids to a harmful level. While this subset of people who meet criteria for cannabis use disorder is a minority of all users, the absolute number of people in the United States with cannabis use disorder is quite large—in the millions—due to the fact that over 22 million Americans used cannabis in the last year.

While the number of Americans meeting criteria for cannabis use disorder is on the rise,[1] it is likely that the estimates are low for several reasons. The polarizing nature of the cannabis debate has contributed to a lack of clarity about the risks of cannabis use. One of those risks around which a lack of clarity exists is cannabis use disorder. Even at this stage of the debate, there are many who do not believe that cannabis is addictive. Of note, both pro- and anti-cannabis groups have contributed to this confusion at times. While most have heard pro-cannabis advocates claim that cannabis is not addictive, flawed drug awareness campaigns crafted by anti-cannabis groups in the 1990s stated that cannabis could be psychologically addictive but not physically addictive. The science shows clearly that heavy cannabis use—daily or near daily—may cause physical dependence marked by tolerance and withdrawal. Cannabis withdrawal symptoms often make it very difficult for a heavy user to stop. As a result of this lack of clarity about the risks of cannabis addiction, there are likely many more people who would meet criteria but have not been diagnosed with cannabis use disorder in part due to the large gap between the science of cannabis and the public perception of it.

Cannabis use disorder, according to DSM-5, is marked by tolerance, withdrawal, and several other clinical characteristics. Tolerance refers to the need to use more and more of a substance to get the same effect. In patients with cannabis use disorder, they may use more cannabis than before or they may transition to more potent forms of cannabis (eg, flower to concentrates). Despite popular belief, patients who use significant amounts of cannabis, often multiple times a day, feel withdrawal symptoms such as anxiety, irritability, and difficulty sleeping when they stop using cannabis abruptly. This is the cannabis withdrawal syndrome. In addition to tolerance and withdrawal, there are nine other criteria. Hazardous use of the substance, social or interpersonal problems related to use, neglecting major responsibilities in order to use, using larger amounts than intended over longer periods of time than intended, repeated attempts to stop using, spending a lot of time using or acquiring the substance, physical or psychological problems related to use, giving up activities that one used to enjoy, and craving.

DSM-5 divides substance use disorders into three categories: mild, moderate, and severe. A person must meet two to three of the criteria mentioned above to meet criteria for a mild substance use disorder, four to five criteria for moderate, and six or more to meet criteria for a severe substance use disorder. Few people with cannabis use disorder seek help on their own. Most are encouraged to seek treatment by a loved one or employer. Due to the subtleties of detecting the presence of a cannabis use disorder, most people who end up seeing a health care provider with cannabis use as part of a chief complaint have a severe form of cannabis use disorder.

Behavioral interventions and medications have been studied as treatments for cannabis use disorder.[2] Multiple behavioral interventions, such as cognitive-behavior therapy and relapse prevention strategies, have been shown to be effective components of comprehensive treatment plans for cannabis use disorder. None of these interventions, however, have been shown to be significantly better than the others, however, so the choice of behavioral intervention depends on the clinical picture and the skill set of the clinician.

There are no FDA-approved medications for the treatment for cannabis use disorder. This is in stark contrast to opioid use disorder, for which three effective medications (buprenorphine, methadone, and naltrexone) are FDA-approved on the strength of multiple randomized controlled clinical trials (RCTs) demonstrating robust effect sizes. As a result, a host of medications with varying mechanisms have been used as pharmacotherapy for cannabis use disorder including N-acetylcysteine, gabapentin, and all of the FDA-approved cannabinoids. Investigators have taken three approaches to developing medications for cannabis use disorder: (1) treatment of cravings related to cannabis use disorder, (2) treatment of cannabis-related withdrawal symptoms, and (3) treatment of comorbid psychiatric disorders that may contribute to ongoing cannabis use.

All three FDA-approved cannabinoids have been studied as treatments for cannabis use disorder. Both dronabinol and nabilone have been studied in RCTs whose results have been published, while cannabidiol (CBD) has been studied in at least one small pilot study whose results have yet to be published.[3]

In a 12-week trial of dronabinol (40 mg) daily for cannabis use disorder, dronabinol pharmacotherapy led to significantly better treatment retention and less withdrawal symptoms than placebo.[4] There was no difference between dronabinol and placebo, however, on the main outcome measure that was the proportion of participants who achieved 2 weeks of abstinence from cannabis at the end of the treatment phase. Dronabinol demonstrated promise in this study, raising questions about its potential effectiveness at higher doses or when added to other medications or behavioral interventions.

In a small pilot RCT of another cannabinoid, nabilone 2 mg daily over 10 weeks proved to be safe and well tolerated as pharmacotherapy for cannabis use disorder.[5] There was no difference in adverse events in the nabilone group compared to placebo in this piloting and feasibility study. Cannabis use as measured by self-report and creatinine-adjusted cannabinoid levels declined in both groups during this study, although there was no significant difference between groups.

Finally, nabiximols, a cannabinoid agonist not available in the United States that contains Δ-9-tetrahydrocannabinol (THC) and CBD in approximately a 1:1 ratio, reduced cannabis use in patients with cannabis use disorder (CUD).[6] In this RCT, 128 participants who has previously failed treatment for CUD received either nabiximols or placebo in conjunction with cognitive-behavioral therapy over a 12-week treatment period. While only half of the participants completed the trial, the nabiximols group used cannabis 35 of 84 days compared with 53.1 of 84 days in the placebo group. There were no differences between groups on measures of withdrawal, cravings, general health, and psychological outcomes. There were no differences in adverse events as well. The trial showed the promise of nabiximols as a treatment for CUD and that, as evidenced by the fact that cannabis was used in 41.7% of possible days, abstinence from cannabis is difficult to achieve.

REFERENCES

[1]Hasin DS. US epidemiology of cannabis use and associated problems. *Neuropsychopharmacology*. 2018;43(1):195-212.

[2]Williams AR, Hill KP. Cannabis and the current state of treatment for cannabis use disorder. *Focus (Am Psychiatr Publ)*. 2019;17(2):98-103. doi: 10.1176/appi.focus.20180038.

[3]Hill KP. Results from NCT03102918. https://clinicaltrials.gov/ct2/show/NCT03102918?term=cannabidiol&cond=cannabis+use+disorder&draw=2&rank=1. Accessed January 28, 2020.

[4]Levin FR, Mariani JJ, Brooks DJ, Pavlicova M, Cheng W, Nunes EV. Dronabinol for the treatment of cannabis dependence: a randomized, double-blind, placebo-controlled trial. *Drug Alcohol Depend*. 2011;116(1-3):142-150. doi: 10.1016/j.drugalcdep.2010.12.010.

[5]Hill KP, Palastro MD, Gruber SA, et al. Nabilone pharmacotherapy for cannabis dependence: a randomized, controlled pilot study. *Am J Addict*. 2017;26(8):795-801. doi: 10.1111/ajad.12622.

[6]Lintzeris N, Bhardwaj A, Mills L, et al. Nabiximols for the treatment of cannabis dependence: a randomized clinical trial. *JAMA Intern Med*. 2019;179(9):1242-1253. doi: 10.1001/jamainternmed.2019.1993.

22

Adverse Effects

- The adverse effects of cannabis use often depend on the dose used and duration of use.
- While there are acute and chronic effects, we know far more about the chronic effects of cannabis use, particularly in those who use heavily.
- Cannabis use may worsen existing psychiatric disorders, and it could potentially increase the incidence of depressive disorders and psychotic disorders in some patients.

As cannabis is evaluated as pharmacotherapy and its use becomes more widespread, its significant side effects remain. Like other substances, there are potential adverse effects with acute and chronic use. Although the acute effects of cannabis use, on driving, for example, have received increasing attention with the implementation of medical and recreational cannabis policies, the effects of chronic use are better described.[1] Regular cannabis use, especially while the brain is under development, is associated with an increased risk of anxiety, depression, and psychotic illness, and cannabis can worsen the courses of these disorders.[2] Keep in mind that the majority of cannabis available these days is Δ-9-tetrahydrocannabinol (THC)-rich cannabis. These associations are especially important given the common co-occurrence of chronic pain and psychiatric conditions.[3] The implementation of medical and recreational cannabis policies offer an opportunity to collect longitudinal data on the effects of cannabis use, although we have yet to capitalize on this opportunity.

22.1 Acute Effects

Acute cannabis use is associated with impaired learning, memory, attention, and motor coordination, areas that can affect important activities of daily living like driving. The wide-ranging effects of cannabis make sense given the presence of CB1 receptors in many different areas of the brain. (See Chapter 6, The Endocannabinoid System.) Acute cannabis use can also affect executive functioning, including the ability to plan, organize, solve problems, and make decisions.[4] This may potentially result in users making risky decisions that they would not otherwise make. Our society is more familiar with the idea of alcohol causing impaired judgment and decision-making, but this is common problem among those who use cannabis regularly. In social situations where poor decisions are possible, cannabis users are more likely to be using their drug of choice as opposed to alcohol, and many patients describe regrettable decisions where cannabis may lower inhibitions, resulting in bad choices that we more customarily associate with alcohol. While there is consensus that acute cannabis use results in cognitive deficits, residual cognitive effects—persisting after acute intoxication—are still debated, especially for those who used cannabis regularly as adolescents.[5]

Overdosing on cannabis is also possible. Of course, the overdose in the case of cannabis is not a fatal overdose, yet rather an unpleasant experience that can bring about feelings of anxiety, paranoia, and even lead to cannabis-induced psychosis. Overdoses occur more often in recreational cannabis use than medicinal cannabis use, often when someone not experienced with cannabis wants to try an edible cannabis product in states where cannabis has been made legal. These users often do not fully understand typical serving sizes for cannabis or the onset of action for orally-consumed cannabis. For example, a typical cannabis brownie contains 100 mg of THC and a standard serving size is 10 mg of THC. Most of us do not eat 1/10 of a brownie when it is time for dessert, so it is easy to understand how one may ingest a much higher dose of cannabis than intended. Similarly, if one takes a bite of an edible and they do not feel any effect within minutes, the user is tempted to take another bite, and so on. This is how a naive user may ingest 4-5 times the intended dose when they experience the effects 30 minutes after ingestion. Either one of these scenarios can lead to a visit to the local emergency department for a nonfatal cannabis overdose.

22.2 Cannabis and Driving

The effect of cannabis on driving has been a major topic of debate in the context of changing cannabis policy. Studies of the impact of those cannabis policies upon cannabis-related traffic outcomes have been mixed so far. The first three states to legalize recreational cannabis have seen a combined 5.2% increase in police-reported crashes as well as a 6% increase in auto insurance collision claims since legalization compared to neighboring states where cannabis is illegal.[6] Since 2013, Washington state has experienced a doubling of drivers killed in car accidents with THC in their blood, although

States like Colorado are doing the best they can to measure cannabis impairment given the available technology. If suspected of driving in Colorado under the influence of cannabis, a person may have their blood drawn by law enforcement, and they can undergo field sobriety testing. This testing may be carried out by a Drug Recognition Expert, an officer specially trained to detect driver impairment by cannabis or other drugs. The *per se* blood level indicating impairment is 5 ng/mL of THC. The problem is that the kinetics of cannabis metabolism mean that blood levels of THC are not accurate predictors of impairment.

Colorado uses the combination of the blood level and field sobriety testing to determine whether an individual can be charged with driving under the influence of cannabis. So it is possible to be found guilty of this offense and to be held accountable for making a reckless decision. The science of cannabis, however, makes it possible for defense attorneys to poke holes in cannabis impairment charges because blood levels are not good proxies for impairment.

Consider the Commonwealth of Massachusetts and its data concerning convictions for driving under the influence of alcohol. The science of breathalyzers and alcohol impairment is strong. Massachusetts couples blood alcohol content with field sobriety testing when developing driving under the influence of alcohol charges. However, a recent study conducted by the Boston Globe in 2011 showed that almost 80% of drivers charged with driving under the influence who opted for a judge-only trial were acquitted of their charges.[14] Therefore, if it is difficult to hold drivers accountable for driving under the influence of alcohol, where the technology and science is strong, it will prove exceedingly difficult to hold those driving under the influence of cannabis accountable. This is a major concern in states that have or are considering medical cannabis or recreational cannabis policies.

22.3 Chronic Effects

As we discussed previously, there are distinct camps in the cannabis debate. At times, both sides are guilty of spinning the data in order to support their preferred narrative. One example of this is the lack of discussion of dose when detailing the effects of chronic cannabis use. The problems stemming from chronic cannabis use that we will summarize in the rest of this chapter are associated with heavy cannabis use at a level that is likely to qualify the user as meeting criteria for a cannabis use disorder (CUD). We are learning more about sporadic cannabis use—there have been recent studies showing that even limited cannabis use may result in structural brain changes—but overall data are limited about the effects of sporadic or limited cannabis use.[15]

Cannabis use differs from alcohol use in which people describe problem drinking in many different patterns. People may drink once a week, every day, or any number of days in between. They binge drink on some of these days, or they may always drink the same number of drinks when they drink. Any one of these patterns may be associated with problem use—for example, binge drinking and daily drinking may constitute an alcohol use disorder.[16] This does not appear to be the case with cannabis. People usually report either liking it a lot, using it if it is available, or not liking it at all. The result is that most people who experience problems related to their cannabis use are using cannabis almost every day and multiple times a day. There is less variability than with patterns of alcohol use.

Chronic cannabis use is associated with an increased risk of cognitive difficulties, psychiatric illness, and addiction. These associations depend upon the amount of cannabis used as well as the age of initiation. Heavy use started at a young age is more likely to contribute to the problems we will discuss.

22.4 Cognitive Effects

We discussed previously the polarizing nature of the cannabis debate. Thus, it is not a surprise that the effects of cannabis use upon cognition continue to be argued with zeal. Several studies have described the adverse effects of regular cannabis use upon the frontal lobe and executive function. Gruber et al. (2012) showed that those who initiate regular cannabis use before the age of 16 years do poorly on many neurocognitive tests and that same group uses cannabis at a greater amount and frequency than those who start using cannabis later in life.[17] Gruber's group has also shown that young cannabis users employ different parts of their brain in order to match the cognitive output of those who do not use cannabis.[18] While there are fewer studies examining the relationship between cannabis use and nondeveloping brains, it appears that the negative effects of chronic adolescent extend into later life. One study of recent users older than

35 years demonstrated significantly worse performance than nonusers across cognitive domains of attention/working memory, information processing speed, and executive functioning.[19] An imaging study of adults in their mid-60s with a history of chronic cannabis use in their early lives showed decreased hippocampal cortical thickness in this group compared to nonusers.[20] This is concerning as hippocampal cortical loss exacerbates age-related cognitive decline.

These studies appear to support possibly the most controversial finding in the area of cannabis and cognition—that early and regular use of cannabis leads to a significant decline in IQ. In perhaps the most-cited study in this area, Meier et al. (2012) followed over 1000 participants longitudinally with these participants undergoing neuropsychological testing at ages 13 and 36.[21] Those that began using cannabis regularly at a young age lost up to 8 IQ points over time. This decrement represents over a standard deviation in IQ and is therefore clinically significant. Furthermore, participants did not experience an increase in IQ upon stopping their use of cannabis. Stopping cannabis use stopped the decline, but it did not lead to a reversal, demonstrating the importance of potentially harmful behaviors during the developmental period.

22.5 Addiction

Cannabis use can lead to addiction. Like alcohol, most people who use cannabis do not develop an addiction, but a subset of cannabis users develops addiction or a CUD in which their frequent use of cannabis leads to problems in multiple key spheres of their lives such as work, school, or relationships. A simple definition of addiction is "repeated use despite harm," but we can also utilize the DSM-5 definition of a CUD marked by tolerance, withdrawal symptoms such as anxiety, irritability, and difficulty sleeping, and a host of psychosocial factors that mostly involve eschewing responsibilities while using or pursuing cannabis. Estimates vary from 9% of adult users developing a CUD to more than 30%.[22,23] For young people, the proportion is higher: about 1 in 6, or ~17%, young people who use cannabis will go on to develop a CUD. From a clinical perspective, though, the fact that only 1 in 6 will go to develop a CUD is comforting neither for parents nor clinicians. Unfortunately, we have not been able to reliably predict which users will go to more problematic use. As a result, any use or suspected use by a young person warrants a significant response.

22.6 Anxiety

The relationship between cannabis and anxiety is an excellent example of the complexities of many cannabis issues. As a reminder, cannabis contains both THC and CBD. CBD alone appears to have anxiolytic properties, but the studies below refer to the use of cannabis with both THC and CBD. Patients often say that they use cannabis in order to manage anxiety. It is understandable that they feel this, especially considering that most people do not feel anxious when under the influence of cannabis. While we continue to learn more about this complicated topic, at this point it appears that initiating cannabis use does not increase the incidence of any anxiety disorder other than panic disorder.[24] Reviews have shown, however, that cannabis use worsens existing anxiety.[25] Thus, using cannabis does not appear to increase the likelihood that one develops an anxiety disorder, perhaps with the exception of panic disorder, but cannabis use will exacerbate symptoms of an existing anxiety disorder. In a related investigation, a reduction in cannabis use was associated with improvement in anxiety symptoms (as well as reduced mood symptoms and improved sleep quality.[26]

22.7 Posttraumatic Stress Disorder

Several investigations have looked at the relationships of cannabis and cannabinoids and posttraumatic stress disorder (PTSD), and the results have been mixed. One observational study evaluated the effects of cannabis use upon 2276 United States Veterans with PTSD and found that cannabis use was associated with increased PTSD symptom severity, violent behavior, drug use, and alcohol use. This study also showed that initiating cannabis use during the observational period worsened overall outcomes.[27] Two observational studies in Veteran populations associated increased cannabis use with increased PTSD symptom severity.[28,29] Oral THC added to current medications in patients with chronic PTSD resulted in measures of sleep and PTSD symptoms but an overall improvement in functioning as measured by the Clinician Global Impressions scale.[30]

There is a hypothetical rationale for cannabis and cannabinoids as being effective pharmacotherapy for PTSD, but it is stronger for CBD than cannabis because of CBD's anxiolytic properties.[31] There are some generally positive studies of nabilone as pharmacotherapy for PTSD as well. Two retrospective chart reviews of patients with PTSD prescribed nabilone in addition to their usual medications suggests that nabilone was associated with a significant improvement in duration of sleep, reduction of nightmares; one of the reviews also showed nabilone to be associated with improvement in PTSD symptom severity.[32,33] A double-blind, crossover study of 10 male soldiers with PTSD and nightmares showed that nabilone pharmacotherapy resulted in a significant reduction in nightmares by no change in PTSD symptoms.[34]

22.8 Depression

Regular cannabis use increases the likelihood that an individual will develop a depressive disorder. Studies have shown the relationship between cannabis use and the development of depression to be dose dependent. A meta-analysis by Lev-Ran et al. calculated an increased odds ratio of 1.17 for those using cannabis regularly and that odds ratio increased to 1.62 with heavy use (daily or near-daily use at the level of CUD). Cannabis has also been shown to worsen existing depression.[35,36] The Degenhardt review shows a strong association between heavy cannabis use and depressive disorders, demonstrating that they often cooccur while offering potential explanations. Feingold et al. used NESARC data to show that the level of cannabis use was associated with an increased number of depressive symptoms at follow-up, although they allowed that sociodemographic and clinical factors complicate this relationship.[36]

22.9 Bipolar Disorder

The relationship between cannabis use and bipolar disorder has been studied less than the relationship between cannabis and unipolar depression. Those with lifetime bipolar disorder have a 7.2% past-year rate of CUD vs 1.2% in the general population. Those with an earlier onset of bipolar disorder are also more likely to have CUD.[37] In addition, those with bipolar disorder are more likely to use cannabis more frequently and in higher quantities than those without.[38] Cannabis use also worsens existing symptoms of bipolar disorder and increases the likelihood of cooccurring disorders such as nicotine use disorder, alcohol use disorder, non-cannabis substance use disorders, and any personality disorder.[37]

22.10 Psychotic Disorders

While it is possible to trigger a psychosis with heavy use of cannabis for medicinal purposes, such instances have been exceedingly rare. However, the adverse effects of cannabis use should be part of the risk/benefit conversation in any patient using medical cannabis. If a young person with epilepsy or irritable bowel syndrome was starting a course of cannabis to treat symptoms of these disorders, such a discussion would be imperative.

There is a significant association—possibly a causal relationship—between cannabis use and the development of psychotic disorders such as schizophrenia, particularly among heavy users who have a family history of psychotic disorders. Several large observational studies have demonstrated this strong association to the degree where experts in the area have discussed the extent of a relationship necessary for it to be termed causal— we appear to be getting closer to a causal relationship.[39] The consensus appears to be that "strong association" is the appropriate terminology here, but the level of discussion about causality underscores the strength of the relationship.

These are unfortunate clinical scenarios. Frequently, initial involvement of an addiction psychiatrist may occur after a young person who has never seen a psychiatrist before, begins using cannabis and develops psychotic symptoms a few months later. These symptoms, usually positive psychotic symptoms, may trigger an inpatient psychiatric hospitalization and a trial of antipsychotic medication. The addiction psychiatrist is forced to answer questions from the family about whether their son or daughter will ever return to their baseline level of function. The unfortunate answer appears to be "no." I have followed some of these patients for years and, if they take their medication, they can work, live alone, and have relationships. Some of the patients I have worked with graduated from elite universities in the Northeast United

States though, and they clearly are not enjoying the same level of success as their classmates. Sadly, if they are taking medication and doing well, they also are able to recognize that they are not as successful in some ways as their peers and that is an ongoing source of frustration for them.

THC causes acute psychotic symptoms in a dose-dependent manner and also worsens outcomes in patients who do not stop using cannabis.[40,41] There are 10 large observational trials of examining the relationship between cannabis and the development of psychosis, and the odds ratios are typically between 1.1 and 2.9, but others have put the odds ratio as high as 5.4.[42] With so many studies showing this relationship, it is critical that we do a better job of educating young people, especially those with a family history of a psychotic disorder, about the risks involved with cannabis use.

22.11 Sleep

Like anxiety, sleep is another reason cited by many for cannabis, and more recently, CBD use. Cannabis has similar effects on sleep as alcohol does. It reduces sleep latency but causes harmful effects in the form of increased slow wave sleep and decreased REM sleep. While it appears that tolerance may develop to the chronic effects of cannabis on sleep, it does not improve sleep quality.[43] Similarly, many CBD products available now tout their ability to improve sleep. There are limited investigations in this area, but at least one expert in the field feels that the effects of CBD on sleep have more to do with what else CBD is "packaged" with in a given formulation than the compound itself.[44]

22.12 Cardiovascular Risks

Studies show tachycardia and slight elevation in supine blood pressure immediately after inhalation and last up to an hour after use.[45,46] While multiple case reports describe acute coronary syndrome after cannabis use, there have been no prospective studies that have shown a strong association between cannabis and long-term cardiovascular outcomes.[47] Case reports and one retrospective study have described arrhythmias in the setting of cannabis use. Desai et al. showed that the all-cause hospital mortality of cannabis users with arrhythmias increased from

3.7% to 4.4% from 2010 to 2014, respectively ($P < .001$).[48] Aside from case reports and the aforementioned retrospective study, however, there have been no robust published studies looking at the association between cannabis use and arrhythmias.

Similarly, some studies suggest that cannabis use is associated with stroke, particularly at a young age. These data are not uniform but point toward such an association. For example, a recent study by Parekh et al. demonstrated that young people who used cannabis regularly were 2.45 times more likely than those who do not use cannabis to suffer a stroke.[49] These young cannabis users were also more likely to use cigarettes and e-cigarettes, although the analyses adjusted for those variables. Two studies using the National Inpatient Sample dataset also showed the incidence of acute ischemic strokes to be greater in cannabis users than the nonusers.[50,51] However, a population-based cohort study of Swedish men found no such association.[52]

22.13 Risks of Prenatal Exposure

For many years, most physicians counseled pregnant mothers against using cannabis during pregnancy based upon the expectation that in utero exposure would adversely affect development of the fetus. In part due to the challenges of studying this type of question, there were little data to support those recommendations. In the context of increased adult cannabis use as states and countries implemented cannabis policies, the need for evidence in this area has grown. While there remains a dire need for more research on prenatal exposure, a pair of recent studies has added to the knowledge base. A recent retrospective cohort study published in JAMA in 2019 demonstrated that 12% of women using cannabis while pregnant experienced preterm births compared to only 6.1% of births by women who were not using cannabis while pregnant (relative risk 1.41).[53] In this study, cannabis use while pregnant was also associated with babies who were small for gestational age, placental abruption, admissions to the Neonatal Intensive Care Unit, and APGAR scores <4.

Another recent preclinical study raises the question of teratogenicity from CBD exposure. Fish et al. (2019) exposed zebrafish to a variety of cannabinoids including CBD and THC and found that even a single exposure to CBD or THC increased the likelihood of facial abnormalities.[54] While it is hard to know whether such findings are translational to humans, this concerning animal work underscores the need for additional research in this area.

22.14 Cannabis Hyperemesis Syndrome

Some regular users of cannabis experience cannabinoid hyperemesis syndrome (CHS), a syndrome characterized by cyclic vomiting in the setting of high-dose cannabis use that is frequently associated with compulsive hot baths or showers used in an attempt to control symptoms.[55] An estimated 2.75 million Americans suffer from CHS each year.[56] The pathophysiology of CHS is unclear, but evidence suggests a dynamic relationship between cannabinoid metabolism and pharmacodynamics at the CB1 receptor. CHS is usually seen in a setting of chronic high-potency cannabis use; patients often describe taking compulsive hot baths or showers in an attempt to stave off symptoms. Fortunately, symptoms abate when users are able to abstain from cannabis.

22.15 Functional Outcomes

There are adverse functional outcomes resulting from chronic cannabis use as well. Almost 20% of lifetime cannabis users met criteria for DSM-5 CUD, of whom 23% were symptomatically severe ($\geq$6 criteria). Of those with CUD, 48% were not functioning in *any* major role in their lives (work, school, or relationships).[57] Regular cannabis use at levels associated with CUD (near-daily use of more than 1/8 ounce of cannabis per week) is associated with worsening functional status including lower income, greater need for socioeconomic assistance, criminal behavior, unemployment, and decreased life satisfaction.[2] Overall, it is imperative to understand that while the majority of cannabis users do not experience the problems described in this chapter, there is a subset of users who can experience significant sequelae resulting from their use. These individuals can escalate their use of a less harmful substance to an extremely harmful level.

REFERENCES

[1]Hill KP. Medical use of cannabis in 2019. *JAMA*. 2019. doi: 10.1001/jama.2019.

[2]Volkow ND, Baler RD, Compton WM, Weiss SR. Adverse health effects of marijuana use. *N Engl J Med*. 2014;370:2219-2227.

[3]Hill KP, Johnson B, Palastro MP, Ditre JW. Cannabis and pain: a clinical review. *Cannabis Cannabinoid Res*. 2017;2(1):96-104. doi: 10.1089/can.2017.0017.

[4]Crean RD, Tapert SF, Minassian A, Macdonald K, Crane NA, Mason BJ. Effects of chronic, heavy cannabis use on executive functions. *J Addict Med*. 2011;5(1):9-15.

[5]Scott JC, Slomiak ST, Jones JD, et al. Association of cannabis with cognitive functioning in adolescents and young adults. *JAMA Psychiat*. 2018;75(6):585-595. doi: 10.1001/jamapsychiatry.2018.0335.

[6]Monfort SS. *Effect of Recreational Marijuana Sales on Police-Reported Crashes in Colorado, Oregon, and Washington*. Arlington, VA: Insurance Institute for Highway Safety; October 2018.

[7]Washington Traffic Safety Commission, May 2019. Accessed January 27, 2020.

[8]*Impacts of Marijuana Legalization in Colorado: A Report Pursuant to Senate Bill 13-283*. Colorado Department of Public Safety; October 2018. Accessed January 27, 2020.

[9]Arkell TR, Lintzeris N, Kevin RC, et al. Cannabidiol (CBD) content in vaporized cannabis does not prevent tetrahydrocannabinol (THC)-induced impairment of driving and cognition. *Psychopharmacology (Berl)*. 2019;236(9):2713-2724. doi: 10.1007/s00213-019-05246-8.

[10]Robbe HWJ, O'Hanlon JF. *Marijuana and Actual Driving Performance*. Maastricht, Netherlands: U.S. Department of Transportation, National Highway Traffic Safety Administration; 1993.

[11]Grotenhermen F, Leson G, Berghaus G, et al. Developing limits for driving under cannabis. *Addiction*. 2007;102(12):1910-1917. doi: 10.1111/j.1360-0443.2007.02009.x.

[12]Asbridge M, Hayden JA, Cartwright JL. Acute cannabis consumption and motor vehicle collision risk: systematic review of observational studies and meta-analysis. *BMJ*. 2012;344:e536. doi: 10.1136/bmj.e536.

[13]Neavyn MJ, Blohm E, Babu KM, Bird SB. Medical marijuana and driving: a review. *J Med Toxicol*. 2014;10(3):269-279. doi: 10.1007/s13181-014-0393-4.

[14]Farragher T. For drunk drivers, a habit of judicial leniency. *The Boston Globe*, October 30, 2011.

[15]Gilman JM, Kuster JK, Lee S, et al. Cannabis use is quantitatively associated with nucleus accumbens and amygdala abnormalities in young adult recreational users. *J Neurosci*. 2014;34(16):5529-5538. doi: 10.1523/JNEUROSCI.4745-13.2014.

[16]American Psychiatric Association. *Diagnostic and Statistical Manual of Mental Disorders: Diagnostic and Statistical Manual of Mental Disorders*. 5th ed. Arlington, VA: American Psychiatric Association; 2013.

[17]Gruber SA, Sagar KA, Dahlgren MK, Racine M, Lukas SE. Age of onset of marijuana use and executive function. *Psychol Addict Behav*. 2012;26(3):496-506. doi: 10.1037/a0026269.

[18]Gruber SA, Dahlgren MK, Sagar KA, Gönenc A, Killgore WD. Age of onset of marijuana use impacts inhibitory processing. *Neurosci Lett*. 2012;511(2):89-94. doi: 10.1016/j.neulet.2012.01.039.

[19]Thames AD, Arbid N, Sayegh P. Cannabis use and neurocognitive functioning in a non-clinical sample of users. *Addict Behav*. 2014;39(5):994-999. doi: 10.1016/j.addbeh.2014.01.019.

[20]Burggren AC, Siddarth P, Mahmood Z, et al. Subregional hippocampal thickness abnormalities in older adults with a history of heavy cannabis use. *Cannabis Cannabinoid Res*. 2018;3(1):242-251. doi: 10.1089/can.2018.0035. eCollection 2018.

[21]Meier MH, Caspi A, Ambler A, et al. Persistent cannabis users show neuropsychological decline from childhood to mid-life. *Proc Natl Acad Sci USA*. 2012;17:642-649.

[22]Lopez-Quintero C, Perez de los Cobos J, Hasin DS, et al. Probability and predictors of transition from first use to dependence on nicotine, alcohol, cannabis, and cocaine: results of the National Epidemiologic Survey on Alcohol and Related Conditions (NESARC). *Drug Alcohol Depend*. 2011;115:120-130.

[23]Hasin DS, Saha, TD, Kerridge BT, et al. Prevalence of marijuana use disorders in the United States between 2001-2002 and 2012-2013. *JAMA Psychiat*. 2015;72:1235-1242.

[24]Feingold D, Weiser M, Rehm J, Lev-Ran S. The association between cannabis use and anxiety disorders: Results from a population-based representative sample. *Eur Neuropsychopharmacol.* 2016;26(3):493-505. doi: 10.1016/j.euroneuro.2015.12.037.

[25]Crippa JA, Zuardi AW, Martín-Santos R, et al. Cannabis and anxiety: a critical review of the evidence. *Hum Psychopharmacol.* 2009;24(7):515-523. doi: 10.1002/hup.1048. Review.

[26]Hser YI, Mooney LJ, Huang D, et al. Reductions in cannabis use are associated with improvements in anxiety, depression, and sleep quality, but not quality of life. *J Subst Abuse Treat.* 2017;81:53-58. doi: 10.1016/j.jsat.2017.07.012.

[27]Wilkinson ST, Stefanovics E, Rosenheck RA. Marijuana use is associated with worse outcomes in symptom severity and violent behavior in patients with posttraumatic stress disorder. *J Clin Psychiatry.* 2015;76(9):1174-1180. doi: 10.4088/JCP.14m09475.

[28]Bonn-Miller MO, Babson KA, Vandrey R. Using cannabis to help you sleep: heightened frequency of medical cannabis use among those with PTSD. *Drug Alcohol Depend.* 2014;136:162-165. doi: 10.1016/j.drugalcdep.2013.12.008.

[29]Boden MT, Babson KA, Vujanovic AA, Short NA, Bonn-Miller MO. Posttraumatic stress disorder and cannabis use characteristics among military veterans with cannabis dependence. *Am J Addict.* 2013;22(3):277-284. doi: 10.1111/j.1521-0391.2012.12018.x.

[30]Roitman P, Mechoulam R, Cooper-Kazaz R, Shalev A. Preliminary, open-label, pilot study of add-on oral Δ9-tetrahydrocannabinol in chronic post-traumatic stress disorder. *Clin Drug Investig.* 2014;34(8):587-591. doi: 10.1007/s40261-014-0212-3.

[31]Haney M, Evins AE. Does cannabis cause, exacerbate or ameliorate psychiatric disorders? An oversimplified debate discussed. *Neuropsychopharmacology.* 2016;41(2):393-401. doi: 10.1038/npp.2015.251.

[32]Cameron C, Watson D, Robinson J. Use of a synthetic cannabinoid in a correctional population for posttraumatic stress disorder-related insomnia and nightmares, chronic pain, harm reduction, and other indications: a retrospective evaluation. *J Clin Psychopharmacol.* 2014;34(5):559-564.

[33]Fraser GA. The use of a synthetic cannabinoid in the management of treatment-resistant nightmares in posttraumatic stress disorder (PTSD). *CNS Neurosci Ther.* 2009;15(1):84-88.

[34]Jetly R, Heber A, Fraser G, et al. The efficacy of nabilone, a synthetic cannabinoid, in the treatment of PTSD-associated nightmares: a preliminary randomized, double-blind, placebo-controlled cross-over design study. *Psychoneuroendocrinology.* 2015;51:585-588.

[35]Degenhardt L, Hall W, Lynskey M. Exploring the association between cannabis use and depression. *Addiction.* 2003;98(11):1493-1504. Review.

[36]Feingold D, Rehm J, Lev-Ran S. Cannabis use and the course and outcome of major depressive disorder: a population based longitudinal study. *Psychiatry Res.* 2017;251: 225-234. doi: 10.1016/j.psychres.2017.02.027.

[37]Lev-Ran S, Le Foll B, McKenzie K, George TP, Rehm J. Bipolar disorder and co-occurring cannabis use disorders: characteristics, co-morbidities and clinical correlates. *Psychiatry Res.* 2013;209(3):459-465. doi: 10.1016/j.psychres.2012.12.014.

[38]Feingold D, Weiser M, Rehm J, Lev-Ran S. The association between cannabis use and mood disorders: a longitudinal study. *J Affect Disord.* 2015;172:211-218. doi: 10.1016/j. jad.2014.10.006.

[39]Gage SH, Hickman M, Zammit S. Association between cannabis and psychosis: epidemiologic evidence. *Biol Psychiatry.* 2016;79(7):549-556. doi: 10.1016/j.biopsych.2015.08.001. Review.

[40]Wilkinson ST, Radhakrishnan R, D'Souza DC. Impact of cannabis use on the development of psychotic disorders. *Curr Addict Rep.* 2014;1(2):115-128.

[41]Tarricone I, Braca M, Allegri F, et al. First-episode psychosis and migration in Italy (PEP-Ita migration): a study in the Italian mental health services. *BMC Psychiatry.* 2014;14:186. doi: 10.1186/1471-244X-14-186.

[42]Di Forti M, Marconi A, Carra E. Proportion of patients in south London with first-episode psychosis attributable to use of high potency cannabis: a case-control study. *Lancet Psychiatry*. 2015;2(3):233-238. doi: 10.1016/S2215-0366(14)00117-5.

[43]Angarita GA, Emadi N, Hodges S, Morgan PT. Sleep abnormalities associated with alcohol, cannabis, cocaine, and opiate use: a comprehensive review. *Addict Sci Clin Pract*. 2016;11(1):9. doi: 10.1186/s13722-016-0056-7. Review.

[44]Russo EB. Cannabidiol claims and misconceptions. *Trends Pharmacol Sci*. 2017;38(3): 198-201. doi: 10.1016/j.tips.2016.12.004.

[45]Singh A, Saluja S, Kumar A, et al. Cardiovascular complications of marijuana and related substances: a review. *Cardiol Ther*. 2018;7(1):45-59. doi: 10.1007/s40119-017-0102-x. Review.

[46]Ponto LL, O'Leary DS, Koeppel J, et al. Effect of acute marijuana on cardiovascular function and central nervous system pharmacokinetics of [(15)O]water: effect in occasional and chronic users. *J Clin Pharmacol*. 2004;44(7):751-766.

[47]Ghosh M, Naderi S. Cannabis and cardiovascular disease. *Curr Atheroscler Rep*. 2019;21(6):21. doi: 10.1007/s11883-019-0783-9. Review.

[48]Desai R, Shamim S, Patel K, et al. Primary causes of hospitalizations and procedures, predictors of in-hospital mortality, and trends in cardiovascular and cerebrovascular events among recreational marijuana users: a five-year nationwide inpatient assessment in the United States. *Cureus*. 2018;10(8):e3195. doi: 10.7759/cureus.3195.

[49]Parekh T, Pemmasani S, Desai R. Marijuana use among young adults (18-44 years of age) and risk of stroke: a behavioral risk factor surveillance system survey analysis. *Stroke*. 2020;51(1):308-310. doi: 10.1161/STROKEAHA.119.027828.

[50]Rumalla K, Reddy AY, Mittal MK. Recreational marijuana use and acute ischemic stroke: a population-based analysis of hospitalized patients in the United States. *J Neurol Sci*. 2016;364:191-196. doi: 10.1016/j.jns.2016.01.066.

[51]Kalla A, Krishnamoorthy PM, Gopalakrishnan A, Figueredo VM. Cannabis use predicts risks of heart failure and cerebrovascular accidents: results from the National Inpatient Sample. *J Cardiovasc Med (Hagerstown)*. 2018;19(9):480-484. doi: 10.2459/JCM.0000000000000681.

[52]Falkstedt D, Wolff V, Allebeck P, Hemmingsson T, Danielsson AK. Cannabis, tobacco, alcohol use, and the risk of early Stroke: a population-based cohort study of 45 000 Swedish men. *Stroke*. 2017;48(2):265-270. doi: 10.1161/STROKEAHA.116.015565.

[53]Corsi DJ, Walsh L, Weiss D, et al. Association between self-reported prenatal cannabis use and maternal, perinatal, and neonatal outcomes. *JAMA*. 2019;322(2):145-152. doi: 10.1001/jama.2019.8734.

[54]Fish EW, Murdaugh LB, Zhang C, et al. Cannabinoids exacerbate alcohol teratogenesis by a CB1-hedgehog interaction. *Sci Rep*. 2019;9(1):16057. doi: 10.1038/s41598-019-52336-w.

[55]Sorensen CJ, DeSanto K, Borgelt L, Phillips KT, Monte AA. Cannabinoid hyperemesis syndrome: diagnosis, pathophysiology, and treatment—a systematic review. *J Med Toxicol*. 2017;13(1):71-87. doi: 10.1007/s13181-016-0595-z. Review.

[56]Habboushe J, Rubin A, Liu H, Hoffman RS. The prevalence of cannabinoid hyperemesis syndrome among regular marijuana smokers in an urban public hospital. *Basic Clin Pharmacol Toxicol*. 2018;122(6):660-662. doi: 10.1111/bcpt.12962.

[57]Hasin DS, Kerridge BT, Saha TD, et al. Prevalence and correlates of DSM-5 cannabis use disorder, 2012-2013: findings from the National Epidemiologic Survey on alcohol and related conditions-III. *Am J Psychiatry*. 2016;173(6):588-599. doi: 10.1176/appi.ajp.2015.15070907.

APPENDIX

Glossary

Term	Meaning
Autoflower	A trait in some strains of drug-type cannabis characterized by the entry into the plant's flowering stage regardless of the extent of light or darkness to which it is exposed. Nonautoflowering plants enter into the flowering stage when exposed to long periods of darkness, typically 12 hours or more.
Bhang	A preparation of drug-type cannabis consisting mostly of cannabis leaves that can be smoked, eaten, or mixed with spices, milk, sugar, and tea to create an intoxicating beverage. Bhang has been and continues to be very popular in South Asia.
Blunt	A cigar that has been emptied of tobacco and refilled with cannabis.
Bong	A water pipe.
Bowl	A pipe used for smoking cannabis. It may also refer to the amount of cannabis contained in the bowl of the pipe. "I smoked a bowl" would mean that the individual filled the pipe with cannabis and then smoked its contents.
Bud	The female flower of drug-type cannabis. Often used to distinguish herbal cannabis from cannabis distillates or concentrates, but sometimes used to refer to all preparations of drug-type cannabis.
Budtender	A cannabis specialist who works in a dispensary. Budtenders may have passed an online certification program, but they are not technically a pharmacist or a medical professional, and they are not qualified to provide medical advice.

Joint	A cigarette containing drug-type cannabis.
Kif (a/k/a kaif) (1)	A preparation of drug-type cannabis popular in Morocco. The cannabis is mixed with tobacco and smoked in a pipe known as a sebsi.
Kif (a/k/a kief) (2)	Trichomes that have been separated from dried leaflets and flowers of cannabis.
Marihuana	Alternate and archaic spelling of "marijuana." Obsolete and potentially offensive to some.
Marijuana (1)	A generic term for a preparation of drug-type cannabis made of the dried flowers and leaves of the female cannabis plant that contains enough THC to produce an intoxicating effect when consumed. The etymology of the word is unclear, but it is believed to have originated in Mexico during the 1800s.
Marijuana (2)	A legal definition meaning any cannabis plant or its derivatives, extracts, isomers, acids, salts, or isomers of salts, whether growing or not, that produces or contains a concentration of THC > 0.3% on a dry weight basis.
Munchies	The feeling of hunger that often arises when one is experiencing cannabis intoxication.
Nugget (a/k/a nugs)	The female flower of drug-type cannabis. Often used to distinguish herbal cannabis from cannabis distillates, concentrates, or other preparations. Whole dried flowers are often nugget-shaped
Number	A cigarette containing drug-type cannabis. The term is largely obsolete.
Preroll	A cannabis cigarette purchased in a dispensary.
Reefer	A cigarette containing drug-type cannabis. The term is obsolete and is often used in a sarcastic manner.
Regs	Drug-type cannabis of medium or "regular" quality.
Sativa	An informal classification of a cannabis strain thought to produce a more social kind of intoxication.
Schwag	Drug-type cannabis of low quality.
Seeds and stems	Drug-type cannabis of low quality.

Set and setting | The mindset and social environment in which one consumes cannabis.

Shatter | A highly concentrated form of cannabis that resembles glass.

Sinsimilla | Spanish for "without seeds." Refers to a preparation of drug-type cannabis that solely includes the unpollinated flower of the female cannabis plant. Unpollinated (seedless) drug-type cannabis plants produce more THC than do pollinated plants.

Spliff | A cigarette containing both cannabis and tobacco.

Strain | The term for different varieties of cannabis. Although the proper term for such a variety is "cultivar," usage of "strain" is ubiquitous.

Sugar leaves | The trichome-rich unifoliolate leaves of the female cannabis plant that grow among the bracts

Terps | Short for terpenes or terpenoids, which are organic hydrocarbons found in plants, including cannabis, that give them their unique smell and taste. Different strains of cannabis have different terpene and terpenoid profiles.

Vape pen | An instrument used to vaporize distilled and liquid cannabis. These devices resemble pens.

Wax | A highly concentrated form of cannabis that resembles wax.

Weed | A generic term for drug-type cannabis.

B

Current Regulations as of Early 2020

Below are the rules and regulations regarding the recreational and medicinal use of cannabis in each state and U.S. territory as of April 2020. For each state, we have provided a description of the laws regulating possession and cultivation, as well as the penalties for violating these laws. For states that have created a medicinal program, we have noted who is legally allowed to recommend cannabis, what qualifying conditions patients must have to be eligible for the program, whether the state allows patients from out of state to participate in the program or to legally possess cannabis, and if there are any unique regulations that exist (eg, a rule allowing only extracts or a limit on THC concentration). We have also provided links to each state's medicinal program, provided one exists.

Before acting on the information below, we ask that you visit this book's Web site, cannabistextbook.com, to ensure that no changes to the law have been made. State laws and regulations regarding cannabis have a tendency to change with an almost maddening level of frequency.

Another important note is that we have chosen to use the word "marijuana" throughout this section, which some may feel is a strange departure from the rest of the book. Though "cannabis" is the preferred word to use when referring to the plant, we have decided to use the word "marijuana" for two reasons. The first is that most states—with the exceptions of Hawaii, Illinois, Maryland, Minnesota, New Hampshire, New Mexico, Utah, and West Virginia (as well as the territories of Guam, Puerto Rico, and the U.S. Virgin Islands)—have a medical "marijuana" (or "marihuana" in Michigan) program. Secondly, when discussing the penalties for possession or cultivation, we are referring to the possession or cultivation of "marijuana" as defined by the federal government— cannabis products that contain more than 0.3% THC.

Alabama

Recreational marijuana is not legal in Alabama. Possession of flower marijuana for personal use is a misdemeanor that may result in punishment of up to 1 year of incarceration and a maximum fine of $6000. This is not necessarily the case in Jefferson County, where personal use has been decriminalized.[1] Possession of marijuana concentrates is a felony that could result in a term of imprisonment from 1 to 10 years and a fine of $15 000. Manufacturing, selling, or distributing marijuana is a felony. Cultivating may be treated as simple possession or it may be treated as possession with intent to distribute depending on circumstances.[2]

Alabama does not currently have a medical marijuana program, but some patients and their caretakers can possess, administer, and consume cannabis formulations containing up to 3% THC under Leni's Law, which was passed in 2016. Physicians in good standing with a license to practice medicine in Alabama and a bona fide physician-patient relationship with patients may recommend such formulations. Only patients with "specific debilitating conditions that produce seizures" are covered by this law.[3]

Senate Bill 225 was signed into law on June 10, 2019, and allows the sale of CBD products in Alabama, provided they are hemp derived and contain <0.3% THC. The law became effective immediately following its passage.[4]

No cannabis formulations containing more than 0.3% are currently available in Alabama.

Alaska

Recreational and medical marijuana are both legal in Alaska. Adults aged 21 and older may possess up to 1 oz of flower marijuana or 7 g of concentrate and can cultivate 6 plants, though only 3 plants may be mature and flowering at any time. Possession of 1-4 oz of marijuana is a misdemeanor punishable by up to 1 year of incarceration and a maximum fine of $10 000. Possession of more than 4 oz is a felony punishable by up to 5 years of imprisonment and a fine of $50 000. It remains illegal to consume marijuana in public places or to drive under the influence of THC. Public consumption may result in a fine of $100.[5]

Physicians in good standing with a license to practice medicine in Alaska who have a bona fide physician-patient relationship with patients may recommend marijuana for the following conditions:

- Cachexia
- Cancer
- Glaucoma
- HIV/AIDS

- Multiple sclerosis
- Muscle spasms
- Seizures
- Severe nausea
- Severe pain

Alaska does not offer reciprocity to patients of participating in the medical programs of other states.

For more information, see the Alaska Department of Health and Social Services' site on marijuana at http://dhss.alaska.gov/dph/Director/Pages/marijuana/default.aspx. For legal specifics, see Alaska Statutes 2019— Sec. 17.37.040.[6]

American Samoa

No form of cannabis is legal in American Samoa. First-time possession is a felony, and the American Samoan government has stated that violators will receive a mandatory minimum sentence of 5 years of imprisonment, a $5000 fine, or both. This includes cannabis that has been obtained legally in another jurisdiction.[7]

American Samoa does not have a medical marijuana program. More importantly, CBD products are not legal in the territory. Though hemp-derived CBD that contains <0.3% THC is legal under federal law, a judge in American Samoa ruled in 2019 that "CBD oil is marijuana regardless of whether or not it is psychoactive and unless and until the Fono [the Legislature of American Samoa] tells us otherwise."[8]

Arizona

Recreational marijuana is not legal in Arizona, and possession of marijuana in either flower form or concentrated form is a felony. However, courts have been directed to offer probation to individuals arrested for first- and second-time possession, provided they are in possession of <2 lb of marijuana and have no prior convictions for violent crimes.[9] Possession or cultivation of more than 2 lb of marijuana can result in felony charges, steep fines, and years of imprisonment.[10]

Arizona does have a medical marijuana program, and allopathic (MD), osteopathic (DO), homeopathic (MD(H) or DO(H)), or naturopathic (NMD or ND) physicians can recommend it to patients, provided they hold a valid Arizona license and have a physician-patient relationship with the patient. Qualifying patients may purchase no more than 2.5 oz in any 2-week period. To grow marijuana at home, patients must live more than 25 miles away from the nearest dispensary and receive approval from the state.[11] Those who can grow marijuana at home are only allowed to grow 12 plants at one time.

Medical marijuana may be recommended for the following conditions:

- Alzheimer disease
- ALS (amyotrophic lateral sclerosis)
- Cancer
- Crohn disease
- Glaucoma
- Hepatitis C
- HIV/AIDS

It may also be recommended to alleviate the following symptoms associated with a debilitating medical condition:

- Cachexia
- Seizures
- Severe and chronic pain
- Severe or persistent muscle spasms[12]

Arizona does offer reciprocity to patients of participating in the medical programs of other states, provided these patients are not residents of Arizona, have been diagnosed with a condition recognized as eligible for Arizona's medical marijuana program, and have their medical card or its equivalent with them. However, out-of-state patients are not allowed to purchase marijuana in an Arizona dispensary.[13]

The Arizona medical marijuana program Web site can be found here: https://www.azdhs.gov/licensing/medical-marijuana/index.php.

Arkansas

Recreational marijuana is not legal in Arkansas. State law describes it as a Schedule VI substance. Despite marijuana being a controlled substance, possession of small amounts of marijuana have been decriminalized in Fayetteville, Eureka Springs, and Jacksonville.[14] In the rest of the state, those found in possession of <4 oz of marijuana could be found guilty of a misdemeanor offense, and those who are convicted may face upwards of 1 year in jail and/or a maximum fine of $2500. Second-time and subsequent offenders, provided they are in possession of more than 1 oz of marijuana, may face felony charges and a punishment of up to 6 years in prison and/or a fine of $6000.[15]

Despite such harsh laws against recreational marijuana, Arkansas does have a medical marijuana program. Patients are not allowed to cultivate plants, but they may purchase up to 2.5 oz or 71 g of marijuana every 14 days. Any MD or DO licensed to practice in Arkansas with a current Drug Enforcement Agency number is authorized to sign the form authorizing a patient to obtain medical marijuana. Authorized medical professionals may recommend it for the following conditions:

- ALS (amyotrophic lateral sclerosis)

- Alzheimer disease
- Cachexia
- Cancer
- Chronic or debilitating diseases
- Crohn disease
- Fibromyalgia
- Glaucoma
- Hepatitis C
- HIV/AIDS
- Intractable pain
- Multiple sclerosis
- Peripheral neuropathy
- PTSD (posttraumatic stress disorder)
- Seizures
- Severe arthritis
- Severe nausea
- Severe and persistent muscle spasms
- Tourette syndrome
- Ulcerative colitis

Additional conditions may qualify, subject to approval by the Department of Health.

For out-of-state patients visiting Arkansas or for patients who have recently moved to Arkansas, the state does have a program that allows you to purchase marijuana from Arkansas dispensaries. Patients can register through the following portal: https://ammsys.adh.arkansas.gov/.

For more information, visit the Web site for the Arkansas Department of Health: https://www.healthy.arkansas.gov/programs-services/topics/medical-marijuana.

California

Recreational and medical marijuana are both legal in California. Medical patients over the age of 18 may possess or grow as much as is deemed necessary. Though the state does not limit the amount of plants that patients can grow to treat their condition, local ordinances may impose limits on cultivation. For recreational users over the age of 21, it is legal to possess only up 28.5 g of plant material or 8 g of concentrate at one time. Possession of more than the legal limit is a misdemeanor punishable by up to 6 months of incarceration and a maximum fine of $500.[16] Cultivation is also limited for recreational users; they may only grow up to 6 plants.[17] For medical and recreational users, it remains illegal to consume marijuana in public places or to drive under the influence of THC.

An MD or DO licensed to practice in California may recommend marijuana to a patient, provided he or she is said patient's "attending physician." Assembly Bill 71, which was passed in 2018, allows physicians, pharmacists, or others authorized in the healing arts to prescribe, furnish, or dispense cannabis products that are high in CBD and below 0.3% THC at their discretion.[18] Marijuana, meanwhile, may be recommended for any debilitating illness where it has been deemed appropriate and recommended by a physician. Specific examples include

- Anorexia
- Arthritis
- Cachexia
- Cancer
- Chronic pain
- HIV/AIDS
- Glaucoma
- Migraines
- Nausea
- Persistent muscle spasms
- Seizures

California does not have a reciprocity program to accommodate medical marijuana patients from out of state.

For more information, please see the state's marijuana portal: https://www.cdph.ca.gov/Programs/CHSI/Pages/MMICP.aspx.

Colorado

Recreational marijuana is legal in Colorado. The state is also home to a medical marijuana program. For recreational use, Coloradans and tourists over the age of 21 are allowed to possess or purchase 1 oz at a time.[19] Individuals may also grow 6 plants, with as many as 3 of those plants flowering at one time.[20] For medicinal use, Coloradans can purchase 2 oz of marijuana at once.

Possession of between 1 and 2 oz of marijuana for nonmedicinal users is a petty offense punishable by a fine no more than $100. Possession of 2-12 oz is a misdemeanor. Possession of between 2 and 6 oz may result in a punishment of up to 12 months of incarceration and a fine of $700, while between 6 and 12 oz may result in a punishment of up to 18 months of incarceration and a fine of $5000. Possession of more than 12 oz of marijuana is a felony punishable by a maximum term of imprisonment of 2 years and a fine of $100 000. Cultivation of 6-30 plants is a felony that may result in a penalty of 6-24 months of incarceration and a maximum fine of $100 000, while cultivation of more than 30 plants may result in a sentence of 2-6 years of imprisonment and a fine of $500 000. Use is public places is still illegal, as is drugged driving.[21]

MDs, DOs, or advanced practice practitioners (dentists, physician assistants, advanced nurse practitioners, podiatrists, optometrists) who are licensed to practice medicine in Colorado with valid, unrestricted DEA certification, and an online account with the Colorado Department of Public Health & Environment can recommend marijuana for either disabling or debilitating conditions. To register, physicians should visit the following site: https://www.colorado.gov/pacific/sites/default/files/CHED_MMR_Physician-Certification_6_28_17.pdf.

Disabling medical conditions include

- Autism spectrum disorder
- PTSD (posttraumatic stress disorder)
- Any condition for which a physician could provide an opioid

Debilitating medical conditions include

- Cachexia
- Cancer
- Chronic pain
- Chronic nervous system disorders
- Glaucoma
- HIV/AIDS
- Nausea
- Persistent muscle spasms
- Seizures

Colorado does not have a reciprocity program to accommodate medical marijuana patients from out of state.

For more information, please see Colorado's Department of Public Health & Environment: https://www.colorado.gov/pacific/cdphe/medicalmarijuana.

Connecticut

Recreational marijuana is not legal in Connecticut, but it has been decriminalized. Possession of 0.5 oz or less results in a civil penalty of $150-$500. Possession of more than 0.5 oz is a misdemeanor that may result in up to 1 year in jail and/or a fine of up to $2000. Cultivation is a felony. For first-time offenders, cultivating enough plants to produce <1 kg of marijuana may result in up to 7 years of imprisonment and a fine of $25 000, while cultivating enough plants to produce 1 kg or more may result in up to a 15-year sentence and a fine of $100 000. Subsequent offenders face similar fines, but more severe terms of imprisonment. Growing <1 kg of marijuana is punishable by a minimum of 5 years of incarceration and a maximum of 20 years, while 1 kg or more will result in a minimum term of imprisonment of 10 years and a maximum of 25 years.[22]

Connecticut does have a medical marijuana program, and participants can possess a supply that can last for 1 month, though patients are not allowed to grow their own plants. To recommend marijuana, physicians or advanced practice registered nurses (APRNs) must have an active Connecticut medical license and DEA registration not subject to limitation with a bona fide physician-patient relationship with the patient. Additionally, authorized physicians must register with the Connecticut Department of Consumer Protection through their portal: https://portal.ct.gov/DCP/Medical-Marijuana-Program/How-to-Register#Physician.

Marijuana may be recommended for the following conditions:

- ALS (amyotrophic lateral sclerosis)
- Cachexia
- Cancer
- Cerebral palsy
- Chronic neuropathic pain
- Complex regional pain syndrome
- Crohn disease
- Cystic fibrosis
- Epilepsy
- Glaucoma
- Hydrocephalus
- HIV/AIDS
- Interstitial cystitis
- Intractable headache syndromes
- Irreversible spinal cord injury
- MALS (medial arcuate ligament syndrome)
- Multiple sclerosis
- Muscular dystrophy
- Neuropathic pain
- Osteogenesis imperfecta
- Parkinson disease
- Neuralgia
- Persistent muscle spasms
- Postlaminectomy syndrome
- PTSD (posttraumatic stress disorder)
- Severe psoriasis and psoriatic arthritis
- Rheumatoid arthritis
- Sickle cell disease
- Tourette syndrome
- Ulcerative colitis
- Vulvodynia

Additional medical conditions are pending approval by Connecticut's Department of Consumer Protection.

- From 20 g to 25 lb: Maximum punishment of 5 years of incarceration and a fine of up to $5000
- 25-2000 lb: Minimum sentence of 3 years in prison; maximum sentence of 15 years and a fine of up to $25 000
- 2-10 000 lb: Minimum sentence of 7 years in prison; maximum sentence of 30 years and a fine of up to $50 000
- 10 000 lb or more: Minimum sentence of 15 years in prison; maximum sentence of 30 years and a fine of up to $200 000

Cultivation of marijuana is a felony and has a similar punishment structure:

- <25 plants: Maximum punishment of 5 years of incarceration and a fine of up to $5000
- 25-300 plants: Maximum sentence of 15 years and fine of up to $10 000
- 300-2000 plants: Minimum sentence of 3 years in prison; maximum sentence of 15 years and a fine of up to $25 000
- 2000-10 000 plants: Minimum sentence of 7 years in prison; maximum sentence of 30 years and a fine of up to $50 000
- 10 000 or more plants: Minimum sentence of 15 years in prison; maximum sentence of 30 years and a fine of up to $200 000

Additionally, possession of hash or concentrates is a felony. Those convicted of possession of hash or concentrates may face up to 5 years in prison and/or a $5000 fine.[28]

In some jurisdictions, possession of small amounts of marijuana (20 g or less) has been decriminalized and may result in a fine. These jurisdictions include

- Alachua County
- Broward County
- Cocoa Beach
- Hallandale Beach
- Key West
- Miami Beach
- Miami-Dade County
- Orlando
- Osceola County
- Palm Beach County
- Port Richey
- Tampa
- Volusia County
- West Palm Beach County

Florida does have a medical marijuana program and strongly encourages the use of concentrates over flower, though flower marijuana is available. Authorized patients may possess upwards of 4 oz of flower marijuana or a 70-day supply of concentrates. Home cultivation is prohibited.[29] Properly licensed MDs or DOs may recommend marijuana to patients, provided they have registered with the state. To register, go to Florida's medical marijuana use registry: https://mmuregistry.flhealth.gov/.

Physicians may recommend marijuana for the following qualifying conditions:

- ALS (amyotrophic lateral sclerosis)
- Cancer
- Crohn disease
- Chronic pain due to a qualifying medical condition
- Epilepsy
- Glaucoma
- HIV/AIDS
- Multiple sclerosis
- Parkinson disease
- PTSD (posttraumatic stress disorder)
- Seizures
- Terminal illnesses (defined as <12 months to live)

Florida does not have a reciprocity program to accommodate medical marijuana patients from out of state.

For more information, please see the Web site for the Florida Department of Health Office of Medical Marijuana Use: https://knowthefactsmmj.com/.

Georgia

Georgia has relatively strict laws against the recreational use of marijuana. Possession of under 1 oz of flower marijuana is a misdemeanor punishable by incarceration of up to 1 year or a fine of $1000. Possession of more than 1 oz may result in a fine of $5000 and a prison sentence between 1 year (the state's mandatory minimum sentence) and 10 years. These penalties are similar for those who sell, cultivate, or intend to distribute under 10 lb of marijuana. Possession of any form of THC concentrate is a felony punishable by a minimum of 1 year of incarceration and a fine of up to $5000.[30]

Despite these harsh penalties at the state level, certain places across the state have decriminalized possession of 1 oz or less. Violators face a fine. The following jurisdictions have decriminalized marijuana:

- Atlanta
- Clarkston
- Forest Park
- Fulton County
- Kingsland
- Macon-Bibb County

- Savannah
- South Fulton

Georgia does have a medical marijuana program that allows qualifying individuals to possess no more than 20 fl oz of cannabis oil, provided the oil contains <5% THC.[31] Oil containing more than 5% is not legal, nor is flower cannabis containing more than 0.3% THC.

To obtain a card allowing one to obtain low THC oil, a physician with whom the patient has a doctor-patient relationship must determine that the patient has one of the qualifying conditions. Qualifying conditions include

- Autism spectrum disorder
- Alzheimer disease
- ALS (amyotrophic lateral sclerosis)
- Cancer
- Crohn disease
- Epidermolysis bullosa
- HIV/AIDS
- Intractable pain
- Mitochondrial disease
- Multiple sclerosis
- Parkinson disease
- PTSD (posttraumatic stress disorder)
- Severe or end-stage peripheral neuropathy
- Seizures
- Sickle cell disease
- Tourette syndrome

Additionally, some patients in hospice care may also qualify for Georgia's Low THC Oil Registry.

To apply, the physician must then fill out a waiver form and a certification form and then have the patient or the patient's legal guardian countersign. The information from these forms must then be entered into Georgia's Low THC Registry portal. Prior to entering this information, physicians must create an account with the Georgia Department of Public Health at this site: https://sendss.state.ga.us/sendss/!thc.thc_login.

Georgia does not have a reciprocity program to accommodate medical marijuana patients from out of state, but patients from other jurisdictions will be exempt from prosecution if they are found in possession of cannabis oil that contains 5% or less of THC, provided they have a registration card from their home state.[32]

For more information, please see the Web site for the Georgia Department of Health: https://dph.georgia.gov/low-thc-oil-faq-general-public.

Guam

Both recreational and medicinal marijuana are legal in Guam. For recreational users, possession is limited to 1 oz or 8 g of THC concentrate for individuals over the age of 21. These adults are also allowed to grow 6 plants for personal use, but only 3 plants can be flowering at any one time.[33] Guam residents who are over the age of 18 and enrolled in the territory's medical marijuana program are allowed to purchase and possess 2.5 oz and to grow 12 plants, but only 6 plants may be flowering at one time. Despite being legal, marijuana use is prohibited in public places, and it is illegal to drive under the influence of THC.

To recommend marijuana to a patient, physicians must be licensed in Guam to prescribe and administer drugs subject to the Guam Uniform Controlled Substances Act.[34] They must also have a bona fide doctor-patient relationship, and the patient must have a condition for which the physician feels medical marijuana may provide relief. Such conditions include

- Cancer
- Epilepsy
- Glaucoma
- HIV/AIDS
- Multiple sclerosis
- PTSD (posttraumatic stress disorder)
- Rheumatoid arthritis
- Spinal cord injury

For more information, visit the Web site for Guam's medical cannabis program: https://dphss.guam.gov/medical-cannabis-information-2/.

Hawaii

Medicinal marijuana is legal in Hawaii, but recreational use is not. Possession of small amounts of marijuana (3 g or less) has been decriminalized and is punishable by a violation of $130. Possession of amount >3 g but <1 lb is a misdemeanor, while possession of more than 1 lb of marijuana is a felony. Possession of <0.125 oz of concentrate is a misdemeanor, while possession of that amount or more is a felony. Misdemeanor and felony possession charges carry the following punishments:

Flower marijuana:
- More than 3 g; <1 oz: Maximum jail sentence of 30 days and $1000 fine

- 1 oz to 1 lb: Maximum period of incarceration of 1 year and up to a $2000 fine
- 1 lb or more: Maximum period of incarceration of 5 years and up to a $10 000 fine

Concentrated THC:

- 0.125-1 oz: Maximum period of incarceration of 10 years and up to a $25 000 fine
- 1 oz or more: Maximum period of incarceration of 20 years and up to a $50 000 fine

Cultivation of more than 25 cannabis plants or any number of plants on property that is not your own is also a felony. Punishment may include the following:

- 25-49 plants on your property: A maximum of 5 years of imprisonment and a fine of $10 000
- 50-99 pants on your property: A maximum of 10 years of imprisonment and a fine of $25 000
- 100 plants or more on your property: A maximum of 20 years of imprisonment and a fine of $50 000
- 24 or fewer plants not on your property: A maximum of 10 years of imprisonment and a fine of $25 000
- 25 or more plants not on your property: A maximum of 20 years of imprisonment and a fine of $50 000[35]

Patients who are enrolled in the state's medical cannabis program can possess up to 4 oz of usable marijuana at one time. Additionally, home cultivation is allowed for patients who have registered. They may grow up to 7 plants—whether mature or immature—at one time.[36]

Hawaii-licensed physicians (MDs and DOs) and APRNs who are allowed to prescribe controlled substances are allowed to certify, in writing, that it is their professional opinion that a patient with whom they have a doctor-patient relationship has a debilitating illness and their use of medical cannabis outweighs any health risks associated with the use of the drug. Qualifying debilitating illnesses include

- ALS (amyotrophic lateral sclerosis)
- Cachexia
- Cancer
- Chronic pain
- Crohn disease
- Epilepsy
- Glaucoma
- HIV/AIDS
- Lupus
- Multiple sclerosis
- Nausea

- Persistent muscle spasms
- PTSD (posttraumatic stress disorder)
- Rheumatoid arthritis
- Seizures

Out-of-state patients who are visiting Hawaii may apply for two 60-day permits per calendar year, which will allow them access to the state's dispensaries. Eligible patients must have a valid card from their home state and a valid government-issued means of identification. The portal to apply for the permit can be found here: https://health.hawaii. gov/medicalcannabisregistry/travel/.

For more information about the state's program or the registration process for in-state patients, please see the site for the Medical Cannabis Registry Program on the Hawaii Department of Health's Web site: https:// health.hawaii.gov/medicalcannabisregistry/providers/.

Idaho

Idaho does not have a medicinal marijuana program, and the use of virtually any cannabis product is illegal, though cannabis-based medications that have received FDA approval can be prescribed to patients. Even CBD products that would be legal under federal law as specified in the 2018 Farm Bill—that is, hemp derived and <0.3% THC— are prohibited under Idaho law. A 2015 opinion from Idaho's Attorney General Lawrence G. Wasden states that CBD products, to be legal, must:

1. Contain 0.0% THC
2. "Be derived or produced from (a) mature stalks of the plant, (b) fiber produced from the stalks, (c) oil or cake made from the seeds or the achene of such plant, (d) any other compound, manufacture, salt, derivative, mixture, or preparation of the mature stalks, or (e) the sterilized seed of such plant which is incapable of germination"[37]

Patients from other states should note that there are major penalties for possession of cannabis. Possession of 3 oz or less is a misdemeanor. Offenders could be incarcerated for up to 1 year and may be fined $1000. Possession of more than 3 oz is a felony, and violators could be incarcerated for up to 5 years and fined $10 000.

Cultivation is also a felony that carries a potential fine of up to $50 000 and mandatory minimum sentencing ranging from 1 to 5 years. For <50 plants, the mandatory minimum sentence is 1 year. For 50-99 plants, the mandatory minimum sentence is 3 years. For 100 or more plants, the mandatory minimum sentence is 5 years.[38]

Illinois

Illinois has a robust medicinal cannabis program. For patients over the age of 21, they may purchase 2.5 oz of flower marijuana in a 14-day period. Patients over 18, but under 21, are prohibited from purchasing cannabis preparations meant to be smoked or vaped. Home cultivation, however, is allowed, though patients enrolled in the state's medicinal program may only grow 5 plants for personal use.

For adults over the age of 21 who are not participating in the state's medical cannabis program, they may possess 30 g of flower marijuana, 5 g of THC concentrate, or 500 mg of THC that has been infused into a product (edible, lozenge, tincture, etc.), while residents of other states may possess half of these amounts—15 g, 2.5 g, and 250 mg, respectively. Residents who are not part of the medical program are prohibited from cultivating marijuana, though cultivation for 5 plants or less is a violation that results in a $200 fine.

Despite these liberal policies, failing to abide by the law can result in imprisonment and steep fines. A first-time offender who is found to be in possession of more than the state's legal limit for possession but under 100 g—that is, 30-100 g—will face misdemeanor charges that could result in a maximum fine of $2500 and a term of imprisonment of up to 1 year. A subsequent possession charge within the same range (30-100 g) is a felony that could result in up to 3 years of incarceration and a $25 000 fine. Individuals found in possession of larger amounts will face felony charges and could see more serious ramifications:

- 100-500 g: Up to 3 years of incarceration and a maximum fine of $25 000
- 500-2000 g: Up to 5 years of incarceration and a maximum fine of $25 000
- 2000-5000 g: Up to 7 years of incarceration and a maximum fine of $25 000
- More than 5000 g: Up to 15 years of incarceration and a maximum fine of $25 000

It is also a felony to grow more than 5 plants. Violators face similarly harsh consequences:

- 5-20 plants: Up to 3 years of incarceration and a maximum fine of $25 000
- 21-50 plants: Up to 5 years of incarceration and a maximum fine of $50 000
- 51-200 plants: Up to 7 years of incarceration and a maximum fine of $150 000
- More than 200 plants: A minimum sentence of 6 years and up to 30 years of incarceration, as well as a maximum fine of $200 000[39]

It remains illegal to consume marijuana in public places or to drive under the influence of THC.

Properly licensed MDs, DOs, APNS, and physician assistants may recommend cannabis so long as they have a bona fide physician-patient relationship with the patient, they complete an in-person assessment of the patient, and the patient has one of the following debilitating conditions:

- Autism
- Alzheimer disease
- ALS (amyotrophic lateral sclerosis)
- Anorexia nervosa
- Arnold-Chiari malformation
- Cancer
- Cachexia/wasting syndrome
- Causalgia
- Chronic inflammatory demyelinating polyneuropathy
- Chronic pain
- Crohn disease
- CRPS (complex regional pain syndrome Type II)
- Dystonia
- Ehlers-Danlos syndrome
- Epilepsy
- Fibrous dysplasia
- Glaucoma
- Hepatitis C
- HIV/AIDS
- Hydrocephalus
- Hydromyelia
- Interstitial cystitis
- IBD (inflammatory bowel disease)
- Lupus
- Migraines
- Multiple sclerosis
- Muscular dystrophy
- Myasthenia gravis
- Myoclonus
- Nail-patella syndrome
- Neuro-Behcet autoimmune disease
- Neurofibromatosis
- Neuropathy
- Osteoarthritis
- Parkinson disease
- PKD (polycystic kidney disease)
- Postconcussion syndrome
- PTSD (posttraumatic stress disorder)
- Reflex sympathetic dystrophy

- Residual limb pain
- Rheumatoid arthritis
- Seizures
- Severe fibromyalgia
- Sjögren syndrome
- Spinal cord diseases
- Spinal cord injuries
- Spinocerebellar ataxia
- Superior canal dehiscence syndrome
- Syringomyelia
- Tarlov cysts
- Tourette syndrome
- Traumatic brain injury
- Ulcerative colitis

Illinois does not have a reciprocity program to accommodate medical marijuana patients from out of state.

For more information about the state's medicinal cannabis program, please visit the Illinois Department of Public Health Web site and the page for physicians specifically: http://www.dph.illinois.gov/topics-services/prevention-wellness/medical-cannabis/physician-information.

Indiana

Indiana does not have a medicinal cannabis program, and the adult use of any cannabis product with a THC content >0.3% is illegal. Possession of <30 g of flower marijuana or <5 g of concentrate is a misdemeanor punishable by up to 180 days in jail and a fine of $1000. If one has a prior offense, possession of the same amount could lead to incarceration for up to 1 year and a fine of $5000. Possession of 30 g or more of flower marijuana or 5 g or more of concentrate, as well as a prior drug offense, or cultivation of more than 30 g without a prior offense, is a felony that could be punishable of up to 30 months of incarceration and a fine of $10 000. Cultivation of more than 10 lb is also a felony that could be punishable by up to 6 years of incarceration and a fine of $10 000.[40]

CBD products sold in compliance with the 2018 Farm Bill—that is, hemp derived and containing <0.3% THC—were legalized by Governor Eric Holcomb in 2018 to provide treatment to patients with treatment-resistant epileptic conditions, including such as Dravet syndrome and Lennox-Gastaut syndrome.[41]

Iowa

Iowa is home to a medicinal marijuana program, but the state's program prohibits the use of flower cannabis as a medicine and has limited the amount of THC concentrations in extracts to 3%.[42] Use of cannabis that contains more than 3% THC, meanwhile, is universally a misdemeanor. First-time offenders can receive a maximum sentence of up to 6 months imprisonment and a fine of $1000. Second-time offenders can receive a maximum sentence of up to 1 year of imprisonment and a fine of $1875. Subsequent offenders can receive a maximum sentence of up to 2 years of imprisonment and a fine of $6250.

The unlicensed cultivation of marijuana is a felony. The maximum penalties are as follows:

- 50 kg or less: 5 years of incarceration and up to $7500 in fines
- 50-100 kg: 10 years of incarceration and up to $50 000 in fines
- 100-1000 kg: 25 years of incarceration and up to $100 000 in fines
- More than 1000 kg: 50 years of incarceration and up to $1 000 000 in fines[43]

For physicians, there are no specific training courses that must be completed to recommend cannabis to patients. Physicians must only be properly licensed MDs and DOs and provide information to the patient about the risks/benefits of cannabis use. Additionally, physicians may only recommend cannabis to patients with the following qualifying conditions:

- Amyotrophic lateral sclerosis
- Autism spectrum disorder
- Cachexia
- Cancer
- Chronic pain
- Crohn disease
- Epilepsy
- Multiple sclerosis
- Cancer-related nausea
- Parkinson disease
- Terminal illnesses
- Ulcerative colitis

For more information, please see the medical cannabidiol page for physicians on the Iowa Department of Public Health's Web site: https://idph.iowa.gov/omc/For-Physicians.

Residents of other states who have enrolled in their home state's cannabis program may not procure cannabis from dispensaries in Iowa; they are merely allowed to possess cannabis preparations containing <3% THC obtained through their state's program. Patients and caregivers are both allowed to register with Iowa's medicinal cannabis program and in the state of Minnesota as a visiting qualified patient or primary caregiver.[44]

For patients interested in learning more about the state's program, direct them to the Department's site for the public: https://idph.iowa.gov/omc/Patient-Registration.

of possession for <2.5 lb for the third time may be punished by up to 2 years of imprisonment and a maximum fine of $2500. Those convicted of possession for <2.5 lb for any instance subsequent to the third time may be punished by up to 8 years of imprisonment and a maximum fine of $5000. Possession of more than 2.5 lb and <60 lb is still not a felony and is punishable by a fine of $30 000 and 8 years of imprisonment. Possession of more than 60 lb of marijuana is a felony. The punishment is severe.

Similarly, the penalties for the unlicensed cultivation of marijuana are extreme. A first-time offender for any amount will receive a mandatory minimum sentence of 5 years of incarceration. The maximum is 30 years and a fine of $30 000. Second-time offenders face a minimum of 10 years of incarceration and a maximum punishment of 60 years and a fine of $100 000.[48]

In the city of New Orleans, simple possession of marijuana has been largely decriminalized by New Orleans City Ordinance 31148. According to the ordinance, first-time offenders receive a verbal warning, second-time offenders receive a written warning, third-time offenders receive a fine of $50, and subsequent offenses result in fines of $100. The ordinance does not define "simple possession," but it seems reasonable to assume that 14 g or less qualifies as such.[49]

Maine

Both recreational and medicinal marijuana are legal in Maine for adults over the age of 21. As in all jurisdictions, public use is prohibited, as is drugged driving. Patients under the age of 21, but 18 years of age or older, may participate in the state's medical marijuana program only. For recreational users, possession of up to 2.5 oz of flower marijuana or 5 g of concentrate is allowed. Possession of larger amounts of marijuana is a crime resulting in:

- 6 months of incarceration and a $1000 fine (2.5-8 oz flower marijuana)
- 1 year of incarceration and a $2000 fine (0.5-1 lb flower marijuana or more than 5 g concentrate)
- 5 years of incarceration and a $5000 fine (1-20 lb)
- 10 years of incarceration and a $20 000 fine (more than 20 lb)

Up to 3 plants may be grown for personal use. Cultivating larger amounts is a crime resulting in:

- 1 year of incarceration and a $2000 fine (4-99 plants)
- 5 years of incarceration and a $5000 fine (100-500 plants)
- 10 years of incarceration and a $20 000 fine (more than 500 plants)

Aggravated circumstances, like prior convictions, may increase penalty severity.[50]

Mainers participating in the state's medical marijuana program may possess up to 2.5 oz and are authorized to cultivate up to 6 mature plants. Medical providers who are in good standing with the appropriate state licensing board can recommend marijuana at their discretion.

Maine does have a reciprocity program to accommodate some medical marijuana patients from out of state. To learn which states have been approved or for more information about medical marijuana in Maine, please see the Web site for the Office of Marijuana Policy: https://www.maine.gov/dafs/omp/medical-use.

Maryland

Maryland does have a medical cannabis program, and participants can possess a 30-day supply of marijuana. Flower and infused products, defined as oil, wax, ointment, salve, tincture, capsule, suppository, dermal patch, cartridge, or other product, but *not food items*, are allowed under Maryland law.[51] For recreational users, possession of small amounts of marijuana (<10 g) has been decriminalized and may result in a $100 fine. The possession of larger amounts of marijuana (provided it is under 50 lb) is a misdemeanor offense punishable by imprisonment of up to 1 year and a fine of $1000. Possession of more than 50 lb is a felony punishable by a mandatory minimum sentence of 5 years and a fine of $100 000.

Cultivation of marijuana is illegal, even for patients enrolled in the state's medicinal program. The punishment is based on the total weight of the plants.[52]

To recommend cannabis, MDs (including dentists, podiatrists) and registered nurses (RNs) must have an active, unrestricted license and be in good standing with state boards. Properly licensed RNs must also have unrestricted licenses to practice as nurse practitioners or nurse midwives.[53] Additionally, medical professionals must register with the Maryland Medical Cannabis Commission at the following site: https://mmcc.maryland.gov/Pages/physicians.aspx.

Cannabis may be recommended to treat the following qualifying conditions:

- Anorexia
- Cachexia or wasting syndrome
- Chronic pain
- Glaucoma
- Nausea
- PTSD (posttraumatic stress disorder)
- Seizures

- Severe or persistent muscle spasms

Additionally, cannabis may be used to treat severe conditions for which other treatment options have been ineffective.

Maryland does not have a reciprocity program to accommodate some medical marijuana patients from out of state.

To learn more about the state's program, see the Maryland Medical Cannabis Commission Web site: https://mmcc.maryland.gov/Pages/home. aspx.

Massachusetts

Both recreational and medicinal marijuana are legal in Massachusetts for adults over the age of 21. Patients under the age of 21, but 18 years of age or older, may participate in the state's medical marijuana program only. For recreational users, possession of 1 oz or 5 g of concentrate is allowed. Possession of more than 5 g but <1 oz of concentrate is a civil offense resulting in a $100 fine. Within a residence, one may have 10 oz and grow up to 6 plants for personal use.

Possession of more than 1 oz of flower marijuana in public is a misdemeanor. First-time offenders may be incarcerated for up to 6 months and/or face fines of up to $500. Second-time offenders face significantly harsher penalties and may be incarcerated for up to 2 years and fined up to $2000. Possession of more than 1 oz of concentrate is a crime punishable by up to 1 year of incarceration and a fine of up to $1000. Public use is prohibited, as is drugged driving.[54]

Participants in Massachusetts' medical marijuana program can purchase/possess no more than 10 oz of marijuana every 2 months. Patients or caregivers may also cultivate a limited number of plants, "sufficient to maintain a 60-day supply of marijuana and shall require cultivation and storage only in an enclosed, locked area."[55] To participate in the program, patients must have one of the following qualifying conditions:

- ALS (amyotrophic lateral sclerosis)
- Cancer
- Crohn disease
- Glaucoma
- HIV/AIDS
- Hepatitis C
- Multiple sclerosis
- Parkinson disease

A qualifying physician may also determine that patients not afflicted by one of the conditions noted above could benefit from the use of marijuana.

Only MDs, DOs, and CNPs with active full licenses with no prescribing restrictions, a Massachusetts Controlled Substances Registration, and at least one established place to practice in the state can recommend marijuana to patients. CNPs must hold board authorization by the Massachusetts Board of Registration in Nursing to practice as a CNP in the state.[56] Additionally, all practitioners must register with the state's Medical Use of Marijuana Program at the following site: https://www.mass.gov/how-to/register-as-a-certifying-health-care-provider-with-the-medical-use-of-marijuana-program.

Massachusetts does not have a reciprocity program to accommodate medical marijuana patients from out of state.

To learn more about the state's program, see the Massachusetts state Web site, https://www.mass.gov/orgs/medical-use-of-marijuana-program, or visit the site of the Massachusetts Patient Policy Alliance: https://www.compassionforpatients.com/.

Michigan

Both recreational and medicinal marijuana are legal in Michigan for adults over the age of 21. Patients under the age of 21, but 18 years of age or older, may participate in the state's medical marijuana program only. Within the state of Michigan, possession of 2.5 oz of flower marijuana or 15 g of concentrate is allowed in public. Within a residence, one may have 10 oz and grow up to 12 plants for personal use. Public use is prohibited, as is drugged driving. Possession of more than 2.5 oz, but <5 oz, is a civil infraction for first-time violators, who may be fined $500. Second-time violators may be charged with another civil infraction and fined $1000. Third-time violations and all subsequent violations are misdemeanors punishable by a fine of not more than $2000. Possession of more than 5 oz is a misdemeanor. Violators will not be subject to imprisonment unless "the violation was habitual, willful, and for a commercial purpose or the violation involved violence."[57]

To qualify for Michigan's medical marijuana program, patients must receive a recommendation from a licensed physician (either MD or DO) with whom they have a bona fide physician-patient relationship, and they must have one of the following qualifying conditions:

- Alzheimer disease
- ALS (amyotrophic lateral sclerosis)
- Arthritis
- Autism spectrum disorder
- Cachexia
- Cancer
- Cerebral palsy
- Colitis

- Chronic pain
- Crohn disease
- Glaucoma
- Hepatitis C
- HIV/AIDS
- IBD (inflammatory bowel disease)
- Nail-patella syndrome
- Nausea
- OCD (obsessive compulsive disorder)
- Parkinson disease
- PTSD (posttraumatic stress disorder)
- Seizures
- Severe and persistent muscle spasms
- Spinal cord injury
- Tourette syndrome
- Ulcerative colitis

Michigan does offer reciprocity to patients from other jurisdictions, but only if said jurisdiction allows reciprocity.

For more information, please see the Web site for the Michigan Medical Marihuana Program: https://www.michigan.gov/lara/0,4601,7-154-89334_79571_79575_79583---,00.html.

Minnesota

Minnesota does have a medical cannabis program, but recreational use is illegal. It has been decriminalized, however. Possession of marijuana in the amount of 42.5 g or less is a misdemeanor punishable by only a fine of no more than $200, provided one is not in one's vehicle. Possession of more than 1.4 g, but <42.5 g, within the interior of one's vehicle (ie, not the trunk) is a misdemeanor punishable by a fine of $1000 and a 90-day period of incarceration. Possession of more than 42.5 g is a felony, and violators may face the following maximum penalties:

- More than 42.5 g and <10 kg: 5 years of incarceration and a fine of $10 000
- 10-50 kg: 20 years of incarceration and a fine of $250 000
- 50-100 kg: 25 years of incarceration and a fine of $500 000
- 100 kg or more: 30 years of incarceration and a fine of $1 000 000

Cultivation of marijuana is illegal, even for patients enrolled in the state's medicinal cannabis program. The punishment is based on the total weight of the plants.[58]

For patients participating in the state's medical program, they may purchase a 30-day supply of cannabis. However, Minnesota's medical cannabis program limits patients to extracts only; the use of flower marijuana is prohibited.

Those authorized to recommend cannabis include MDs, DOs, APRNs, and physician assistants. On top of having these credentials, they must be licensed to practice in the state of Minnesota, have a bona fide physician-patient relationship with the patient they are treating, and register at the following Web site: https://www.health.state.mn.us/people/cannabis/index.html. Additionally, they can only recommend cannabis to treat the following conditions:

- ALS (amyotrophic lateral sclerosis)
- Cancer
- Cachexia
- Crohn disease
- Glaucoma
- HIV/AIDS
- Multiple sclerosis
- Nausea or severe vomiting
- Seizures
- Severe and persistent muscle spasms
- Severe or chronic pain
- Tourette syndrome
- Terminal illnesses with a probable life expectancy of <1 year, provided the treatment produces cachexia, chronic pain, and nausea

Minnesota does not have a reciprocity program to accommodate patients who have enrolled in the program of another state.

For more information, see the Web site for the Minnesota Department of Health: https://www.health.state.mn.us/people/cannabis/data/index.html.

Mississippi

Recreational marijuana is not legal in Mississippi, but first-time possession of small amounts of flower marijuana (30 g or less) has been decriminalized. Violators face a fine of $250. Second-time possession of a similar amount is a misdemeanor punishable by 5-60 days in jail and a fine of $250. Subsequent offenses are also misdemeanors and result in a jail sentence of between 5 days and 6 months, as well as a $1000 fine. Possession of 30 g or less in one's vehicle (trunk excluded) is a misdemeanor with a maximum penalty of 90 days in jail and a $1000 fine.

Possession of more than 30 g of flower marijuana is a felony punishable in the following way:

- 30-250 g: Maximum term of imprisonment of 3 years and a fine of $1000
- 250-500 g: Minimum term of imprisonment of 2 years, maximum of 8 years; $50 000 fine

- 0.5-1 kg: Minimum term of imprisonment of 4 years, maximum of 16 years; $250 000 fine
- 1-5 kg: Minimum term of imprisonment of 6 years, maximum of 24 years; $500 000 fine
- 5 kg or more: Minimum term of imprisonment of 10 years, maximum of 30 years; $1 000 000 fine

Possession of even 0.1 g of THC concentrate is potentially a felony punishable by up to 1 year of incarceration and a fine of $1000. Possession of more than 0.1 g is a felony punishable the following way:

- 0.1-2 g: Maximum term of imprisonment of 3 years and a fine of $50 000
- 2-10 g: Maximum term of imprisonment of 8 years and a $250 000 fine
- 10-30 g: Maximum term of imprisonment of 20 years; $500 000 fine
- 30 g or more: Maximum term of imprisonment of 30 years and a $1 000 000 fine

Cultivation of marijuana is illegal. The penalty is based on the total weight of the plants.[59]

Mississippi does not currently have a medical cannabis program. Following the passage of Harper Grace's Law in 2014, some patients and their caretakers can possess, administer, and consume low-THC cannabis formulations that contain more than 15% CBD and no more than 0.5% THC. Physicians licensed to practice in Mississippi may obtain formulations that comply with the law through the University of Mississippi's Center for National Production Research and must administer or supervise the administration of the formulation to qualifying patients. Currently, the only conditions for which physicians can provide these formulations of cannabis are epilepsy or seizures.[60]

Mississippi's CBD program is not open to residents of other states, and the state of Mississippi does not recognize the validity of other jurisdictions' medical cannabis programs.

Missouri

Missouri has a medical marijuana program, but recreational use is illegal. Possession of 35 g or less is a misdemeanor; possession of more than 35 g is a felony punishable by incarceration of up to 7 years of imprisonment and a fine of up to $10 000. Possession of more than 10 g, but <35 g, is punishable by up to 7 years of incarceration and a fine of $2000. Possession of 10 g or less is punishable by a $500 fine for first-time offenders and 1 year of incarceration and a fine of up to $2000 for subsequent offenses.

Unless one is participating in the state's medical marijuana program, marijuana cultivation is a felony. The penalty for growing 35 g or less is up to 4 years of imprisonment and a maximum fine of $10 000. The penalty for growing more than 35 g of marijuana is a maximum fine of $10 000 and up to 10 years of incarceration.[61]

The following three cities in Missouri have decriminalized marijuana possession of 35 g or less: Columbia, Kansas City, and St. Louis. Violators face fines of $250, $25, and $100-$500, respectively.

Patients participating in Missouri's medical marijuana program can buy up to 4 oz of flower at one time or its equivalent in a 30-day period. They may also choose to grow up to 6 of their own plants. There is an additional $100 fee for this privilege, and patients must abide by security regulations outlined in 19 CSR 30-95.030(4).[62]

Patients with the following conditions may be eligible for Missouri's medicinal marijuana program:

- ALS (amyotrophic lateral sclerosis)
- Alzheimer disease
- Autism spectrum disorder
- Cachexia
- Cancer
- Crohn disease
- Chronic pain or neuropathy
- Epilepsy
- Glaucoma
- Hepatitis C
- HIV/AIDS
- Huntington disease
- IBD (inflammatory bowel disease)
- Intractable migraines
- Multiple sclerosis
- Opioid substitution
- Parkinson disease
- PTSD (posttraumatic stress disorder) or other debilitating psychiatric disorders
- Tourette syndrome
- Sickle cell anemia
- Seizures

Additionally, qualifying physicians may recommend marijuana should they feel it will ameliorate symptoms or conditions associated with any terminal illness or with any chronic, debilitating medical condition. At this time, only MDs and DOs licensed to practice and in good standing in the state of Missouri may choose to recommend marijuana to patients.

Missouri does not have a reciprocity program to accommodate medical marijuana patients from out of state.

For more information, see the Missouri Department of Health & Senior Service's page on Medical Marijuana Regulation here: https://health.mo.gov/safety/medical-marijuana/index.php.

Montana

It is not legal to consume marijuana in Montana unless it has been recommended by a medical professional. For those who are not participating in Montana's medical program, possession of 60 g or less of flower marijuana or 1 g or less of THC concentrate is a misdemeanor that may result in a maximum fine of $500 and incarceration for up to 6 months for first-time offenders. Subsequent violations may lead to fines of up to $1000 and 3 years of incarceration. In Missoula County, first-time possession for under 60 g of flower marijuana or 1 g or less of concentrate has been decriminalized and violators may face fines of up to $500. Possession of larger amounts of marijuana is a felony punishable by up to 5 years of imprisonment and $50 000 in fines. Cultivation of any number of plants is also a felony that may result in a $50 000 fine. Terms of imprisonment vary depending on the number of plants.[63]

Patients participating in the state's medicinal program may possess 1 oz of usable marijuana, provided they have named a provider. Those who have not named a provider may possess up to 4 mature plants, 4 immature plants, and 1 oz of usable marijuana. MDs or DOs with a license to practice medicine in Montana must have a bona fide physician-patient relationship with patients to recommend marijuana, and may only do so for the following qualifying conditions:

- Cachexia
- Cancer
- Crohn disease
- Epilepsy
- Glaucoma
- HIV/AIDS
- Intractable nausea or vomiting
- Peripheral neuropathy
- PTSD (posttraumatic stress disorder)
- Severe and chronic pain
- Severe and persistent muscle spasms

Patients who are under hospice care may also qualify.

Montana does not have a reciprocity program to accommodate medical marijuana patients from out of state.

For more information, see the Montana Medical Marijuana Program page: https://dphhs.mt.gov/marijuana.

Nebraska

There is no medical cannabis program of any kind in Nebraska, but Legislative Bill 657 brings state law into compliance with federal law regarding hemp-derived CBD containing <0.3% THC.[64]

Cannabis defined as "marijuana" (containing more than 0.3% THC) is considered a controlled substance in the state of Nebraska. First-time possession of <1 oz of flower marijuana, while illegal, has been decriminalized and may result in a fine of $300. Subsequent instances of possession of <1 oz of marijuana count as a misdemeanor and may result in a few days in jail and a fine of $500. Possession of more than 1 oz but <1 lb is also a misdemeanor and may result in a maximum term of imprisonment of 3 months and a fine of $500. Possession of more than 1 lb of marijuana is a felony and may result in a maximum term of imprisonment of 5 years and a fine of $10 000. Possession of any amount of THC concentrate is also a felony and may result in a maximum term of imprisonment of 5 years and a fine of $10 000.

Cultivation of marijuana is illegal. The penalty is based on the total weight of the plants.[65]

Nevada

Recreational and medical marijuana are both legal in Nevada. Adults aged 21 and older may possess up to 1 oz of marijuana (or up to 3.5 g of concentrate). It remains illegal to consume marijuana in public places or to drive under the influence of THC. Additionally, possession of more than the allowed amount is a misdemeanor offense punishable by a $600 fine.[66]

Individuals who are not enrolled in the state's medical marijuana program can cultivate 6 plants, provided they reside 25 miles or more from an operating dispensary, but plants must be grown in a secure, indoor location. Individuals who are enrolled in the state's medical program may grow up to 12 plants, provided they reside 25 miles or more from an operating dispensary with the following two caveats: New patients may be authorized to grow their own 12 plants even if they reside within 25 miles of a dispensary if no dispensary within their county of residence carries a specific cultivar for their illness or if they are incapable of traveling due to illness or lack of transportation, according to Chapter 453A.718.2(b) of the Nevada Administrative Code.[67] As is the case with individuals cultivating marijuana for nonmedicinal reasons, all plants must be grown in a secure, indoor location. Failure to adhere to these laws is a felony with following penalty structure:

- 12 plants or more: Minimum of 1 year of incarceration, maximum of 4 years; $5000 maximum fine
- 100-2000 lb: Minimum of 1 year of incarceration, maximum of 5 years; $25 000 maximum fine
- 2000-10 000 lb: Minimum of 2 year of incarceration, maximum of 10 years; $50 000 maximum fine
- 10 000 lb or more: Minimum of 5 year of incarceration, maximum of life in prison; $200 000 maximum fine[68]

Any health care provider who is currently licensed to write a prescription for a chronic or debilitating medical condition and who is in good standing with his or her state Board may recommend marijuana for any of the following conditions:

- Anorexia
- Anxiety
- Autism spectrum disorder
- Autoimmune disorders
- Cachexia
- Cancer
- Chronic pain
- Glaucoma
- HIV/AIDS
- Opioid dependency
- Muscle spasms
- Neuropathic conditions
- PTSD (posttraumatic stress disorder)
- Seizures
- Severe nausea
- Severe pain

Patients may petition the Division to include additional conditions beyond those listed above, pursuant to Nevada Revised Statute 453A.710.[69] The Division will approve or deny this petition within 180 days.

Out-of-state patients with valid medical cannabis cards may purchase marijuana in a Nevada medical dispensary, provided they are enrolled with programs from the following jurisdictions:

- Alaska
- Arizona
- Arkansas
- California
- Connecticut
- District of Columbia
- Delaware
- Ely Shoshone Tribe
- Hawaii
- Illinois

- Maine
- Maryland
- Massachusetts
- Michigan
- Minnesota
- Montana
- New Hampshire
- New Jersey
- New York
- New Mexico
- Ohio
- Oregon
- Pennsylvania
- Pyramid Lake Paiute Tribe
- Rhode Island
- Vermont
- Washington
- Yerington Paiute Tribe
- Winnemucca Indian Colony[70]

For more information on the state's medicinal marijuana program, please see the Department of Health and Human Services Nevada Division of Public and Behavioral Health Web site: http://dpbh.nv.gov/Reg/Medical_Marijuana/.

New Hampshire

New Hampshire is home to a medical cannabis program, but the recreational use of marijuana is not legal even if it has been decriminalized for offenders who are found in possession of 0.75 oz or less of flower marijuana or 5 g or less of THC concentrate. First- and second-time offenders face a fine of $100. Third-time offenders face a fine of $300, provided the period of time between the first violation and the third violation is <3 years. Fourth-time offenders face misdemeanor charges and a fine of $1200, but no jail time, provided all four violations occur within 3 years. Possession of more than 0.75 oz or more than 5 g of concentrate is a misdemeanor punishable by 1 year of incarceration and a maximum fine of $350.

Cultivation of marijuana is illegal, even for patients enrolled in the state's medicinal cannabis program. The punishment is based on the total weight of the plants.[71]

Patients who have enrolled in the state's program can possess 2 oz of cannabis that can be purchased at a medicinal dispensary. Any physician, PA, or APRN who is licensed to practice in New Hampshire is permitted to issue a patient written certification for the state's medical cannabis program. Qualifying conditions include

- ALS (amyotrophic lateral sclerosis)
- Alzheimer disease
- Cachexia
- Cancer
- Chemotherapy-induced anorexia
- Chronic pain
- Chronic pancreatitis
- Crohn disease
- Ehlers-Danlos syndrome
- Elevated intraocular pressure
- Epilepsy
- Glaucoma
- Hepatitis C
- HIV/AIDS
- Lupus
- Multiple sclerosis
- Muscular dystrophy
- Nausea or vomiting
- Parkinson disease
- Persistent muscle spasms
- PTSD (posttraumatic stress disorder)
- Seizures
- Severe pain
- Spinal cord injury or disease
- Traumatic brain injury or disease

New Hampshire does have a reciprocity program. Out-of-state patients may not purchase cannabis at dispensaries in the state, but they will not be charged for possession if they have one of the above qualifying conditions and a valid card authorizing them to possess medical cannabis from another jurisdiction.

For more information, see the state's Therapeutic Cannabis Program Web site: https://www.dhhs.nh.gov/oos/tcp/index.htm.

New Jersey

New Jersey is home to a medical marijuana program, but recreational use is prohibited. Possession of 50 g or less of flower marijuana or 5 g or less of THC concentrate may result in disorderly person charges, fines up to $1000, and a term of incarceration of up to 6 months. Individuals found to be in possession of larger amounts may be charged with a crime and could face fines of up to $25 000. The maximum period of imprisonment for possession of more than 50 g of flower marijuana is 1.5 years, while the maximum for possession of more than 5 g of THC concentrate is 6 months. Cultivation is a crime, and punishment may be as follows:

- <10 plants: Mandatory minimum term of imprisonment of 3 years and up to 5 years; $25 000 fine
- 10-50 plants: Mandatory minimum term of imprisonment of 5 years and up to 10 years; $150 000 fine
- More than 50 plants: Mandatory minimum term of imprisonment of 10 years and up to 20 years; $300 000 fine[72]

The law prohibiting cultivation extends to those enrolled in New Jersey's medical marijuana program. There is no exception.

Patients may purchase up to 3 oz of marijuana per month at state-operated dispensaries. To enroll, patients must be recommended marijuana by an MD or DO in good standing and licensed to practice in the state of New Jersey with whom the patient has a bona fide physician-patient relationship. Additionally, physicians must register with the New Jersey Medicinal Marijuana Program. To register, follow the instructions found through the state's portal here: https://njmmp.nj.gov/njmmp/jsp/physRegistration.jsp.

Physicians can recommend marijuana to patients with terminal illnesses, so long as the physician has determined that the patient has less than a year to live. Additionally, physicians can recommend marijuana for the following qualifying conditions:

- ALS (amyotrophic lateral sclerosis)
- Anxiety
- Cancer
- Chronic pain
- Crohn disease
- Dysmenorrhea
- Epilepsy
- Glaucoma
- HIV/AIDS
- IBD (inflammatory bowel disorder)
- Migraines
- Multiple sclerosis
- Muscular dystrophy
- Opioid dependency
- PTSD (posttraumatic stress disorder)
- Seizure disorders
- Spasticity disorders
- Tourette disorder

The state of New Jersey allows out-of-state patients to bring marijuana into the state, provided they have a valid card authorizing them to possess medical marijuana from another jurisdiction.

For more information, visit the Web site for the state's Division of Medical Marijuana: https://www.nj.gov/health/medicalmarijuana/.

New Mexico

It is not legal to consume marijuana in New Mexico unless it has been recommended by a medical professional. Despite being illegal, decriminalization efforts have made the possession of small amounts of flower marijuana (under 0.5 oz) a violation that results in a $50 fine. In the cities of Albuquerque and Santa Fe, marijuana has been decriminalized further, and possession of up to 1 oz of marijuana is punishable by a $25 fine.

Possession of between 0.5 and 1.0 oz of marijuana is a misdemeanor. First-time offenders may be incarcerated for up to 15 days and fined $100, while subsequent offenders could be jailed for upwards of 1 year and fined as much as $1000. Any offender found to be in possession of more than 1.0 oz but <8 oz will face a similar punishment—1 year of incarceration and a $1000 fine. Possession of more than 8 oz is a felony. The punishment for possession of concentrated THC is uniform. Violators will be charged with a misdemeanor and could be incarcerated for up to 1 year and fined a maximum of $1000.

Cultivation is a felony. First-time offenders could be incarcerated for up to 9 years and fined up to $10 000. Subsequent offences could result in up to 18 years of incarceration and fines of $15 000.[73]

Patients participating in the state's medicinal cannabis program may procure up to 8 oz over a 90-day period. Patients may also grow up to 16 of their own cannabis plants, but only four can be mature at one time.

To recommend cannabis, practitioners must have a physician-patient relationship with the patient and be licensed in New Mexico to prescribe and administer drugs that are subject to the Controlled Substances, provided the patient has one of the following qualifying conditions:

- ALS (amyotrophic lateral sclerosis)
- Alzheimer disease
- Anorexia
- Arthritis
- Autism spectrum disorder
- Cancer
- Cachexia
- Crohn disease
- Epilepsy
- Friedrich ataxia

- Glaucoma
- Hepatitis C
- HIV/AIDs
- Huntington disease
- Inclusion body myositis
- Intractable nausea/vomiting
- LBD (Lewy body disease)
- Multiple sclerosis
- Obstructive sleep apnea
- Opioid use disorder
- Peripheral neuropathy
- Parkinson disease
- PTSD (posttraumatic stress disorder)
- Severe chronic pain
- Spasmodic torticollis
- Spinal cord injury
- Spinal muscular atrophy
- Ulcerative colitis

Patients who are under hospice care may also qualify.

New Mexico does allow patients from other jurisdictions who hold proof of authorization to participate in the state's medicinal cannabis program.[74]

For more information, please see the Medical Cannabis Program page on the New Mexico Department of Health Web site: https://nmhealth.org/about/mcp/svcs/.

New York

New York has a medical marijuana program, but it has not legalized recreational marijuana at this time. However, possessing small amounts of marijuana has been decriminalized and may only result in a violation and a fine ($50 for 28 g or less, $200 for between 28 g and 2 oz). Possession of more than 2 oz and <8 oz, or <0.25 oz of THC concentrate, is a misdemeanor punishable by up to 1 year of incarceration and a fine of $1000. Possession of anything more than either 8 oz of flower marijuana or 0.25 oz of concentrate is a felony punishable by:

- 8 oz-1 lb flower: Up to 4 years of incarceration and a maximum fine of $5000
- 1-10 lb flower/0.25-1 oz concentrate: Up to 7 years of incarceration and a maximum fine of $5000
- More than 10 lb flower/1 oz concentrate: Up to 15 years of incarceration and a maximum fine of $51 000

Under current case law, cultivation is possession. Offenders may face additional charges of cultivation for any number of plants.

Cultivation is a misdemeanor punishable by up to 1 year of incarceration and a fine of $1000.[75]

Patients participating in the state's medicinal marijuana program are authorized to acquire and possess at 30-day supply of THC-infused, nonsmokable products to treat the following conditions:

- ALS (amyotrophic lateral sclerosis)
- Cancer
- Chronic pain
- Epilepsy
- HIV/AIDS
- Huntington disease
- IBD (inflammatory bowel disorder)
- Multiple sclerosis
- Neuropathies
- Opioid substitution
- Parkinson disease
- PTSD (posttraumatic stress disorder)
- Spinal cord damage

For physicians to take part in New York's medical marijuana program, one must be an MD, DO, CNP, or physician assistant in good standing who has completed a course approved by the Commissioner of the Department of Health and registered with the New York State Department of Health Medical Marijuana Program. To begin the registration process, follow these instructions: https://www.health.ny.gov/regulations/medical_marijuana/practitioner/.

New York does not have a reciprocity program to accommodate medical marijuana patients from out of state.

For more information, see the Web site for the state's Medical Marijuana Program here: https://www.health.ny.gov/regulations/medical_marijuana/.

North Carolina

Recreational marijuana is not legal in North Carolina, but possession of small amounts of flower marijuana (0.5 oz or less) is treated as a minor misdemeanor. Those found guilty face a fine of $200 only. Possession of <0.05 oz of THC concentrate is also a misdemeanor, and those found guilty face a $200 fine, as well as up to 10 days of incarceration. Possession of 0.5-1.5 oz of flower marijuana or 0.05-0.15 oz of concentrate is also a misdemeanor, but the penalties for this are more severe. Those found guilty of possessing this amount of flower marijuana could be punished with between 1 and 45 days incarceration and a fine of $200.

Possession of larger amounts of marijuana is a felony, especially if one intends to sell or distribute. Simple possession of more than 1.5 oz but <10 lb of flower marijuana is punishable by up to 8 months of incarceration and a fine of $1000. Simple possession of more than 0.15 oz of THC concentrate is punishable by up to 6 months in jail and a fine of $200.

Cultivation is also a felony with the following penalty structure:

- <10 lb: Up to 8 months of incarceration and a maximum fine of $1000
- 10-50 lb: A mandatory minimum sentence of 2 years and a maximum sentence of up to 2.5 years of incarceration, as well as a maximum fine of $5000
- 50-2000 lb: A mandatory minimum sentence of 3 years and a maximum sentence of up to 3.5 years of incarceration, as well as a maximum fine of $25 000
- 2000-10 000 lb: A mandatory minimum sentence of 6 years and a maximum sentence of up to 7 years of incarceration, as well as a maximum fine of $50 000
- More than 10 000 lb: A mandatory minimum sentence of 14.5 years and a maximum sentence of up to 18 years of incarceration, as well as a maximum fine of $200 000[76]

North Carolina does not currently have a medical marijuana program. According to the North Carolina Epilepsy Alternative Treatment Act, only individuals with intractable epilepsy as determined by a board-certified neurologist affiliated with a hospital licensed in North Carolina may possess or consume low-THC cannabis formulations that contain at least 5% CBD and no more than 0.9% THC. Their caretakers are protected from prosecution for possession of a controlled substance.[77]

North Dakota

North Dakota does have a medical marijuana program, but recreational marijuana remains illegal. It has been decriminalized, however. Possession of <0.5 oz of marijuana is a criminal infraction that carries a punishment of a $1000 fine. Possession of more than 0.5 oz but <500 g is a misdemeanor punishable by incarceration of no more than 30 days and a fine of up to $1500. Larger amounts are still a misdemeanor and could result in punishment of up to 1 year in jail and/or a $3000 fine. Consuming hash or THC concentrates carries a similar punishment. Possession of hash or concentrates is a felony that could result in a sentence of 5 years of incarceration and/or a $10 000 fine.

Cultivation of marijuana is illegal, even for patients enrolled in the state's medicinal marijuana program. The punishment is based on the total weight of the plants.[78]

For patients participating in the state's medical program, they may not purchase a cumulative amount of concentrates that exceeds 2000 mg of THC in a 30-day period or more than 3 oz of flower marijuana. Edible products are prohibited under North Dakota's medical marijuana law, while flower may only be purchased from state-run dispensaries if a patient's physician formally certifies that the patient is permitted to use such a preparation.

Only physicians who have a bona fide physician-patient relationship with the patient and are properly licensed to practice in North Dakota may recommend marijuana for the following conditions:

- Alzheimer disease
- ALS (amyotrophic lateral sclerosis)
- Anorexia
- Arthritis
- Autism spectrum disorder
- Brain injury
- Bulimia
- Cachexia
- Cancer
- Chronic or debilitating diseases
- Crohn disease
- Ehlers-Danlos syndrome
- Endometriosis
- Epilepsy
- Fibromyalgia
- Glaucoma
- Hepatitis C
- **HIV/AIDS**
- Interstitial cystitis
- Intractable nausea
- Neuropathy
- Migraine
- Multiple sclerosis
- PTSD (posttraumatic stress disorder)
- Seizures
- Severe and persistent muscle spasms
- Severe debilitating pain
- Spinal injury
- Spinal stenosis
- Tourette syndrome

If a patient's debilitating condition is PTSD, the physician recommending the marijuana must be a licensed psychiatrist.

North Dakota does not have a reciprocity program to accommodate medical marijuana patients from out of state.

For more information, see the Web page for the state's Division of Medical Marijuana here: https://www.health.nd.gov/mm.

Northern Mariana Islands

There is no formal medical marijuana program in the Northern Mariana Islands, but adults over the age of 21 are free to possess various forms of cannabis, regardless of THC content. They may also gift certain amounts of cannabis to other adults over the age of 21. These amounts include

- 1 oz of flower marijuana
- 16 oz of cannabis products in solid form
- 72 oz of cannabis products in liquid form
- 5 g of cannabis extract
- 6 immature cannabis plants

It should be remembered that, while marijuana has been legalized, it may not be consumed in public, and drugged driving is strictly prohibited.

The Northern Mariana Islands are unique because there are no dispensaries as of this time. House Bill 20-178 allows registered adults to cultivate no more than 6 mature and 12 immature plants per household, but individuals cannot possess more than 8 oz of home-grown marijuana.[79] Individuals may be allowed to double the amount of plants they are allowed to grow if their physician deems that larger quantities of marijuana are necessary. Patients, including those under the age of 21, may be recommended marijuana by a physician if they have a debilitating condition, including one of the following:

- ADD/ADHD (attention deficit disorder/attention deficit hyperactive disorder)
- ALS (amyotrophic lateral sclerosis)
- Alzheimer disease
- Asthma
- Cancer
- Cerebral palsy
- Crohn disease
- Diabetes
- Glaucoma
- HIV/AIDS
- Hepatitis C
- Multiple sclerosis
- Muscular dystrophy
- Parkinson disease
- PTSD (posttraumatic stress disorder)
- Traumatic brain injury
- Ulcerative colitis
- Wilson disease

It may also be recommend to treat symptoms associated with chronic or debilitating diseases. These symptoms include:

- Cachexia
- Severe nausea
- Severe pain
- Severe and persistent muscle spasms
- Seizures

Ohio

Recreational marijuana is not legal in Ohio, but the possession of small amounts has been decriminalized at the state level and within individual jurisdictions. The following municipalities have decriminalized possession of up to 200 g:

- Athens
- Bellaire
- Bremen
- Columbus
- Fremont
- Logan
- Nelsonville
- Newark
- Norwood
- Oregon
- Roseville
- Toledo
- Windham

Dayton, meanwhile, has decriminalized the possession of 100 g or less, while Northwood has decriminalized the possession of 20 g of less. At the state level, possession of larger amounts of marijuana may result in imprisonment or fines of increasing severity depending on how much one has on one's possession and the type of cannabis one possesses.

For flower marijuana:

- <100 g: Misdemeanor offense and a $150 fine
- 100-200 g: Misdemeanor offense with a maximum punishment of 30 days imprisonment and a fine of $250
- 200-1000 g: Felony offense with a maximum punishment of 1 year of imprisonment and a fine of $2500
- 1-20 kg: Felony offense with a maximum punishment of 5 years of imprisonment and a fine of $10 000.
- 20-40 kg: Felony offense with a minimum term of imprisonment of 5 years and a maximum term of 8 years, as well as a fine of $15 000
- Over 40 kg: Felony offense with a minimum term of imprisonment of 8 years and a maximum fine of $20 000

For solid concentrate:

- <5 g: Misdemeanor offense and a $150 fine
- 5-10 g: Misdemeanor offense with a maximum punishment of 30 days imprisonment and a fine of $250
- 10-50 g: Felony offense with a maximum punishment of 1 year of imprisonment and a fine of $2500
- 50-1000 g: Felony offense with a maximum punishment of 3 years of imprisonment and a fine of $10 000
- Over 1 kg: Felony offense with a maximum punishment of 8 years and a fine of $15 000

For liquid concentrate:

- <1 g: Misdemeanor offense and a $150 fine
- 1-2 g: Misdemeanor offense with a maximum punishment of 30 days imprisonment and a fine of $250
- 2-10 g: Felony offense with a maximum punishment of 1 year of imprisonment and a fine of $2500
- 10-200 g: Felony offense with a maximum punishment of 3 years of imprisonment and a fine of $10 000
- Over 200 g: Felony offense with a maximum punishment of 8 years and a fine of $15 000

The penalties for cultivation are the same as possession of flower marijuana, though the state does allow an affirmative defense should the amount grown be <1 kg. In this case, an individual may be able to plead guilty to a misdemeanor rather than a felony.[80]

Ohio does have a medical marijuana program, and MDs and DOs with a license to practice medicine in Ohio who have a bona fide physician-patient relationship with a patient may recommend marijuana for the following conditions:

- ALS (amyotrophic lateral sclerosis)
- Alzheimer disease
- Cancer
- Chronic traumatic encephalopathy
- Crohn disease
- Fibromyalgia
- Glaucoma
- Hepatitis C
- HIV/AIDS
- IBD (inflammatory bowel disorder)
- Multiple sclerosis
- Chronic or intractable pain
- Parkinson disease
- PTSD (posttraumatic stress disorder)
- Sickle cell anemia
- Spinal cord injury or disease
- Tourette disease

- Traumatic brain injury
- Ulcerative colitis

Ohio does not have a reciprocity program to accommodate medical marijuana patients from out of state.

For more information, please see the Ohio Medical Marijuana Control Program Web site: https://www.medicalmarijuana.ohio.gov/.

Oklahoma

In 2015, Oklahoma passed legislation allowing patients with pediatric epilepsy to be treated with low-THC preparations of cannabis largely consistent with the Farm Bill of 2018, which set a limit on THC concentration at 0.3%. In 2018, the state created a medical marijuana program that allows patients to possess up to 3 oz of flower marijuana, 1 oz of concentrate, or 72 oz of edible cannabis on their person. (8 oz of flower marijuana may be stored in their home.) Patients are authorized to grow up to 12 plants, but only 6 can be mature at any given time. Individuals who claim to have a medical condition but have not obtained a state-issued license to possess marijuana will only face a misdemeanor offense and a fine not to exceed $400, provided they are found in possession of under 1.5 oz.[81]

MDs or DOs with a license to practice medicine in Oklahoma who have a bona fide physician-patient relationship with a patient may recommend marijuana. The state allows the attending physician to use their discretion when making the recommendation.

Oklahoma does not have a reciprocity program to accommodate medical marijuana patients from out of state.

For more information about the state's medical marijuana program, please see the Web site for the Oklahoma Medical Marijuana Authority: http://omma.ok.gov/.

Possession of marijuana for nonmedicinal reasons is a misdemeanor punishable by incarceration for 1 year and a fine of $1000. Cultivation is a felony. For <1000 plants, the penalty is a minimum of 2 years of imprisonment and a maximum of life in prison, as well as a fine of $25 000.[82] For more than 1000 plants (or 1000 kg), the fine is $50 000 and violators face a minimum sentence of 20 years in prison and a maximum sentence of life in prison.[83]

Oregon

Recreational and medical marijuana are both legal in Oregon, but it is illegal to consume marijuana in public places or to drive under the influence of THC. Adults aged 21 and older may possess 1 oz or less of marijuana on their person or have up to 8 oz in their residence.

Possession of between 1 and 2 oz on one's person is a violation punishable by a fine of up to $650. Possession of between 2 and 4 oz on one's person or between 1 and 2 lb in one's home is a misdemeanor punishable by a $2500 fine and imprisonment of up to 6 months. Possession of more than 4 oz on one's person or over 2 lb in one's home is a misdemeanor punishable by a maximum fine of $6250 and incarceration of up to 1 year.

Individuals may cultivate up to 4 plants. The unlicensed growing of 4-8 plants is a misdemeanor punishable by 6 months of incarceration and a fine of $2500. Unlicensed growers who cultivate more than 8 plants may face felony charges, which entails a possible punishment of 5 years of incarceration and a fine of $125 000. Individuals in possession of more than 0.25 oz of high THC concentrate not purchased from a licensed retailer may face a similar punishment.[84]

Patients who are enrolled in Oregon's medical marijuana program can possess 24 oz of usable marijuana and to have 6 mature plants and 18 immature seedlings. To enroll, patients must receive a recommendation from a properly licensed MD or DO who currently provides the patient with primary care. Patients with the following conditions may qualify for the program:

- Alzheimer disease
- Cancer
- Glaucoma
- HIV/AIDS
- PTSD (posttraumatic stress disorder)

Practitioners may recommend marijuana for patients whose treatment or condition results in:

- Cachexia
- Persistent muscle spasms
- Severe nausea
- Severe pain
- Seizures

Oregon does not have a reciprocity program to accommodate medical marijuana patients from out of state.

For more information about the program, please see the Oregon Medical Marijuana Program Web site: https://www.oregon.gov/oha/ph/DiseasesConditions/ChronicDisease/MedicalMarijuanaProgram/Pages/index.aspx.

Pennsylvania

Pennsylvania has a medical marijuana program. Participants are authorized to possess a 30-day supply of marijuana. Home cultivation is prohibited, as are combustible forms of cannabis.

Medical professionals in the state of Pennsylvania must be either MDs or DOs with active medical licenses if they would like to recommend marijuana to patients. Additionally, all qualifying practitioners are required to create a profile by following the instructions on the Pennsylvania Department of Health portal: https://padohmmp. custhelp.com/app/login. They then must complete a 4-hour training program.

Patients with the following conditions may qualify as participants in Pennsylvania's program:

- ALS (amyotrophic lateral sclerosis)
- Anxiety disorders
- Autism spectrum disorder
- Cancer
- Crohn disease
- Dyskinetic/spastic movement disorder
- Epilepsy
- Glaucoma
- HIV/AIDS
- Huntington disease
- IBD (inflammatory bowel disorder)
- Intractable pain
- Intractable seizures
- Intractable spasticity
- Multiple sclerosis
- Neurodegenerative disorders
- Neuropathies
- Parkinson disease
- PTSD (posttraumatic stress disorder)
- Sickle cell anemia
- Tourette disease
- Terminal illnesses

Pennsylvania does not have a reciprocity program to accommodate medical marijuana patients from out of state. More importantly, the law allowing parents or legal guardians to obtain marijuana from out of state for patients under the age of 18 is no longer in effect. It has since lapsed.

For more information about Pennsylvania's program, please see the Web site for the state's Department of Health: https://www.health.pa.gov/ topics/programs/Medical%20Marijuana/Pages/Medical%20Marijuana. aspx.

Recreational marijuana is not legal in the state of Pennsylvania, but the following jurisdictions have decriminalized possession of up to 30 g, and only issue a fine for violators:

- Allentown ($25 fine)
- Erie ($25 fine)
- Harrisburg ($75-$150 fine)

- Norristown ($25 fine)
- Phoenixville ($25-$100 fine)
- Philadelphia ($25 fine)
- Pittsburgh ($25 fine)
- State College ($250 fine)
- York ($100 fine)

The city of Lancaster has decriminalized up to 1 oz of marijuana. The penalty for possessing this amount is $25-$75.

In the rest of the state, possession is a misdemeanor. Possession of 30 g or less of flower marijuana or 8 g or less of THC concentrate may result in a fine of $500 and a period of incarceration of up to 30 days. Possession of more than 30 g of flower marijuana or more than 8 g of concentrate may result in a fine of $5000 and up to 1 year of incarceration. Cultivation is a felony punishable by 2.5-5 years of incarceration and a fine no more than $15 000.[85]

Puerto Rico

Despite having a medical cannabis program, Puerto Rico strictly prohibits the use of marijuana if it is not sanctioned by a medical professional. Possession is a felony. For first-time offenders, the penalties are 2-5 years of incarceration and fines of up to $5000. The penalties for subsequent offenses are 4-10 years of incarceration and fines of up to $5000.[86] Cultivating marijuana is also a felony. Penalties for cultivating any amount are severe: 12 years in prison and a maximum fine of $20 000. Aggravating circumstances may make the penalties even more serious.[87]

Patients who have been recommended cannabis to treat a qualifying condition can purchase up to a 30-day supply, but dispensaries only carry extracts, as the use of herbal cannabis is prohibited. Only medical professionals licensed to practice medicine and to prescribe controlled Class II drugs in Puerto Rico may recommend cannabis to patients. They may recommend it for the following conditions:

- ALS (amyotrophic lateral sclerosis)
- Alzheimer disease
- Anorexia
- Anxiety
- Arthritis
- Cachexia
- Cancer
- Crohn disease
- Epilepsy
- Fibromyalgia
- Hepatitis C

- HIV/AIDS
- Migraines
- Multiple sclerosis
- Parkinson disease
- PTSD (posttraumatic stress disorder)
- Severe pain
- Spinal cord injury

Additionally, qualifying practitioners must complete an 8-hour certified training course created by the Department of Health on Medical Cannabis. To register for this course, see the DHMC Web site: http://www.salud.gov.pr/Dept-de-Salud/Pages/Cannabis-Medicinal.aspx.

Puerto Rico does not have a reciprocity program to accommodate medical marijuana patients from other jurisdictions.

Rhode Island

Medical marijuana was legalized in Rhode Island in 2006. Though the state has not legalized recreational marijuana, possession of <1 oz is a civil violation that carries a $150 fine. Possession of between 1 oz and 1 kg of marijuana is a misdemeanor offense punishable by incarceration of up to 1 year and a $500 fine.

Possession or cultivation of more than 1 kg is a felony.[88] Possession or cultivation of 1-5 kg of marijuana carries a minimum sentence of 10 years in prison, a maximum sentence of 50 years, and a maximum fine of $500 000. Possession or cultivation of more than 5 kg carries a mandatory minimum sentence of 25 years in prison, a maximum sentence of life, and a fine of $1 000 000.[89]

Despite these extremely stern penalties, participants in Rhode Island's medical marijuana program can possess up to 2.5 oz and to grow 12 plants and 12 seedlings, provided it is all grown in one location and stored in an indoor facility.

To recommend marijuana in Rhode Island, medical professionals must be licensed to practice in Rhode Island, Massachusetts, or Connecticut; have a practitioner-patient relationship with the patient; and provide written certification to the patient. They can recommend marijuana for the following qualifying conditions:

- Alzheimer disease
- Autism spectrum disorder
- Cachexia
- Cancer
- Chronic pain
- Crohn disease
- Glaucoma
- Hepatitis C

- HIV/AIDS
- Nausea
- Persistent muscle spasms
- PTSD (posttraumatic stress disorder)
- Seizures

Rhode Island allows patients from other jurisdictions to possess and even purchase marijuana from the state's dispensaries.

For more information about Rhode Island's program, please see the state's Department of Health Web site: https://health.ri.gov/licenses/detail.php?id=280.

South Carolina

Recreational marijuana is not legal in South Carolina. First-time offenders caught in possession of flower marijuana in the amount of 1 oz or less may be charged with a misdemeanor and face incarceration of up to 30 days and a fine of $200. Subsequent instances of possession involving 1 oz or less of flower marijuana will also be considered misdemeanors, but individuals may face more severe punishments of up to 1 year of incarceration and a maximum fine of $2000. Possession of more than 1 oz of flower marijuana is a felony.

Those found in possession of 10 g or less of THC concentrate could be charged with misdemeanor charges and may face incarceration of up to 30 days and a fine of $200. If one is found in possession of larger amounts of concentrate, the punishment could include up to 5 years of imprisonment and a maximum fine of $5000.

Cultivation is a felony with the following penalty structure:

- <100 plants: Maximum of 5 years of imprisonment and a fine of $5000
- 100-1000 plants: Minimum sentence of 25 years in prison and a fine of $25 000
- 1000-10 000 plants: Minimum sentence of 25 years in prison and a fine of $50 000
- More than 10 000 plants: Minimum sentence of 25 years in prison and a fine of $200 000[90]

The only medicinal use of cannabis allowed in the state includes OTC preparations of hemp-derived CBD that contain <0.3% THC, as well as preparations containing 15% CBD and no more than 0.9% THC for which the only qualifying conditions are certain forms of childhood epilepsy. The law authorizing the recommendation of the latter formulation, known as Julian's Law, allows MDs and DOs who are licensed by the South Carolina Board of Medical Examiners to recommend cannabis for Dravet syndrome, Lennox-Gastaut syndrome, and refractory epilepsy. However, the law did not create a medical cannabis program; it merely allows qualifying individuals and their caretakers to possess preparations containing up to 0.9% THC without fear of prosecution.[91]

South Dakota

South Dakota does not have a medicinal cannabis program, and the adult use of any cannabis product is illegal, though cannabis-based medications that have received FDA approval can be prescribed to patients. Even CBD products that would be legal under federal law as specified in the 2018 Farm Bill—that is, hemp derived and <0.3% THC— may be considered illicit substances under South Dakota law. At the time of this writing, the status of these products remains an open question.

Patients from other states should note that there are major penalties for possession of cannabis. Possession of 2 oz or less is a misdemeanor. Offenders could be incarcerated for up to 1 year and may be fined $2000. Possession of more than 2 oz is a felony. If the quantity possessed is under 0.5 lb, the punishment can be incarceration of up to 1 year and a fine of up to $4000. If it is between 0.5 and 1.0 lb, violators may be incarcerated up to 5 years and fined $10 000. If it is between 1 and 10 lb, violators may be incarcerated up to 10 years and fined $20 000. If it is over 10 lb, the term of imprisonment may be up to 15 years and the maximum fine could be $30 000. The punishment for cultivation is based on the total weight of the plants.

Possession of concentrated cannabis is a felony punishable by up to 10 years in prison and a fine of $20 000.[92]

Tennessee

Recreational marijuana is illegal in Tennessee, and the punishment for possession is strict. Possession of more than 0.5 oz of flower is a felony under Tennessee law, as is possession of more than 14.75 g of THC concentrate. Offenders may face upwards of 6 years of incarceration and fines of $5000, provided they are found in possession of <10 lb of flower marijuana or 2 lb. of concentrate.

First-time offenders found in possession of 0.5 oz or less of flower marijuana will face misdemeanor charges and be punished by a mandatory fine of $250 and up to 1 year of incarceration. For subsequent offenses the fine is increased to $500. Those found guilty of first-time possession of <14.75 g of THC concentrate face misdemeanor charges and could be punished with incarceration of up to 11 months and 29 days, as well as a fine no greater than $2500. A second or subsequence conviction is punishable as a felony, which may result in a 6-year term of imprisonment and a fine of up to $3000.

Cultivation is a felony in the state of Tennessee with the following penalty structure:

- 10 plants or less: Maximum sentence of 6 years of imprisonment; maximum fine of $5000
- 10-19 plants: Maximum sentence of 12 years of imprisonment; maximum fine of $50 000
- 20-99 plants: Maximum sentence of 15 years of imprisonment; maximum fine of $100 000
- 100-499 plants: Maximum sentence of 30 years of imprisonment; maximum fine of $200 000
- 500 or more plants: Maximum sentence of 60 years of imprisonment; maximum fine of $500 000[93]

Tennessee does not currently have a formal medical cannabis program, but the state did create a pathway to allow caregivers and individuals with intractable epilepsy or another uncontrolled seizure disorder the ability to possess formulations that contain no more than 0.9% THC without fear of prosecution. However, on top of having a qualifying disorder, patients must be enrolled in an approved clinical research study and be under the care of a physician practicing at a hospital or associated clinic affiliated with a Tennessee university's college or school of medicine.[94]

At this time, these are the only medical professionals allowed to recommend any formulation of cannabis with more than 0.3% THC.

Texas

The use of cannabis is prohibited in the state of Texas, though some extracts that contain no more than 0.5% THC are legal if one is enrolled in the state's Compassionate Use/Low-THC program. Possession of <4 oz of flower cannabis that is classified as marijuana under federal law (having THC content >0.3%) is a misdemeanor. Possession of 2 oz or less is punishable by a maximum fine of $2000 and a period of incarceration no longer than 180 days. Possession of more than 2 oz, but <4 oz, is punishable by a maximum fine of $4000 and a period of incarceration no longer than 1 year.

Possession of more than 4 oz of flower or any cannabis concentrates that contain more than 0.3% THC, provided one is not participating in the state's Compassionate Use/Low-THC program and is in possession of extract that contains no more than 0.5% THC, is a felony. The punishment for possessing more than 4 oz of flower is as follows:

- 4 oz to 5 lb: Minimum of 180 days of incarceration and a maximum of 2 years; maximum fine of $10 000
- 5-50 lb: Minimum of 2 years of incarceration and a maximum of 10 years; maximum fine of $10 000

and chiropractors. The Virgin Islands Medical Cannabis Patient Care Act recognizes that cannabis may alleviate, and may therefore be recommended for, any condition that either requires hospice care or causes cachexia, nausea, seizures, or severe muscle spasms. It also specifically mentions that the following debilitating conditions may be treated with cannabis:

- Alzheimer disease
- ALS (amyotrophic lateral sclerosis)
- Arthritis
- Cancer
- Crohn disease
- Diabetes
- Epilepsy
- Hepatitis C
- HIV/AIDS
- Huntington disease
- Multiple sclerosis
- Neuropathy
- Parkinson disease
- PTSD (posttraumatic stress disorder)
- Spinal cord injury
- Traumatic brain injury

There are no state-run dispensaries open as of this time, unfortunately. Once they are open, they will be allowed to provide cannabis to patients from other jurisdictions, provided they have proof of enrollment. As stated in the Virgin Islands Medical Cannabis Patient Care Act, nonresidents may possess 3 oz.

Utah

Though it is one of the most socially conservative states in the United States, Utah has passed two distinct medicinal cannabis laws. The first allowed MDs, DOs, APRNs, and physician assistants who are licensed to prescribe a controlled substance to recommend cannabis extracts with THC concentrations below 0.3% to patients with intractable epilepsy and individuals with terminal illnesses who have <6 months to live. This law has since been superseded after Utahans voted in favor of Proposition 2 in 2018, which expanded the state's medical cannabis program.

The resultant legislation, HB3001, created a state program that came online in 2020 and will become fully operational in 2021. Once operational, it will allow patients over the age of 18 (though patients under the age of 21 must have their application approved by the Compassionate Use Board) to acquire a card authorizing them to purchase cannabis from a medical cannabis pharmacy. Within any 28-day period, these pharmacies may only sell either an amount sufficient to provide 30 days of treatment to a patient or a processed form of cannabis, excluding anything resembling candy, containing no more than 20 g of THC, whichever is less.[98] Under the law, smokable forms of cannabis and home cultivation remain illegal.

Prior to the time the program comes online, patients will be offered an affirmative defense if they have been recommended cannabis by a physician.[99]

To be considered for the program, patients must have one of the following qualifying conditions:

- Alzheimer disease
- ALS (amyotrophic lateral sclerosis)
- Autism
- Cancer
- Cachexia
- Crohn disease
- Epilepsy
- HIV/AIDS
- Multiple sclerosis
- Persistent and severe muscle spasms
- Persistent nausea
- PTSD (posttraumatic stress disorder)
- Severe pain
- Terminal illnesses when the patient has <6 months to live

Additionally, patients in hospice are also eligible to enroll in the program, as are patients approved by the Compassionate Use Board and patients suffering from some diseases that affect <200 000 individuals in the United States.[100]

Utah does not and does not intend to have a reciprocity program to accommodate medical marijuana patients from out of state.

MDs, DOs, APRNs, and physician assistants who are licensed in the state of Utah may receive approval from the Department of Health to recommend cannabis but must first register through an electronic verification system here: https://medicalcannabis.utah.gov/providers/become-a-qualified-medical-provider/.

For more information on the program, please visit the Utah Medical Cannabis Program Web site: https://medicalcannabis.utah.gov/.

The recreational use of cannabis that is classified as marijuana (containing a concentration of THC above 0.3%) is prohibited for individuals who are not enrolled in the state's cannabis program. Possession of under 1 lb is a misdemeanor offense. For possession of <1 oz, the punishment is a maximum of 6 months of incarceration and a fine of $1000. For the possession of 1 oz or more, but <1 lb, the punishment is a maximum of 1 year of incarceration and a fine of

$2500. Possession of between 1 and 100 lb is a felony punishable by a maximum fine of $5000 and a maximum term of imprisonment of 5 years. Possession of over 100 lb is punishable by a maximum fine of $10 000 and a period of imprisonment between 1 and 15 years.

Cultivation of marijuana is illegal. Punishment is based on the total weight of the plants.[101]

Vermont

Recreational marijuana is legal in Vermont. However, H.511 of 2018, which ended total prohibition and made it permissible for individuals 21 years of age or older to possess 1 oz or less of flower marijuana, 5 g or less of THC concentrate, or 2 mature plants and 4 immature plants, did not create a regulatory framework to oversee a commercial market. Consequently, there are no dispensaries where one can purchase recreational marijuana.

Possessing or growing more than what is allowed by H.511 is against the law. Possession of between 1 and 2 oz is a misdemeanor. First-time offenders may face a maximum punishment of incarceration for 6 months and a fine of $500. Subsequent offences may result in a maximum punishment of incarceration for 2 years and a fine of $2000. Possession of more than 5 g of concentrate is a misdemeanor. First-time offenders face a maximum fine of $500 and a term of imprisonment up to 6 months. Subsequent offences may result in fines of up to $2000 and terms of imprisonment of up to 2 years.

It is a felony to cultivate more than the number of plants allowed by H.511 or to possess more than 2 oz of marijuana, and the penalty structure for these offenses is the same.

The maximum punishment for cultivating 3-10 mature plants or possessing between 2 oz and 1 lb of marijuana is a term of imprisonment of 3 years and a fine of $10 000. The punishment for cultivating 11-25 plants or possessing between 1 and 10 lb is a term of imprisonment of 5 years and a fine of $100 000. The punishment for cultivating more than 25 plants or possessing more than 10 lb is a term of imprisonment of 15 years and a fine of $500 000.[102]

Vermont is also home to a medical marijuana program, and there are currently five dispensaries for participating patients. Patients may possess 2 oz of usable marijuana. Home cultivation is also allowed, and patients may grow a maximum of 9 plants, 2 of which may be mature at any one time.

Patients must receive a recommendation from their doctor to possess or grow medicinal marijuana. Medical professionals authorized to recommend it include properly licensed physicians who are authorized and licensed to prescribe drugs, licensed naturopathic physicians, licensed physician assistants, and licensed APRNs who have a bona fide physician-patient relationship with the patient. Qualification extends to physicians who meet the above criteria who are professionally licensed under substantially equivalent provisions in adjacent states (New Hampshire, Massachusetts, and New York). Qualifying conditions include

- Cachexia
- Cancer
- Crohn disease
- Glaucoma
- HIV/AIDS
- Multiple sclerosis
- Parkinson disease
- PTSD (posttraumatic stress disorder)
- Seizures
- Severe or chronic pain
- Severe nausea

Physicians are also authorized to recommend marijuana to patients receiving hospice care.

Vermont does not have a reciprocity program to accommodate medical marijuana patients from out of state.

For more information about the state's program, see the Department of Public Safety's site for the Marijuana Registry: https://medicalmarijuana.vermont.gov/.

Virginia

Virginia's medical marijuana program allows MDs, DOs, physician assistants, or nurse practitioners who have been certified by the state to recommend marijuana to patients. Medical professionals can apply for certification through the Virginia Department of Health Professions portal found here: https://www.license.dhp.virginia.gov/apply/. There are no qualifying conditions. The attending physician has the authority to make the recommendation at his or her discretion.[103]

Under Virginia law, patients who have been recommended marijuana can only possess cannabis formulations that contain no <15% CBD or Δ^9-tetrahydrocannabinolic acid (THC-A) and no more than 5% THC. Additionally, these extracts cannot have a dosage of over 10 mg of THC. These formulations may be procured at specially licensed establishments known as pharmaceutical processors.

Virginia does not have a reciprocity program to accommodate medical cannabis patients from out of state.

For more information about the state's medical marijuana program, please see the Board of Pharmacy site created by the Department

of Health Professions here: https://www.dhp.virginia.gov/pharmacy/
PharmaceuticalProcessing/default.htm.

Recreational marijuana and cannabis extracts are prohibited
by state law. Possession of <0.5 oz flower marijuana or cannabis
concentrate that contains <12% THC is a misdemeanor.[104] First-time
offenders face up to 30 days in jail and a maximum fine of $500.
Subsequent offences may result in up to 1 year of incarceration and
a maximum fine of $2500. Possession of more than 0.5 oz is a felony.
Punishment is dependent upon whether or not one intended to sell
or distribute the marijuana.[105] Cannabis concentrate with a THC
concentration above 12% is not considered "marijuana" by Virginia state
law.[106] Possession is a felony.[107]

Washington

Recreational and medical marijuana are both legal in Washington.
Adults aged 21 and older may possess 1 oz or less of marijuana.
Possession of more than 1 oz, but <40 g is a misdemeanor punishable by
a $1000 fine and a term of imprisonment >24 hours but no more than
90 days. Possession of more than 40 g of marijuana is a felony that could
result in 5 years of imprisonment and $10 000 in fines. It remains illegal
to consume marijuana in public places or to drive under the influence of
THC. Cultivation for recreational use is also prohibited, and growing any
number of plants is a felony that could result in 5 years of imprisonment
and $10 000 in fines.[108]

Patients who are enrolled in Washington's medical marijuana
program may possess 21 g of cannabis concentrate, 3 oz of flower
marijuana, 48 oz of THC-infused product in solid form, or 216 oz of
THC-infused product in liquid form. Patients may grow up to 6 plants
and possess up to 8 oz of useable marijuana from their harvest. In
certain circumstances, patients may be authorized to grow 15 plants
and possess up to 16 oz of useable marijuana from their harvest.
Meanwhile, qualifying patients who have not entered the state's medical
marijuana database may grow up to 4 plants and possess up to 6 oz of
useable marijuana. In all cases, the plants must be grown in the patient's
domicile.[109]

Properly licensed MDs, DOs, APRNs, physician assistants, and
naturopaths who have a documented relationship with the patient may
recommend marijuana for the following conditions:

- Cachexia
- Cancer
- Crohn disease
- Hepatitis C

- HIV/AIDS
- Intractable pain
- Muscle spasms
- Nausea
- PTSD (posttraumatic stress disorder)
- Seizures
- Traumatic brain injury
- Severe pain

Additionally, practitioners may recommend marijuana for patients suffering any terminal or debilitating condition.

Washington does not have a reciprocity program to accommodate medical marijuana patients from out of state.

For more information about the program, see the Washington State Department of Health's Web site: https://www.doh.wa.gov/YouandYourFamily/Marijuana/MedicalMarijuana.

West Virginia

West Virginia passed legislation allowing for the creation of a medical cannabis program several years ago, but the system is still not online as of this time. There is currently no legal means of acquiring cannabis for medicinal purposes except for terminally ill patients who enjoy reciprocity with other states.

Even after the establishment of the state-run program, the use of flower cannabis will continue to be universally prohibited. It is a misdemeanor punishable by up to 6 months imprisonment and a maximum fine of $1000 to possess any amount of flower cannabis, regardless of whether one is enrolled in the state's program or not. Cultivation of marijuana is also illegal, even for patients enrolled in the state's medicinal cannabis program. If one is growing marijuana only for oneself, it is treated as possession. If one is growing marijuana with intent to sell or distribute, it is treated as a felony, and the penalty is a fine of up to $15 000, a mandatory minimum sentence of 1 year in prison, and a maximum term of imprisonment lasting 5 years.[110]

Once the West Virginia medical cannabis program has come online, enrollees will be allowed to possess infused pills, oils, topicals, vaping or nebulizing formulas, tinctures, and dermal patches of an unspecific amount, provided they have one of the following conditions:

- ALS (amyotrophic lateral sclerosis)
- Cancer
- Crohn disease
- HIV/AIDS
- Epilepsy
- Huntington disease

- Intractable seizures
- Multiple sclerosis
- Neuropathies
- Parkinson disease
- PTSD (posttraumatic stress disorder)
- Severe chronic or intractable pain
- Sickle cell anemia
- Spinal cord damage
- Terminal illnesses

To recommend cannabis, a physician will be required to be either an MD or a DO who is fully licensed by the state and who has passed a 4-hour training course on cannabis and registered with the state. Currently, neither the electronic registry nor the training course exists.

For more information, please see the Web site for the West Virginia Office of Medical Cannabis: https://dhhr.wv.gov/bph/Pages/Medical-Cannabis-Program.aspx.

Wisconsin

Wisconsin does not have a medical cannabis program, but physicians may recommend preparations that are high in CBD and currently available over the counter as a treatment akin to how one would recommend any OTC medication. Possession of any cannabis preparations that contain more than 0.3% THC is prohibited.

Possession of any amount of marijuana is a misdemeanor punishable by imprisonment of no more than 6 months and a maximum fine of $1000. Subsequent offenses are felonies that carry a maximum term of 3.5 years of imprisonment and a fine of $10 000. However, the following jurisdictions have decriminalized marijuana at the local level:

- Appleton (amount: <25 g; fine: $200)
- Eau Claire (amount: <25 g; fine: $100-$500)
- Green Bay (amount: <28 g; fine: $1-$500)
- Kenosha (amount: <1 oz; fine: $10-$750)
- La Crosse (amount: <7 g; fine: $338)
- Madison (amount: <10 g; fine: $100)
- Milwaukee (amount: <25 g; fine: $50)
- Monona (amount: <25 g; fine: $200 for public smoking, $0 for possession)
- Oshkosh (amount: <25 g; fine: $200)
- Racine (amount: <25 g on private property; fine: $75)
- Stevens Point (amount: <5 g; fine: $100)
- Superior (amount: <25 g; fine: $100-$500)
- Waukesha (amount: not defined; fine: $1000)
- Wausau (amount: <28 g; fine: $50-$500)

Intent to sell or distribute any amount of marijuana is a felony. Cultivation is a felony, as well, and the penalty structure is severe:

- 1-3 plants: Minimum sentence of 3 years of imprisonment and a maximum fine of $10 000
- 4-20 plants: Minimum sentence of 6 years of imprisonment and a maximum fine of $10 000
- 20-50 plants: Minimum sentence of 10 years of imprisonment and a maximum fine of $25 000
- 50-200 plants: Minimum sentence of 12.5 years of imprisonment and a maximum fine of $25 000
- More than 200 plants: Minimum sentence of 15 years of imprisonment and a maximum fine of $50 000[111]

Wyoming

Wyoming does not have a medical cannabis program. Physicians may recommend cannabis preparations high in CBD that are currently available over the counter as a treatment akin to how one would recommend any OTC medication. Possession of any cannabis preparation that contains more than 0.3% THC, "marijuana" as defined by the 2018 Farm Bill, is a crime.[112]

Being under the influence of THC is a misdemeanor that could result in a maximum term of imprisonment of 6 months and a fine of $750. Possession of 3 oz or less (0.3 g of concentrate or less) is a misdemeanor punishable by imprisonment of no more than 12 months and a maximum fine of $1000. Possession of more than 3 oz (more than 0.3 g of concentrate) is a felony that could lead to 5 years of incarceration and a fine of up to $10 000. Cultivation of any amount of marijuana is a misdemeanor offense with a maximum penalty of 6 months of incarceration and a fine of $1000.[113]

REFERENCES

[1]Associated Press. Jefferson County ends misdemeanor pot arrest. Montgomery Advertiser Web site. April 23, 2019. https://www.montgomeryadvertiser.com/story/news/local/alabama/2019/04/23/jefferson-county-ends-misdemeanor-pot-arrests/3550176002/. Accessed April 7, 2020.

[2]Public Health Laws of Alabama. Alabama Public Health Web site. 2019. https://www.alabamapublichealth.gov/legal/assets/publichealthlawsofalabama.pdf. Accessed April 7, 2020.

[3]Leni's Law—Alabama House Bill 61. Legiscan Web site. https://legiscan.com/AL/text/HB61/id/1320785. Accessed April 7, 2020.

[4]Alabama Senate Bill 225. Legiscan Web site. https://legiscan.com/AL/text/SB225/2019. Accessed April 7, 2020.

[5]Alaska laws & penalties. NORML Web site. https://norml.org/laws/item/alaska-penalties. Accessed April 7, 2020.

[6]Alaska Statutes 2019—Sec. 17.37.040. The Alaska State Legislature Web site. http://www.akleg.gov/basis/statutes.asp#17.37.040. Accessed April 7, 2020.

[7]Information on American Samoa from the American Samoa Government Department of Legal Affairs Office of the Attorney General. Pagopago Web site. https://www.pagopago.com/artsfestival/facts/drugs.htm. Accessed April 7, 2020.

[8]Court says CBD oil is illegal. July 12, 2019. Talanei Web site. https://www.talanei.com/2019/07/12/court-says-cbd-oil-is-illegal/. Accessed April 7, 2020.

[9]Arizona Revised Statutes 13-901.01. Arizona State Legislature Web site. https://www.azleg.gov/viewdocument/?docName=https://www.azleg.gov/ars/13/00901-01.htm. Accessed April 7, 2020.

[10]Arizona Revised Statutes 13-3405. Arizona State Legislature Web site. https://www.azleg.gov/viewdocument/?docName=https://www.azleg.gov/ars/13/03405.htm. Accessed April 7, 2020.

[11]Can I legally grow marijuana in Arizona? Schill Law Group Web site. https://schilllaw-group.com/legally-grow-marijuana-arizona/. Accessed April 7, 2020.

[12]What medical conditions will qualify a patient for medical marijuana? Arizona Department of Health Services Web site. https://www.azdhs.gov/licensing/medical-marijuana/index.php#faqs-patients. Accessed April 7, 2020.

[13]Arizona medical marijuana law. NORML Web site. https://norml.org/legal/item/arizona-medical-marijuana. Accessed April 7, 2020.

[14]Turnage C. City in central Arkansas switches marijuana tactics; officers to cite, not arrest some offenders, chief says. Arkansas Democrat Gazette Web site. June 28, 2018. https://www.arkansasonline.com/news/2018/jun/28/jacksonville-switches-pot-tactics-20180-1/. Accessed April 7, 2020.

[15]2012 Arkansas Code § 5-64-419—Possession of a controlled substance. Justia Web site. https://law.justia.com/codes/arkansas/2012/title-5/subtitle-6/chapter-64/subchapter-4/section-5-64-419. Accessed April 7, 2020.

[16]California Health and Safety Code § 11357. California Legislature Web site. https://leginfo.legislature.ca.gov/faces/codes_displaySection.xhtml?sectionNum=11357.&lawCode=HSC. Accessed April 7, 2020.

[17]California Health and Safety Code § 11358. California Legislature Web site. https://leginfo.legislature.ca.gov/faces/codes_displaySection.xhtml?sectionNum=11358.&lawCode=HSC. Accessed April 7, 2020.

[18]AB-710—Cannabidiol. California Legislature Web site. https://leginfo.legislature.ca.gov/faces/billTextClient.xhtml?bill_id=201720180AB710. Accessed April 7, 2020.

[19]Laws about marijuana use. Colorado Official State Portal. https://www.colorado.gov/pacific/marijuana/laws-about-marijuana-use. Accessed April 7, 2020.

[20]Home grow laws. Colorado Official State Portal. https://www.colorado.gov/pacific/marijuana/home-grow-laws. Accessed April 7, 2020.

[21]Colorado laws and & penalties. NORML Web site. https://norml.org/laws/item/colorado-penalties. Accessed April 7, 2020.

[22]Connecticut General Statutes Chapter 240b, dependency-producing drugs. Connecticut General Assembly Web site. https://www.cga.ct.gov/current/pub/chap_420b.htm. Accessed April 7, 2020.

[23]Delaware laws & penalties. NORML Web site. https://norml.org/laws/item/delaware-penalties. Accessed April 7, 2020.

[24]Chapter 49A. The Delaware Medical Marijuana Act. State of Delaware Web site. https://delcode.delaware.gov/title16/c049a/index.shtml. Accessed April 7, 2020.

[25]District of Columbia laws & penalties. NORML Web site. https://norml.org/laws/item/district-of-columbia-penalties. Accessed April 7, 2020.

[26]District of Columbia Municipal Regulations for the Medical Marijuana Program. District of Columbia Health Web site. January 9, 2018. https://dchealth.dc.gov/sites/default/filesattachments/MEDICAL%20MARIJUANA.2018.updates.pdf. Accessed April 7, 2019.

[27]B21-2010—Medical Marijuana Reciprocity Amendment Act of 2015. Council of the District of Columbia Web site. http://lims.dccouncil.us/Legislation/B21-0210. Accessed April 7, 2020.

[28]Florida laws & penalties. NORML Web site. https://norml.org/laws/item/florida-penalties. Accessed April 7, 2020.

[29]CS/CS/CS/SB 182: Medical Use of Marijuana. The Florida Senate Web site. March 18, 2019. https://www.flsenate.gov/Session/Bill/2019/182/?Tab=BillText. Accessed April 7, 2020.

[30]Georgia medical marijuana law. NORML Web site. https://norml.org/legal/item/georgia-medical-marijuana. Accessed March 27, 2020.

[31]House Bill 324/AP. Georgia Legislature Web site. http://www.legis.ga.gov/Legislation/20192020/187578.pdf. Accessed March 27, 2020.

[32]Senate Bill 16. Georgia Legislature Web site. http://www.legis.ga.gov/Legislation/20172018/170462.pdf. Accessed April 7, 2020.

[33]Guam laws & penalties. NORML Web site. https://norml.org/laws/item/guam-penalties-2#medical. Accessed March 27, 2020.

[34]Draft Guam rules governing medical marijuana. Guam Department of Public Health and Social Services Web site. http://dphss.guam.gov/document/draft-guam-rules-governing-medical-marijuana/. Accessed March 27, 2020.

[35]Hawaii laws & penalties. NORML Web site. https://norml.org/laws/item/hawaii-penalties. Accessed April 7, 2020.

[36]Hawaii medical marijuana law. NORML Web site. https://norml.org/laws/item/hawaii-penaltics. Accessed April 7, 2020.

[37]Idaho Attorney General's Annual Report. Idaho Office of the Attorney General Web site. https://www.ag.idaho.gov/content/uploads/2017/12/2015.pdf. Accessed March 27, 2020.

[38]Idaho laws & penalties. NORML Web site. https://norml.org/laws/item/idaho-penalties. Accessed April 7, 2020.

[39]Illinois laws & penalties. NORML Web site. https://norml.org/laws/item/illinois-penalties. Accessed April 7, 2020.

[40]Indiana laws & penalties. NORML Web site. https://norml.org/laws/item/indiana-penalties-2. Accessed April 7, 2020.

[41]Senate Enrolled Act No. 52. Indiana General Assembly Web site. http://iga.in.gov/legislative/2018/bills/senate/52#document-6a10d137. Accessed April 7, 2020.

[42]Medical Cannabidiol Act. Iowa Legislature Web site. https://www.legis.iowa.gov/docs/code/124e.pdf. Accessed March 31, 2020.

[43]Iowa laws & penalties. NORML Web site. https://norml.org/laws/item/iowa-penalties-2. Accessed April 7, 2020.

[44]House File 524—Enrolled. Iowa Legislature Web site. https://www.legis.iowa.gov/docs/publications/LGE/87/HF524.pdf. Accessed April 7, 2020.

[45]Claire and Lola's Law—Possession of Certain Cannabidiol Treatment Preparations, Actions and Proceedings Prohibited, Affirmative Defense; Grandfathering of Certain Podiatrists; SB28. Kansas Legislature Web site. http://www.kslegislature.org/li/b2019_20/measures/documents/summary_sb_28_2019. Accessed April 2, 2020.

[46]Kentucky laws & penalties. NORML Web site. https://norml.org/laws/item/kentucky-penalties-2. Accessed April 8, 2020.

[47]Senate Bill 124—The Clara Madeline Gilliam Act. Kentucky Legislature Web site. https://apps.legislature.ky.gov/record/14rs/sb124.html. Accessed April 8, 2020.

[48]Louisiana laws & penalties. NORML Web site. https://norml.org/laws/item/louisiana-penalties-2. Accessed April 8, 2020.

[49]Ordinance, City of New Orleans, Calendar No. 31,148. City of New Orleans Web site. http://cityofno.granicus.com/MetaViewer.php?view_id=3&clip_id=2288&meta_id=318863. Accessed April 2, 2020.

[50]Maine laws & penalties. NORML Web site. https://norml.org/laws/item/maine-penalties-2. Accessed April 8, 2020.

[51]Maryland Department of Health Title 10. Miscellaneous health care programs, subtitle 62—Natalie M. LaPrade Medical Cannabis Commission. Maryland Medical Cannabis Commission Web site. January 2020. http://www.dsd.state.md.us/COMAR/subtitle_chapters/10_Chapters.aspx#Subtitle62. Accessed April 1, 2020.

[52]Maryland laws & penalties. NORML Web site. https://norml.org/laws/item/maryland-penalties-2. Accessed April 8, 2020.

[53]Maryland Department of Health Title 10. Miscellaneous health care programs, subtitle 62—Natalie M. LaPrade Medical Cannabis Commission. Maryland Medical Cannabis Commission Web site. January 2020. http://www.dsd.state.md.us/COMAR/subtitle_chapters/10_Chapters.aspx#Subtitle62. Accessed April 1, 2020.

[54]Massachusetts laws & penalties. NORML Web site. https://norml.org/laws/item/massachusetts-penalties-2. Accessed April 8, 2020.

[55]General Laws of the Commonwealth of Massachusetts, Part I, Title XV, Chapter 94I, Section 2. Massachusetts Legislature Web site. https://malegislature.gov/Laws/GeneralLaws/PartI/TitleXV/Chapter94I/Section2. Accessed March 31, 2020.

[56]Guidance for healthcare providers regarding the medical use of marijuana. Commonwealth of Massachusetts Web site. December 1, 2017. https://www.mass.gov/doc/guidance-for-health-care-providers-on-the-medical-use-of-marijuana/download. Accessed November 26, 2019.

[57]Michigan Regulation and Taxation of Marihuana Act. Michigan Legislature Web site. https://www.legislature.mi.gov/(S(rzzqvpcp54ovl4wkfuumnqwk))/documents/mcl/pdf/mcl-Initiated-Law-1-of-2018.pdf. Accessed April 8, 2020.

[58]Minnesota laws & penalties. NORML Web site. https://norml.org/laws/item/minnesota-penalties-2. Accessed April 8, 2020.

[59]Mississippi laws & penalties. NORML Web site. https://norml.org/laws/item/mississippi-penalties-2#medicalcbd. Accessed April 8, 2020.

[60]House Bill 1231. Mississippi Legislature Web site. http://billstatus.ls.state.ms.us/documents/2014/html/HB/1200-1299/HB1231SG.htm. Accessed April 8, 2020.

[61]Missouri laws & penalties. NORML Web site. https://norml.org/laws/item/missouri-penalties-2. Accessed April 8, 2020.

[62]19 CSR 30-95.030 Qualifying Patient / Primary Caregiver. Missouri Legislature Web site. https://health.mo.gov/about/proposedrules/pdf/19CSR-30-95.030.pdf. Accessed April 8, 2020.

[63]Montana laws & penalties. NORML Web site. https://norml.org/laws/item/montana-penalties-2#medical. Accessed April 8, 2020.

[64]Legislative Bill 657. Nebraska Legislature Web site. https://nebraskalegislature.gov/FloorDocs/106/PDF/Slip/LB657.pdf. Accessed April 2, 2020.

[65]Nebraska laws & penalties. NORML Web site. https://norml.org/laws/item/nebraska-penalties-2. Accessed April 8, 2020.

[66]Nevada laws & penalties. NORML Web site. https://norml.org/laws/item/nevada-penalties-2. Accessed April 8, 2020.

[67]Nevada Administrative Code: Chapter 453A—Medical Use of Marijuana. Nevada Legislature Web site. https://www.leg.state.nv.us/NAC/NAC-453A.html. Accessed April 1, 2020.

[68]Nevada laws & penalties. NORML Web site. https://norml.org/laws/item/nevada-penalties-2. Accessed April 8, 2020.

[69]Nevada Revised Statutes: Chapter 453A—Medical Use of Marijuana. Nevada Legislature Web site. https://www.leg.state.nv.us/NRS/NRS-453A.html. Accessed April 1, 2020.

[70]Marijuana establishments. State of Nevada Department of Taxation Web site. https://tax.nv.gov/MME/Marijuana_Establishments_-_Home/. Accessed April 8, 2020.

[71]New Hampshire laws & penalties. NORML Web site. https://norml.org/laws/item/new-hampshire-penalties-2. Accessed April 8, 2020.

[72]New Jersey laws & penalties. NORML Web site. https://norml.org/laws/item/new-jersey-penalties-2. Accessed April 8, 2020.

[73]New Mexico laws & penalties. NORML Web site. https://norml.org/laws/item/new-mexico-penalties-2. Accessed April 8, 2020.

[74]Senate Bill 139 of 2020. New Mexico Legislature Web site. https://www.nmlegis.gov/Legislation/Legislation?chamber=S&legType=B&legNo=139&year=20. Published February 21, 2020. Accessed April 8, 2020.

[75]New York laws & penalties. NORML Web site. https://norml.org/laws/item/new-york-penalties-2. Accessed April 8, 2020.

[76]North Carolina laws & penalties. NORML Web site. https://norml.org/laws/item/north-carolina-penalties-2. Accessed April 8, 2020.

[77]Session Law 2015-154. North Carolina Legislature Web site. https://www.ncleg.gov/Sessions/2015/Bills/House/PDF/H766v6.pdf. Accessed March 30, 2020.

[78]North Dakota laws & penalties. NORML Web site. https://norml.org/laws/item/north-dakota-penalties-2. Accessed April 8, 2020.

[79]House Bill 20-178. Northern Marianas Commonwealth Legislature Web site. http://www.cnmileg.gov.mp/documents/house/hse_bills/20/HB20-178.pdf. Accessed April 2, 2020.

[80]Ohio laws & penalties. NORML Web site. https://norml.org/laws/item/ohio-penalties-2. Accessed April 8, 2020.

[81]63 O.S. § 420 (OSCN 2020), Medical Marijuana. Oklahoma State Courts Network Web site. https://www.oscn.net/applications/oscn/DeliverDocument.asp?CiteID=483199. Accessed March 31, 2020.

[82]Oklahoma laws & penalties. NORML Web site. https://norml.org/laws/item/oklahoma-penalties-2. Accessed April 8, 2020.

[83]Uniform Controlled Dangerous Substances Act—HB2166 of 2004. Oklahoma Legislature Web site. http://www.oklegislature.gov/cf_pdf/2003-04%20INT/hb/HB2166%20int.pdf. Accessed April 8, 2020.

[84]Oregon laws & penalties. NORML Web site. https://norml.org/laws/item/oregon-penalties-2. Accessed April 8, 2020.

[85]Pennsylvania laws & penalties. NORML Web site. https://norml.org/laws/item/pennsylvania-penalties-2. Accessed April 8, 2020.

[86]Puerto Rico laws & penalties. NORML Web site. https://norml.org/laws/item/puerto-rico-penalties-2. Accessed April 8, 2020.

[87]Laws of Puerto Rico, Title 24, Part V, Chapter 111, Subchapter IV - § 2401. Prohibited Acts (A); penalties. Lexis Nexis. https://advance.lexis.com/container?config=0151JABiZDY4NzhiZS1hN2IxLTRlYzUtOTg3Yi1hNzIxN2RlMDM1ZDIKAFBvZENhdGFsb2eo3IN9q6nyuOdhcatJGdcs&crid=e7bf96e6-80ed-4963-91ad-b240466b0e27&prid=90ebf9b6-59b4-428e-8279-c10c7232d42e. Accessed April 8, 2020.

[88]Rhode Island laws & penalties. NORML Web site. https://norml.org/laws/item/rhode-island-penalties-2. Accessed April 8, 2020.

[89]2014 Rhode Island General Laws, § 21-28-4.01.2 Minimum sentence—Certain quantities of controlled substances. Justia Web site. https://law.justia.com/codes/rhode-island/2014/title-21/chapter-21-28/section-21-28-4.01.2/. Accessed April 8, 2020.

[90]South Carolina laws & penalties. NORML Web site. https://norml.org/laws/item/south-carolina-penalties-2. Accessed April 8, 2020.

[91]South Carolina General Assembly 120th Session, Medical Cannabis Therapeutic Treatment Research Act. South Carolina Legislature Web site. https://www.scstatehouse.gov/sess120_2013-2014/bills/1035.htm. Accessed April 1, 2020.

[92]South Dakota laws & penalties. NORML Web site. https://norml.org/laws/item/south-dakota-penalties-2. Accessed April 8, 2020.

[93]Tennessee laws & penalties. NORML Web site. https://norml.org/laws/item/tennessee-penalties-2. Accessed April 8, 2020.

[94]House Bill 2144. Tennessee General Assembly Web site. http://wapp.capitol.tn.gov/apps/ Billinfo/default.aspx?BillNumber=HB2144&ga=109. Accessed March 31, 2020.

[95]Texas laws & penalties. NORML Web site. https://norml.org/laws/item/texas-penalties-2. Accessed April 8, 2020.

[96]Virgin Islands laws & penalties. NORML Web site. https://norml.org/laws/item/virgin-islands-penalties-2. Accessed April 8, 2020.

[97]Bill No. 32-0135, The Virgin Islands Medical Cannabis Patient Care Act. NORML Web site. https://norml.org/pdf_files/Virgin-Islands-Bill-32-0135.pdf. Accessed March 31, 2020.

[98]Title 26, Chapter 61a, Part 5, Section 502 of the Utah Code. Utah Legislature Web site. https://le.utah.gov/xcode/Title26/Chapter61A/26-61a-S502.html?v=C26-61a-S502_2018120320181203. Accessed April 6, 2020.

[99]Utah Medical Cannabis Act. Utah Legislature Web site. https://le.utah.gov/~2018S3/bills/ static/HB3001.html. Accessed April 6, 2020.

[100]Utah Medical Cannabis Act. Utah Legislature Web site. https://le.utah.gov/~2018S3/bills/ static/HB3001.html. Accessed April 6, 2020.

[101]Utah laws & penalties. NORML Web site. https://norml.org/laws/item/utah-penalties-2#medical. Accessed April 8, 2020.

[102]H.511 of 2018, No. 86. An act relating to eliminating penalties for possession of limited amounts of marijuana by adults 21 years of age or older. Vermont Legislature Web site. https://legislature.vermont.gov/Documents/2018/Docs/ACTS/ACT086/ACT086%20As%20 Enacted.pdf. Accessed April 3, 2020.

[103]§ 54.1-3408.3 Certification for use of cannabidiol or THC-A oil for treatment. Virginia Legislature Web site. https://law.lis.virginia.gov/vacode/54.1-3408.3/. Accessed April 6, 2020.

[104]Section 18.2-247 of the Code of Virginia. Virginia Code Web site. https://vacode.org/ 18.2-247/. Accessed on April 6, 2020.

[105]Section 18.2-248.1 of the Code of Virginia. Virginia Code Web site. https://vacode.org/ 18.2-248.1/. Accessed on April 6, 2020.

[106]Section 54.1-3446. of the Code of Virginia. Virginia Code Web site. https://vacode.org/ 54.1-3446/. Accessed on April 6, 2020.

[107]Section 18.2-248 (D) of the Code of Virginia. Virginia Code Web site. https://vacode. org/2016/18.2/7/1/18.2-248/. Accessed on April 6, 2020.

[108]Washington laws & penalties. NORML Web site. https://norml.org/laws/item/washington-penalties-2. Accessed on April 8, 2020.

[109]Certificate of Enrollment—Second Substitute Senate Bill 5052. Washington Legislature Web site. http://lawfilesext.leg.wa.gov/biennium/2015-16/Pdf/Bills/Senate%20Passed%20 Legislature/5052-S2.PL.pdf. Accessed April 1, 2020.

[110]West Virginia laws & penalties. NORML Web site. https://norml.org/laws/item/west-virginia-penalties-2. Accessed April 8, 2020.

[111]Wisconsin laws & penalties. NORML Web site. https://norml.org/laws/item/wisconsin-penalties-2. Accessed April 8, 2020.

[112]Biros AG. Wyoming legalizes hemp, CBD oil. *Cannabis Industry Journal.* https://canna-bisindustryjournal.com/news_article/wyoming-legalizes-hemp-cbd-oil/. Published March 6, 2019. Accessed March 31, 2020.

[113]Wyoming laws & penalties. NORML Web site. https://norml.org/laws/item/wyoming-penalties-2. Accessed April 8, 2020.

Index